Thyroid and Heart Failure

Giorgio Iervasi • Alessandro Pingitore
Editors

Thyroid and Heart Failure

From Pathophysiology to Clinics

Forewords by
Paul W. Ladenson
Attilio Maseri

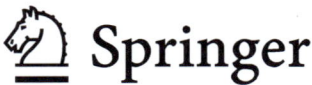
Springer

Editors
Giorgio Iervasi
C.N.R. Clinical Physiology Institute
S. Cataldo Research Campus
Pisa, Italy

Alessandro Pingitore
C.N.R. Clinical Physiology Institute
S. Cataldo Research Campus
Pisa, Italy

ISBN 978-88-470-1142-7

e-ISBN 978-88-470-1143-3

DOI 10.1007/978-88-470-1143-3

Springer Dordrecht Heidelberg London Milan New York

Library of Congress Control Number: 2009925123

Cover illustration: Yuri Kalendarev, "Shma"/Listen, 96 x 96 cm, Ink on paper, 2002

Typesetting: Graphostudio, Milan, Italy
Printing and binding: Printer Trento Srl, Trento, Italy
Printed in Italy

Springer-Verlag Italia S.r.l. – Via Decembrio 28 – I-20137 Milan
Springer is a part of Springer Science+Business Media

Ostinato rigore. Destinato rigore.
No' si volta chi a stella è fisso

Ostinate rigour. To rigour destinated.
Who is fixed to a star will nothing change

Leonardo da Vinci

Foreword

The clinical significance of heart failure is enormous, and the need for novel therapeutic approaches compelling. In the United States alone, almost six million people are affected by the condition and another half million are newly diagnosed annually. Among those older than 65 years, heart failure is the most common indication for hospitalization. It is estimated that heart failure will account for more than $37 billion in U.S. healthcare costs in 2009[1]. Overall, heart failure and other cardiovascular diseases are responsible for more deaths than accidents, cancer, and cerebrovascular accidents combined. Furthermore, in the decades ahead, the impact of heart failure on human health and healthcare economics is bound to increase due to aging of the population. Although the treatment of heart failure with beta-blockers, aldosterone antagonists, angiotensin I converting enzyme inhibitors and angiotensin II receptor blockers, implanted defibrillators, and cardiac resynchronization therapy has led to improvements in mortality and morbidity, the prognosis for patients afflicted with the condition is still poor. Consequently, the search for novel therapeutic targets to improve heart failure outcomes continues.

The earliest reports of patients with myxedema and thyrotoxicosis noted the profound effects of thyroid hormone deficiency and excess, respectively, on the cardiovascular system. Since then, our knowledge of how thyroid hormones regulate cardiac and peripheral vascular functions has progressively advanced from the physiological to the biochemical and molecular levels. Concurrently, our understanding of how systemic illnesses in general, and heart failure in particular, alter thyroid gland function, thyroid hormone metabolism, and triiodothyronine's molecular actions has grown tremendously. Recent animal and pilot clinical studies have begun to examine the potential of thyromimetic agents–some naturally occurring and others in the form of synthetic analogues–with targeted actions that selectively affect or spare cardiovascular functions.

Consequently, a monograph comprehensively describing the interrelationships between thyroid hormones and heart failure is most timely. The distinguished authors recruited by editors Iervasi and Pingitore summarize the state of the art regarding the molecular and physiological actions of thyroid hormones on the heart and peripheral vasculature (Chap. 5); the pathophysiological effects of mild and overt thyroid dysfunction on the cardiovascular system (Chaps. 3, 4, 12, 15, and 19) and cardiovascular risk factors (Chap. 14); the changes in thyroid function and thyroid hormone receptors and actions that accompany heart failure and are associated with its severity

---

[1] Lloyd-Jones D, Adams R, Carnethon M et al (2009) Heart disease and stroke statistics–2009 update: a report from the American Heart Association Statistics Committee and Stroke Statistics Subcommittee. Circulation 119:480-486

(Chaps. 7, 10, 11, 16, 17, and 18); and pilot studies investigating the application of native thyroid hormones (Chaps. 13 and 21), their metabolites (Chap. 6), and their analogs (Chaps. 9 and 20), and their downstream molecular and biochemical actions (Chap. 22) as potential new approaches to heart failure treatment.

As we stand at the threshold of testing the applicability of all of this knowledge about thyroid hormone actions to the enormous and incompletely addressed clinical challenge of heart failure, this monograph represents an important scholarly map, summarizing where we have been and plotting the most promising directions ahead.

Baltimore, April 2009

Paul W. Ladenson, MD
Professor of Medicine, Pathology, Oncology,
and Radiology
John Eager Howard Professor of Endocrinology
and Metabolism
Distinguished Service Professor
Director, Division of Endocrinology and Metabolism
Johns Hopkins University
Baltimore, MD, United States

Foreword

The opportunity to look at old problems from a new angle is always welcome. Today, the possibility of investigating accepted, traditional paradigms in increasingly finer detail has been accompanied by the exponential development of research technologies. These, in turn, have largely been applied in attempts to explain the many and highly variable clinical observations within the already established framework while at the same time adding new information to it. Yet, major breakthroughs in our knowledge often occur by looking at problems from a different perspective, which not infrequently reveals that some long-held and broadly accepted notions are not universally true, such that new, unexpected avenues for research, diagnosis, and treatment are suddenly opened.

The relationship between the thyroid and the cardiovascular system has, until now, received insufficient attention because it remained outside the mainstream of cardiovascular thinking not only in clinical practice but also in research.

This very timely volume offers a unique focus and thereby a clearer understanding of clinical findings with intriguing research potential as well as relevant clinical applications. There is no doubt that this illuminating, very wisely assembled and coordinated volume will stimulate the work of investigators and provide clinicians with inquisitive minds new insights into their daily practice.

The book sets the stage very lucidly with a comprehensive analysis of the general aspects of the interrelationships between thyroid and cardiac failure and, more generally, between thyroid hormones and cardiovascular function. This novel, integrated approach also extends to proposals for new therapeutic strategies. The coordinators of this volume should be wholeheartedly congratulated for their wisdom and foresight in opening a new window of observation into the cardiovascular world. Their efforts will long be appreciated and gratefully acknowledged by all the readers of this volume.

Florence, April 2009

Prof. Attilio Maseri, MD
President Heart Care Foundation
Florence, Italy

Preface

In many fields of biomedicine there has been a virtual explosion of new knowledge over the past few years. Among these, a primary position is occupied by the physiological and pathophysiological neurohormonal control of the cardiovascular system, in which the state of the thyroid has assumed a prominent role. Extensive investigations that have made use of new technologies to study animal and human models of disease have focused on the modulation of cardiovascular function by the thyroid system. These results have supported and coincided with a growing understanding of the interacting biomolecular mechanisms that underlie the complex relationships between the thyroid system and cardiovascular function, although many aspects remain largely undefined.

The planning of this book was initiated at the end of 2007, as researchers and clinicians became aware of the pathophysiological and clinical significance of thyroid function with respect to cardiac failure. At the same time, the implications of this relationship for public health, including the socioeconomic aspects, became clear. The driving considerations behind the book can be summarized as follows:

1) Cardiac failure worldwide represents a major public health problem.
2) Cardiac failure is the only common cardiovascular condition that is increasing in prevalence and incidence; it is responsible for about 1 million hospital admissions and 400,000 deaths annually in the United States and in Europe.
3) The critical role of the neuroendocrine system in the evolution of heart failure and in its prognosis is well defined; there is additional evidence that drugs able to modify the natural course of cardiovascular disease act on the neuroendocrine system, namely β-blockers and inhibitors of the renin-angiotensin-aldosterone system.
4) Thyroid hormones are essential for maintaining cardiovascular homeostasis. An altered thyroid hormone profile (including both the so-called low-T_3 syndrome and mild primary thyroid dysfunction) is observed in more than 30% of the total heart failure population.
5) The relationship between an altered thyroid hormone profile and cardiac failure is nowadays widely accepted: nonetheless, it is controversially interpreted by research scientists and clinicians.

Considering the importance of cardiac failure and its relationship to thyroid function, a traditional monographic publication would have been unable to integrate and give sufficient relevance to all the component inter- and multi-disciplinary issues. Instead, the task of bringing together the many different but equally significant aspects was given to the Institute of Clinical Physiology of the National Research Council of Pisa. The integration and merging of information from different disciplines to form a unified whole has been a particular specialty of the Institute since its founding, in 1968, by Professor Luigi Donato.

This book is therefore the result of a collaborative effort aimed at presenting a broad-ranging discussion of the relationship between thyroid and cardiac (dys)function, from the cellular mechanisms of thyroid-hormone action on the heart and vascular system to the clinical implications of their relatedness.

To facilitate the use of this book as a reference work, the contributions have been organized into four sections. Section one is a general introduction to the problem of heart failure with respect to thyroid function, while section two explores the basic aspects of the thyroid-hormone and cardiovascular systems in the normal and in the failing heart. Section three examines the clinical aspects, and section four the current and future therapeutic options for patients with thyroid and cardiac dysfunction.

Once the topics of the book were decided upon, we set about to identify the authors who could contribute to it by providing state-of-the-art information regarding the complex and widely debated emerging field of cardio-endocrinology. We sought to take into account the needs of medical students, post-graduates in the various medical disciplines (especially cardiology, internal medicine, and endocrinology), researchers working in the relevant fields of study, physicians of general medicine, and specialists who are confronted daily with the problem of heart failure associated with thyroid dysfunction. Accordingly, the scope of the book ranges from the cellular and subcellular mechanisms of thyroid-related cardiac disease to its clinical and epidemiological features. The authors who contributed to the volume are specialists in often very different, at times seemingly unrelated branches of medicine, such as biochemistry, cardiovascular physiology, endocrine physiology, experimental cardiology, experimental endocrinology, clinical cardiology, clinical endocrinology, nephrology, neuropsychiatry and cardiovascular epidemiology. They were invited exclusively on the basis of their internationally recognized authority and leadership, as pioneers and innovators in their areas of expertise. Without exception, they have transmitted their knowledge in a straightforward, exhaustive, and highly readable manner.

Fortunately, what had at first appeared to be a complicated task, joining these seemingly disparate chapters into a book, was greatly facilitated by the enormous enthusiasm and spirit of collaboration of the contributing authors, whom we warmly thank.

The reader of this book will notice that several topics of particular interest have been treated by authors, some from different specialties, with contrasting points of view. Rather than being a source of confusion, these differences prevent the book's uniformity and coherence from becoming synonymous with a static and dogmatic vision. Certainty has no place in the medical sciences, and scientific curiosity represents a first and necessary step in innovation, which derives from a dynamic and critical exchange of ideas. In our opinion, these differences in opinion and interpretation are one of the strong points of the book rather than an element of weakness: they provide the reader with fresh points of view on important topics and reflect the lack of a common interpretation by the most competent authorities in the field. The same can be said for the slight overlaps in content that sometimes occur, as in many cases they present the same information from a different perspective and thus with different emphasis.

Moreover, as Editors of the book, we felt that it was important that the book's individual chapters be able to stand alone in terms of subject matter. To this end, we gave the authors free hand to express their personal points of view and to develop their arguments in the context of their specialties.

The authors are particularly grateful to the Editorial Team of Springer, specifically, Drs. Donatella Rizza, Alessandra Born, and Angela Vanegas, who believed in the goals of the project. Their competence, professionalism, constant support, patience, and kindness have made this book more than just an adventure but also a thoroughly enjoyable and stimulating experience.

If this multi-disciplinary but cohesive book is able to assist the clinician in his or her clinical practice, guide students and post-doctoral students of medicine, and encourage clinical as well as basic researchers towards new initiatives and explorations in the field, it will have certainly fulfilled its function.

Pisa, April 2009   *Giorgio Iervasi*
                                                                                        Alessandro Pingitore

Contents

Section III   Clinical Aspects

Section IV   Treatment: Present and Future Options

Contributors

Reto Auer, MD Department of Ambulatory Care and Community Medicine, University of Lausanne, Lausanne, Switzerland

Peter H. Backx, DVM, PhD Departments of Physiology and Medicine, University of Toronto, Toronto, Canada

Bernadette Biondi, MD Department of Clinical and Molecular Endocrinology and Oncology, University of Naples Federico II, Naples, Italy

Michael R. Bristow, MD Division of Cardiology, University of Colorado, Denver, CO, United States

Robertas Bunevičius, MD, PhD Institute of Psychophysiology and Rehabilitation, Kaunas University of Medicine, Palanga, Lithuania

Anne R. Cappola, MD, ScM Division of Endocrinology, Diabetes and Metabolism, University of Pennsylvania School of Medicine, Philadelphia, PA, United States

Claudio Ceconi, MD, PhD Chair of Cardiology, University of Ferrara, Ferrara, Cardiovascular Research Centre, Salvatore Maugeri Foundation, IRCCS Gussago (BS), Italy

Yuefeng Chen, MD, PhD Cardiovascular Research Center, Sanford Research/ University of South Dakota, Sioux Falls, SD, United States

Grazia Chiellini, PhD Department of Human and Environmental Sciences, University of Pisa, Pisa, Italy; Department of Biochemistry, College of Agriculture and Life Sciences, University of Wisconsin-Madison, Madison, WI, United States

Dennis V. Cokkinos, MD 1st Cardiology Department, Onassis Cardiac Surgery Center, Athens, Greece

Sara Danzi, MD, PhD North Shore University Hospital, Department of Medicine and the Feinstein Institute for Medical Research, Manhasset, NY, United States

Mark Davis, MD Departments of Physiology and Medicine, University of Toronto, Toronto, Canada

Wolfgang H. Dillmann, MD Department of Medicine, University of California, San Diego, CA, United States

Roberto Ferrari, PhD Department of Cardiology, University of Ferrara, Cardiovascular Institute, Arcispedale S. Anna Hospital, Ferrara, Italy

Francesca Forini, PhD C.N.R. Clinical Physiology Institute, S. Cataldo Research Campus, Pisa, Italy

Kate Gaskell, MD Endocrine Clinic, Royal Infirmary, Edinburgh, Scotland, United Kingdom

A. Martin Gerdes, PhD Cardiovascular Research Center, Sanford Research/ University of South Dakota, Sioux Falls, SD, United States

Sandra Ghelardoni, PhD Department of Human and Environmental Sciences, University of Pisa, Pisa, Italy

Giorgio Iervasi, MD C.N.R. Clinical Physiology Institute, S. Cataldo Research Campus, Pisa, Italy

George J. Kahaly, MD, PhD Department of Medicine I, Gutenberg University Hospital, Mainz, Germany

Koichiro Kinugawa, MD, PhD Department of Cardiovascular Medicine, University of Tokyo, Tokyo, Japan

Irwin Klein, MD North Shore University Hospital, Department of Medicine and the Feinstein Institute for Medical Research, Manhasset, NY, United States

Mark Y. Jeong, MD Division of Cardiology, University of Colorado, Denver, CO, United States

Antonio L'Abbate, MD The Sant'Anna School of Advanced Studies of Pisa, and C.N.R. Institute of Clinical Physiology, Pisa, Italy

Vincenzo Lionetti, MD, PhD The Sant'Anna School of Advanced Studies of Pisa, University of Pisa, Pisa, Italy

Carlin S. Long, MD Division of Cardiology, University of Colorado, Denver, CO, United States

Francesca Mallamaci, MD Renal and Transplantation Unit, United Hospitals, and CNR-IBIM Clinical Epidemiology and Pathophysiology of Renal Diseases and Hypertension Unit, Reggio Calabria, Italy

Iordanis Mourouzis, MD 1st Cardiology Department, Onassis Cardiac Surgery Center, Athens, Greece

Giuseppina Nicolini, PhD C.N.R. Clinical Physiology Institute, S. Cataldo Research Campus, Pisa, Italy

Aaron K. Olson, MD Acting Assistant Professor of Pediatrics and Pediatric Cardiology, University of Washington, and Children's Hospital and Regional Medical Center, Seattle, WA, United States

Constantinos Pantos, MD, PhD 1 Department of Pharmacology, University of Athens, School of Medicine, Athens, Greece

Michael A. Portman, MD University of Washington and Seattle Children's Hospital, Seattle, WA, United States

Alessandro Pingitore, MD, PhD C.N.R. Clinical Physiology Institute, S. Cataldo Research Campus, Pisa, Italy

Nicolas Rodondi, MD, MAS Department of Ambulatory Care and Community Medicine, University of Lausanne, Lausanne, Switzerland

Laura Sabatino, PhD C.N.R. Clinical Physiology Institute, S. Cataldo Research Campus, Pisa, Italy

Warner S. Simonides, PhD VU University Medical Center Amsterdam, Institute for Cardiovascular Research, Department of Physiology, Amsterdam, The Netherlands

Anthony Toft, MD Endocrine Clinic, Royal Infirmary, Edinburgh, Scotland, United Kingdom

Maria Giovanna Trivieri, MD Departments of Physiology and Medicine, University of Toronto, Toronto, Canada

Avantika C. Waring, MD Division of Endocrinology, Diabetes and Metabolism, University of Pennsylvania School of Medicine, Philadelphia, PA, United States

Wilmar M. Wiersinga, MD Department of Endocrinology and Metabolism, Academic Medical Center, University of Amsterdam, Amsterdam, The Netherlands

Carmine Zoccali, MD Renal and Transplantation Unit, United Hospitals, and CNR-IBIM Clinical Epidemiology and Pathophysiology of Renal Diseases and Hypertension Unit, Reggio Calabria, Italy

Riccardo Zucchi, MD, PhD Professor of Biochemistry, University of Pisa, Pisa, Italy

Heart Failure: From Epidemiology to Pathophysiology

1

Antonio L'Abbate

Abstract   Heart failure (HF) is the leading cause of hospitalization, giving rise to costs that outrun those of all other causes of disability, illness, and death throughout developed and even developing countries. HF is an enormous health problem, leading to significant morbidity and mortality. The pathogenetic interpretation of HF has radically changed in the last 40 years. Nowadays HF is considered a systemic disease that derives from a "faulty" neurohormonal response by the organism to primary cardiac damage that is able to elicit the activation of powerful, phylogenetically well-established mechanisms against the life-threatening loss of blood volume, such as hemorrhage, hypovolemia, and trauma. The degree of systemic activation is disproportionate to the severity of the primary cardiac damage, and it is this that is responsible for the development of HF and its progression. Early clinical recognition of neurohumoral activation is essential to prevent progression of HF.

Keywords   Renin–angiotensin–aldosterone system • Hemorrhage • Systolic dysfunction • Diastolic dysfunction • Cardiac hypertrophy • Intracellular matrix • Implantable defibrillator • Resynchronization therapy • Myocardial ischemia • Endothelial dysfunction • Myocardial perfusion • Coronary microvascular dysfunction • Positron emission tomography • Multislice CT coronary angiography

1.1 Introduction

According to the American Heart Association, more than 5 million Americans have heart failure (HF); HF is the leading cause of hospitalization and an estimated 550,000 new cases occur each year in the United States [1]. The costs associated with HF outrun those of all other causes of disability, illness, and death in the United States and throughout the developed and even the developing countries, where cardiovascular risk factors and cardiovascular diseases are on the rise. In the Euro Heart survey, 24% of patients discharged from internal medicine, geriatric, cardiology, and cardiac surgery hospital wards in 24 countries were identified as having suspected or confirmed HF [2].

HF is thus an enormous health problem leading to significant morbidity and mortality. Moreover, in spite of evidence of improved survival of HF patients documented in the past few decades [3], the progressive aging of the population, the pandemic of cardiovascular diseases (CVD), and the improved survival from acute cardiovascular events all converge to foster a growing epidemic of HF, presage a progressive rise in its incidence and prevalence, and magnify the paramount importance of its prevention [4].

The challenge of HF involves every part of the

A. L'Abbate (✉)
The Sant'Anna School of Advanced Studies of Pisa and C.N.R.
Institute of Clinical Physiology, Pisa, Italy

G. Iervasi, A. Pingitore (eds.), *Thyroid and Heart Failure*.

community: an aging population increasingly burdened with chronic diseases, particularly of the heart, kidneys, and lungs; the government seeking ways of both preventing the surge in organ failure and controlling the costs of treatment, while assuring a uniform standard of health care; and drug and technology industries tasked with discovering novel methods of prediction, diagnosis, and treatment while keeping the costs of these efforts from spiraling out of control.

The Framingham investigators have estimated that the lifetime risk of developing HF at the age of 40 is 21% for men and 20% for women (11% and 15% in the absence of documented myocardial infarction) [5]. Community-based studies in the United States also show that the prevalence of HF is seven times higher in blacks than in Asians, whites, and Hispanics, with an increasing trend in all groups [6].

1.2 Pathophysiology

As HF is the result of acute and chronic cardiac injury and its pathogenesis is still elusive, it may escape a unifying definition. Thus, the best way of illustrating the advances in our understanding of HF, the changes in conceptual models of HF, and hence the changes in its definition, is to summarize the history of its interpretation and treatment.

Over the last forty years there have been at least three different models for interpreting HF and its signs, all with important correlates in different–and often opposite–ways of treating the syndrome. In the 1970s, HF was interpreted as the clinical manifestation of impaired myocardial contractile force, which was seen as causing a drop in cardiac output and thus in renal flow and urine output. Because of this view, therapy was based on digitalis to potentiate contractile force and on diuretics to limit water retention. At that time β-blocking drugs were already available but were specifically contraindicated in HF because of their negative inotropic effect, while the use of vasoconstrictive drugs was encouraged to counteract arterial hypotension and cardiogenic shock. Thus, according to this view, the entire problem of HF was confined within the heart and HF was interpreted as the direct consequence of impaired contractile cardiac function.

In the 1980s, clinical studies accumulated evidence of the presence of diffuse vasoconstriction in HF, while experimental cardiology was clarifying the crucial role of increased afterload in the deterioration of cardiac output and enforcement of myocardial extra energy demand. As a consequence of this important new information, medical treatment started to include the use of vasodilators in addition to diuretics and digitalis. New drugs were developed–the phosphodiesterase inhibitors amrinone, milrinone, and others, capable of stimulating cardiac inotropism while dilating the vasculature. However, they did not appear to be beneficial in long-term controlled clinical trials.

The third step forward occurred in the 1990s, when vasoconstriction and sodium and water retention were recognized as consequences of the activation of both the adrenergic system and the renin–angiotensin–aldosterone system (RAAS) [7]. From the physiological point of view, it is well established that activation of these systems provides effective protection against the deleterious effects of hemorrhage or dehydration. On this basis, the signs and symptoms of HF have been attributed to phylogenetically well-established mechanisms elicited by the body when faced with life-threatening loss of blood volume–namely, activation of the RAAS and of the sympathetic nervous system–leading to systemic vasoconstriction and fluid retention in the attempt to preserve arterial blood pressure and/or cardiac output (this point is still the subject of debate) and to divert the available blood flow from skeletal muscle and visceral organs towards the heart and brain. In brief, the neurohormonal response observed during HF is interpreted as an activation of the powerful stereotyped response of the body to life-threatening events such as hemorrhage, hypovolemia, and trauma [8].

While such a response is beneficial in the short-term protection from acute loss of blood volume, if continued in the long term it becomes largely adverse. In particular, it should be borne in mind that the natural response evoked by blood volume loss does not imply a diseased heart. In the presence of heart disease, any increase in peripheral vascular resistance increases cardiac afterload and impairs left ventricular ejection of blood [9]. Table 1.1 summarizes the two groups of vasoconstrictive and vasodilator substances that modulate vascular tone and thus resistance to blood flow; in HF, regulation of tone is unbalanced towards vasoconstriction. Efforts to delay disease progression and improve survival are now based on measures aimed at counteracting the above neurohormonal activation and

Table 1.1 Vasoactive substances involved in heart failure

Vasoconstrictors	Vasodilators
Epinephrine–norepinephrine	Atrial natriuretic peptide–brain natriuretic peptide
Endothelins	Bradykinin
Isoprostanes	Calcitonin-gene-related peptide
Renin–angiotensin–aldosterone	Nitric oxide
Vasopressin	Prostaglandins

Table 1.2 Factors triggering and/or modulating heart failure

Circuit	Heart chambers, valves, vessels
Circuit content	Blood volume
Heart muscle	Loss of tissue Contractile force Relaxation Compliance
Time sequence of heart chambers' contractions	Rhythm and sequence of contraction Synchronization of ventricular contraction
Control systems	Neuroendocrine Inflammation

mainly consist in the administration of vasodilators, diuretics, and adrenergic β-blockers, in the careful control of fluid balance, and in tailored physical training. In the same decade, the efficacy and safety of deactivation of the RAAS and the adrenergic system by both pharmacological and physical (exercise) intervention have been extensively proved in controlled clinical trials conducted in large populations.

Meanwhile, additional information has been collected that adds to the modern concept of HF as no longer a cardiac disease but rather a systemic disease involving the main controlling systems of the entire organism, including the nervous, endocrine, and immune systems. In this new view, the heart triggers the activation of a systemic reaction which in turn further damages the heart, thus feeding a vicious cycle leading to progressive cardiovascular dysfunction. The salient points in this scenario are:

– Any alteration affecting the cardiovascular circuit–i.e., the heart or the vascular tree or the blood volume (Table 1.2), either separately or in concert– is signaled, likely through a decrease in arterial blood pressure, to the control systems, in particular the autonomic nervous system and the kidney, thus triggering a systemic reaction aimed at restoring blood pressure.
– The magnitude of the systemic activation is not proportional to the initial cardiac damage. This point is of clinical relevance as it substantiates the common observation of an inconsistent relationship between the clinical manifestation of HF and the instrumental recognition of cardiac damage.
– The magnitude and time course of activation are not the same for the different control systems.
– Over time, an untreated systemic response impairs cardiovascular function. This occurs through a series of effects at cellular and subcellular levels and leads to substantial changes in both the anatomy and the function of the heart and the vasculature (Fig. 1.1).
– Again, this process, called cardiac and vascular remodeling, cannot be clinically predicted by the severity of the primary cardiac damage, but rather by the magnitude of the systemic activation.

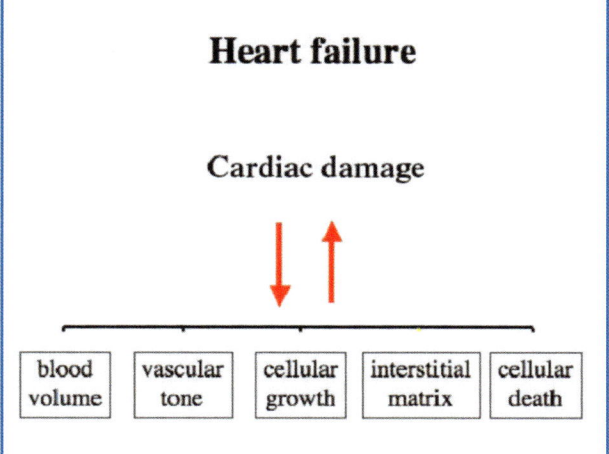

Fig. 1.1 The vicious cycle of heart failure. Any alteration affecting the heart triggers a systemic reaction involving the control systems (autonomic nervous system, kidney, hormones, inflammation) which over time, through a series of effects at cellular and sub-cellular levels, produces substantial changes in both the anatomy and function of the heart as well as of the vessels

– Systolic dysfunction, i.e., impairment of the heart's ability to contract, is not alone responsible for HF. As many as 40% of patients show signs of diastolic dysfunction with normal or near-normal systolic function [10, 11]. This alteration is related to altered relaxation of the myocardium and/or reduced compliance of the ventricular walls (Table 1.2). As to reduced ventricular compliance, myocyte growth (cardiac hypertrophy) and alterations at the level of intracellular matrix (Fig. 1.1) seem to be the major actors [12].

From the above considerations it may be seen that the best approach to counteracting progression of HF is prevention and treatment of neurohormonal and inflammatory activation in addition to interventions aimed at correcting the primary cardiac and/or vascular damage (coronary revascularization, for example), and so interrupt the vicious cycle.

As to direct interventions on the heart to modify the prognosis of overt HF, an important annotation came from technological advances and the introduction of novel devices such as the implantable defib-

rillator and the resynchronizing multisite ventricular electrical stimulator. Both these instruments belong to the category of "permanent devices" and differ widely from others, such as the aortic balloon pump or various types of extracorporeal pumps, whose purpose is the short-term support of blood circulation during acute cardiac failure. The use of "permanent devices" has shown a clear-cut beneficial effect on the prognosis of HF, provided candidate patients are selected carefully [13–16].

1.3 HF and Risk Factors

In the past few decades, clinical research has used prospective epidemiological studies extensively to identify risk factors and risk markers for the development of HF [17], as well as prospective studies in patients with overt HF for the stratification of the risk of cardiac events during follow-up. Table 1.3 outlines the major and minor clinical risk factors identified. From this table, it is evident that many of the major and minor risk factors for HF are also well-known

Table 1.3 Established and hypothesized risk factors for heart failure. (From [4], with permission)

Major clinical risk factors	Toxic risk precipitants
Age, male sex	Chemotherapy (anthracyclines, cyclophosphamide, 5-FU, trastuzumab)
Hypertension, LVH	Cocaine, NSAIDs
Myocardial infarction	Thiazolidinediones
Diabetes mellitus	Doxazosin
Valvular heart disease	Alcohol
Obesity	
Minor clinical risk factors	Genetic risk predictors
Smoking	SNP (e.g., α2CDel322-325, β1Arg389)
Dyslipidemia	
Sleep-disordered breathing	Morphological risk predictors
Chronic kidney disease	Increased LVID, mass
Albuminuria	Asymptomatic LV dysfunction
Homocysteine	LV diastolic dysfunction
Immune activation, IGF1,TNFα, IL-6, CRP	
Natriuretic peptides	
Anemia	
Dietary risk factors	
Increased heart rate	
Sedentary lifestyle	
Low socioeconomic status	
Psychological stress	

5-FU 5-Fluorouracil, *LVH* left ventricular hypertrophy, *NSAIDs* nonsteroidal anti-inflammatory drugs, *SNP* single-nucleotide polymorphism, *LVID* left ventricular internal dimension, *IGF* insulin-like growth factor, *TNF* tumor necrosis factor, *IL* interleukin, *CRP* C-reactive protein risk factors for coronary artery disease (CAD). This overlap is in agreement with the epidemiological finding that CAD is the leading cause of HF in Western countries. Among all the medical trials reported in the *New England Journal of Medicine* over the past 20 years (24 trials involving over 43 000 patients), CAD was the underlying cause of HF in 62% of the patients [18]. The main risk factors for HF and CAD are briefly reported below.

The incidence of HF increases exponentially with age [19, 20] and is greater in men, particularly at younger ages [21, 22]. Arterial hypertension increases the risk of HF two- to threefold [23] and diabetes two- to fivefold [19, 20, 22, 24]. Myocardial infarction is an important risk factor for HF, being associated with a two- to threefold increased risk [17, 22, 23]; obesity [20, 22, 25], albuminuria, and chronic renal insufficiency [26, 27] have recently been demonstrated to be significantly associated with CAD and in turn with HF. The association of dyslipidemia with HF also seems to be at least in part mediated by CAD and myocardial infarction [20, 28].

The type and number of risk factors present in particular individuals differ as well as the combination of their aggregation (Fig. 1.2). Although the aggregation of multiple risk factors is generally associated with a greater likelihood of having the disease, this correlation is neither linear nor particularly significant.

On the basis of the documented large overlap of risk factors for HF and CAD, we may conclude that prevention and treatment of CAD are the major tasks in combating HF. However, several questions on the pathogenesis of CAD and on its relationship with HF remain unanswered. Because of its strategic importance, this topic will now be discussed in further detail.

1.4 CAD and HF: Unanswered Questions

In everyday clinical practice, the main clinical manifestations of ischemic heart disease (IHD) (angina, myocardial infarction, cardiac sudden death, and HF) are attributed to the obstruction of the epicardial (large) coronary arteries (CAD). In this view, stenotic or occluded coronary arteries hamper downstream myocardial perfusion, causing ischemia and contractile dysfunction. Thus, in patients with ischemic symptoms or cardiac dysfunction (either global or regional), the first clinical task is to assess the presence of CAD and reestablish blood flow by mechanical or pharmacological coronary recanalization.

However, the equivalence between IHD and CAD-a paradigm largely accepted in cardiology-does not always fit with the clinical manifestations of IHD and/or with the instrumental signs of myocardial

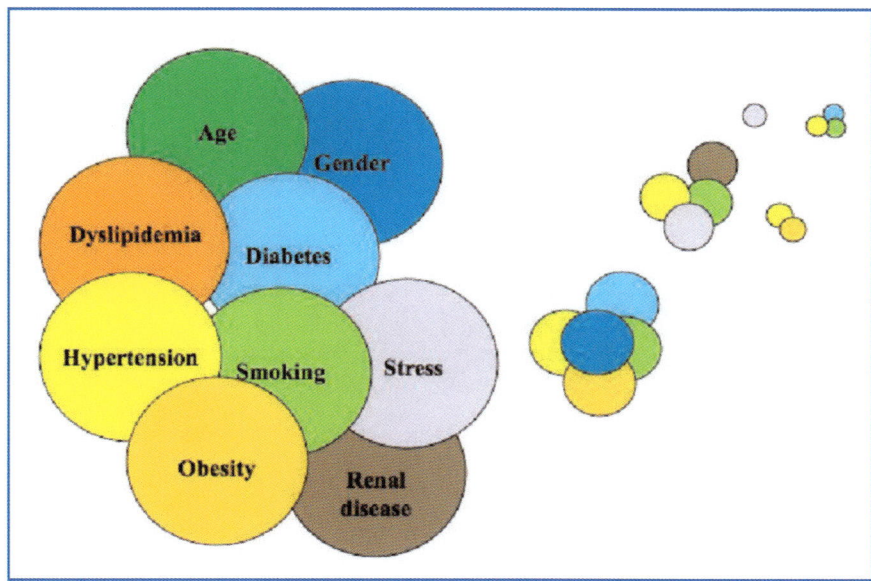

Fig. 1.2 Risk factors aggregate differently in individual patients with heart failure. Although the aggregation of multiple risk factors is generally associated with a higher prevalence of the disease, the correlation is not linear

ischemia or infarction, nor does it allow the progression and response to treatment of IHD to be predicted. In other words, the presence of CAD does not imply IHD, nor is CAD a prerequisite for IHD. Endothelial dysfunction can alter the vasodilating properties of both macro- and microvessels, impair myocardial perfusion, and evoke ischemia even in the absence of CAD [29]. Thus, silent CAD (significant coronary atherosclerosis not followed by any clinical manifestation of IHD) and myocardial ischemia sustained by microvascular rather than macrovascular alterations are the two extreme conditions that contradict the widely accepted equation CAD = IHD. Moreover, to complicate the matter, it should be kept in mind that both macro and micro alterations may coexist in the same heart or even in the same territory [30, 31].

Despite the pathogenetic complexity of myocardial ischemia, the diagnostic work-up of patients with suspected IHD is still mainly oriented towards the detection of "anatomical" CAD. This anatomically oriented approach may lead to suboptimal treatment, additional risks, and increased health costs. Recent results confirm that, in the presence of documented stable CAD, revascularization improves survival rate more than optimal medical therapy does only when significant ischemia can be documented by stress imaging tests [32–34]. In the presence of significant CAD but the absence of inducible myocardial ischemia, coronary revascularization is associated with a worse prognosis than is conservative therapy [35, 36].

According to this conceptualization, CAD and IHD cannot be considered equivalent; as a consequence, an adequate strategy is needed in patients with suspected IHD, which would be aimed at first documenting the presence of ischemia and then defining whether the impairment of myocardial blood perfusion is of micro- or macrovascular origin. In addition, as ischemia results from the imbalance between oxygen supply and demand, factors that may be increasing cardiac work also have to be investigated, as outlined in Fig. 1.3.

In conclusion, coronary microvascular dysfunction leading to impairment of myocardial perfusion may be just as responsible for cardiac ischemia as CAD. This conclusion is of particular clinical relevance in the case of cardiac dysfunction not supported by findings of CAD or valvular or extracardiac disease. In such patients, positron emission tomography (PET) perfusion studies have clearly shown the impairment of absolute myocardial blood flow and coronary flow reserve [37]. Importantly, myocardial perfusion abnormalities in the absence of CAD are able to stratify the long-term prognosis [38, 39]. Thus, in the clinical arena, coronary microvascular dysfunction has gained an important position among the pathogenic factors of cardiac dysfunction [40].

Today, multislice CT (MSCT) coronary angiography can noninvasively detect coronary atherosclerosis. The combination of MSCT with perfusion imaging, either with single-photon-emission computed tomography (SPECT) or PET, can identify coronary stenoses that can limit blood flow during stress and hence require revascularization [41], but can also document impairment of myocardial perfusion that is not directly related to obstructive coronary lesions but which nevertheless requires aggressive medical treatment. Unfortunately, the elevated cost and the exposure to ionizing radiation greatly restrict the clinical application of this approach.

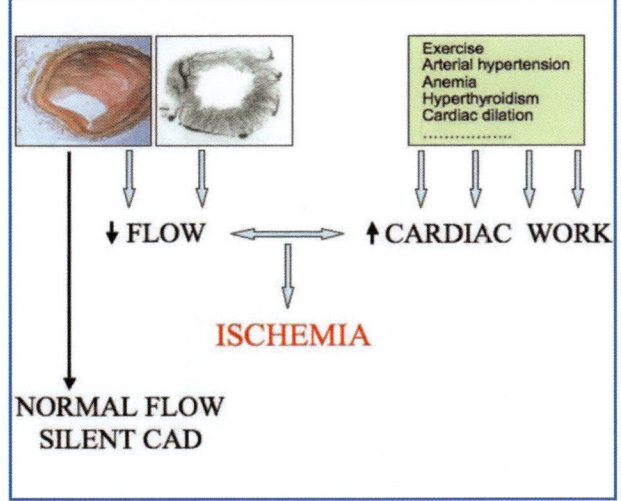

Fig. 1.3 Coronary microvascular alterations in cardiac failure. Myocardial ischemia is the result of imbalance between oxygen supply (blood flow) and oxygen demand (cardiac work). Both stenotic lesions of large coronary arteries and microvascular alterations may impair coronary blood flow (*left*), while cardiac work may be modulated by several factors affecting heat rate, contractility, and/or cardiac loads (*right*). Note that coronary atherosclerotic lesions are not necessarily associated with impaired blood flow; hence, coronary artery disease (*CAD*) is not synonymous with ischemic heart disease

1.5 HF and the Thyroid

The present volume is devoted to HF and the thyroid. The interest in the role of the thyroid in HF is supported by the documentation of changes in thyroid hormones in patients with chronic HF [42]. In addition, recent studies have demonstrated that a reduced serum T_3 concentration has a strong predictive power for cardiovascular mortality in various categories of cardiac patients [43], opening the prospect of new approaches in the treatment of HF based on thyroid hormone replacement. The inclusion of thyroid hormone in the plethora of hormones already involved in the pathogenesis and treatment of HF further enhances the "systemic disease" characterization of HF. However, this should not come as a surprise when one remembers the numerous direct and indirect effects of thyroid hormones on the cardiovascular system and the significant similarities that can be found between the hypothyroid phenotype and the HF phenotype [44]. In addition to the classical "cardiovascular side effects" of primary thyroid dysfunction, such as those on peripheral vascular resistance, heart rate, and myocardial contractility and relaxation, more recent research has identified novel cellular and molecular mechanisms by which thyroid hormone might exert its action in HF. These changes are the net result of decreased serum T_3 levels acting on both genomic and nongenomic mechanisms in the heart and in the vasculature in the setting of congestive HF [45]. In brief, these include erythropoietin synthesis [46], endothelial nitric oxide synthesis [47, 48], protein kinase Akt pathway [49], angiogenesis [47], renin substrate synthesis in the liver [50], and gene expression of natriuretic hormones [51]. Thus, thyroid hormones interact with the other hormones involved in HF and with the main hemodynamic and metabolic variables discussed above in this chapter that can modulate the development and progression of HF.

1.6 Conclusions

Modern medical treatment of HF requires the use of different drugs, each aimed at counteracting a specific mechanism responsible for the development and/or progression of HF. To take advantage of the available armamentarium, each patient has to be carefully characterized from the pathogenetic point of view. After this, daily management relies on relatively simple physical signs such as heart rate, arterial pressure, respiratory rate, O_2 blood saturation, and body weight, which, however, need to be carefully monitored in order to optimize the efficacy of treatment and, just as importantly, to prevent a HF relapse with the need for hospitalization.

The next few decades will offer tremendous opportunities for advances in the prevention and treatment of HF. Genetic research will likely provide insights into the pathophysiology of HF and contribute to risk stratification, while pharmacogenetics will hopefully maximize the efficacy and minimize the side effects of drugs; "personalization" of therapy could be the most effective way to reduce the cost of health care. The challenge of the HF pandemic demands preventive intervention on a formerly unimagined scale.

New results on the systemic response to primary cardiac damage, as appears to occur in the case of the thyroid, might translate into novel treatments for patients with HF [52]–similarly to what has already occurred for other hormones found to be implicated in HF, but hopefully in a shorter time. Brain natriuretic peptide was discovered in 1981, but was only approved as a treatment for HF 20 years later.

Key Points

- Twenty years from now, heart failure and atrial fibrillation will be the most common cause of hospitalization.

- Heart failure is characterized by high morbidity and mortality.

- Ischemic heart disease is the main underlying disease (60%).

- Both systolic and diastolic dysfunction (diastolic 40%) are responsible for heart failure.

(Cont. →)

(*cont.*)

- Heart failure is a systemic disease.

- Beyond the initial cardiac damage, progression of heart failure is the consequence of systemic activation of neurohormonal–immunological systems.

- The systemic activation is disproportionate to the severity of the initial cardiac damage.

- Early clinical recognition of the systemic activation is the basis for preventing the progression of heart failure.

References

1. Rosamond W, Flegal K, Friday G et al; American Heart Association Statistics Committee and Stroke Statistics Subcommittee (2007) Heart disease and stroke statistics–2007 update: a report from the American Heart Association Statistics Committee and Stroke Statistics Subcommittee. Circulation 115:e69–e171

2. Scholte op Reimer WJM, Gitt AK, Boersma E, Simoons ML (eds) (2006) Cardiovascular diseases in Europe. Euro Heart Survey. European Society of Cardiology, Sophia Antipolis. France

3. Roger VL, Weston SA, Redfield MM et al (2004) Trends in heart failure incidence and survival in a community-based population. JAMA 292:344–350

4. Schocken DD, Benjamin EJ, Fonarow GC et al; American Heart Association Council on Epidemiology and Prevention; American Heart Association Council on Clinical Cardiology; American Heart Association Council on Cardiovascular Nursing; American Heart Association Council on High Blood Pressure Research; Quality of Care and Outcomes Research Interdisciplinary Working Group, Functional Genomics and Translational Biology Interdisciplinary Working Group (2008) Prevention of heart failure: a scientific statement from the American Heart Association Councils on Epidemiology and Prevention, Clinical Cardiology, Cardiovascular Nursing, and High Blood Pressure Research; Quality of Care and Outcomes Research Interdisciplinary Working Group; and Functional Genomics and Translational Biology Interdisciplinary Working Group. Circulation 117:2544–2565

5. Lloyd-Jones DM, Larson MG, Leip EP et al; Framingham Heart Study (2002) Lifetime risk for developing congestive heart failure: the Framingham Heart Study. Circulation 106:3068–3072

6. Davis SK, Liu Y, Gibbons GH (2003) Disparities in trends of hospitalization for potentially preventable chronic conditions among African Americans during the 1990s: implications and benchmarks. Am J Public Health 93: 447–445

7. Packer M (1992) The neurohormonal hypothesis: a theory to explain the mechanism of disease progression in heart failure. J Am Coll Cardiol 20:248–254

8. Harris P (1988) Role of arterial pressure in the oedema of heart disease. Lancet 1:1036–1038

9. Schrier RW, Abraham WT (1999) Hormones and hemodynamics in heart failure. N Engl J Med 341:577–585

10. Dauterman KW, Massie BM, Gheorgiade M (1998) Heart failure associated with preserved systolic function: a common and costly clinical entity. Am Heart J 135:S310–319

11. Smith GL, Masoudi FA, Vaccarino V et al (2003) Outcomes in heart failure patients with preserved ejection fraction. J Am Coll Cardiol 41:1510–1518

12. Weber KT, Brilla CG (1991) Pathological hypertrophy and cardiac interstitium: fibrosis and renin-angiotensin-aldosterone system. Circulation 83:1849–1865

13. Owens DK, Sanders GD, Heidenreich PA et al (2002) Effect of risk stratification on cost-effectiveness of the implantable cardioverter defibrillator. Am Heart J 144:440–448

14. Bardy GH, Lee KL, Mark DB et al; Sudden Cardiac Death in Heart Failure Trial (SCD-HeFT) Investigators (2005) Amiodarone or an implantable cardioverter-defibrillator for congestive heart failure. N Engl J Med 352:225–237

15. Cleland JG, Daubert JC, Erdmann E et al; Cardiac Resynchronization-Heart Failure (CARE-HF) Study Investigators (2005) The effect of cardiac resynchronization therapy on morbidity and mortality in heart failure. N Engl J Med 352:1539–1549

16. Bristow MR, Saxon LA, Boehmer J et al; Comparison of Medical Therapy, Pacing, and Defibrillation in Heart Failure (COMPANION) Investigators (2004) Cardiac-resynchronization therapy with or without an implantable defibrillator in advanced chronic heart failure. N Engl J Med 350:2140–2150

17. Kannel WB, D'Agostino RB, Silbershatz H et al (1999) Profile for estimating risk of heart failure. Arch Intern Med 159:1197–1204

18. Gheorghiade M, Sopko G, De Luca L et al (2006) Navigating the crossroads of coronary heart disease and heart failure. Circulation 114:1202–1213

19. Wilhelmsen L, Rosengren A, Eriksson H, Lappas G (2001) Heart failure in the general population of men: morbidity, risk factors and prognosis. J Intern Med 249:253–261

20. Kenchaiah S, Narula J, Vasan RS (2004) Risk factors for heart failure. Med Clin North Am 88:1145–1172

21. Mckee PA, Castelli WP, McNamara PM, Kannel WB (1971) The natural history of congestive heart failure. The Framingham study. N Engl J Med 285:1441–1446

22. He J, Ogden LG, Bazzano LA et al (2001) Risk factors for congestive heart failure in US men and women: NHANES I epidemiologic follow-up study. Arch Intern Med 161:996–1002

23. Levy D, Larson MG, Vasan RS et al (1996) The progression from hypertension to congestive heart failure. JAMA 275:1557–1562

24. Kannel WB, Hjortland M, Castelli WP (1974) Role of diabetes in cogestive heart failure: the Framingham study. Am J Cardiol 34:29–34

25. Kenchainah S, Evans JC, Levy D et al (2002) Obesity and risk of heart failure. N Engl J Med 347: 305–313

26. Chae CU, Albert CM, Glynn RJ et al (2003) Mild renal insufficiency and risk of congestive heart failure in men and women ≥ 70 years of age. Am J Cardiol 92:682–686

27. Fried LF, Shlipak MG, Crump C et al (2003) Renal insufficiency as a predictor of cardiovascular outcomes and mortality in elderly individuals. J Am Coll Cardiol 41:1364–1372

28. Horio T, Miyazato J, Kamide K et al (2003) Influence of low high-density lipoprotein cholesterol on left ventricular hypertrophy and diastolic function in essential hypertension. Am J Hypertens 16(Pt1):938–944

29. L'Abbate A, Sambuceti G, Neglia D (2002) Myocardial perfusion and coronary microcirculation: from pathophysiology to clinical application. J Nucl Cardiol 9:328–337

30. Sambuceti G, Marzullo P, Giorgetti A et al (1994) Global alteration in perfusion response to increasing oxygen consumption in patients with single-vessel coronary artery disease. Circulation 90:1696–1705

31. Sambuceti G, Marzilli M, Mari A et al (2005) Coronary microcirculatory vasoconstriction is heterogeneously distributed in acutely ischemic myocardium. Am J Physiol Heart Circ Physiol 288:H2298–H2305

32. Hachamovitch R, Hayes SW, Friedman JD et al (2003) Comparison of the short-term survival benefit associated with revascularization compared with medical therapy in patients with no prior coronary artery disease undergoing stress myocardial perfusion single photon emission computed tomography. Circulation 107:2900–2907

33. Shaw LJ, Berman DS, Maron DJ et al; COURAGE Investigators. (2008) Optimal medical therapy with or without percutaneous coronary intervention to reduce ischemic burden: results from the Clinical Outcomes Utilizing Revascularization and Aggressive Drug Evaluation (COURAGE) trial nuclear substudy. Circulation 117:1283–1291

34. Boden WE, O'Rourke RA, Teo KK et al; COURAGE Trial Research Group (2007) Optimal medical therapy with or without PCI for stable coronary disease. N Engl J Med 356:1503–1516

35. Picano E, Landi P, Bolognese L et al on behalf of the EPIC Study Group (1993) Prognostic value of dipyridamole-echocardiography early after uncomplicated myocardial infarction: a large scale multicenter trial. Am J Med 11:608–618

36. Hachamovitch R, Hayes SW, Friedman JD et al (2003) Comparison of the short-term survival benefit associated with revascularization compared with medical therapy in patients with no prior coronary artery disease undergoing stress myocardial perfusion single photon emission computed tomography. Circulation 107:2900–2907

37. Neglia D, Parodi O, Gallopin M et al (1995) Myocardial blood flow response to pacing tachycardia and to dipyridamole infusion in patients with dilated cardiomyopathy without overt heart failure. A quantitative assessment by positron emission tomography. Circulation 92:796–804

38. Neglia D, Michelassi C, Trivieri MG et al (2002) Prognostic role of myocardial blood flow impairment in idiopathic left ventricular dysfunction. Circulation 105:186–193

39. Schindler TH, Nitzsche EU, Schelbert HR et al (2005) Positron emission tomography-measured abnormal responses of myocardial blood flow to sympathetic stimulation are associated with the risk of developing cardiovascular events. J Am Coll Cardiol 45:1505–1512

40. Camici PG, Crea F (2007) Coronary microvascular dysfunction. N Engl J Med 356:830–840

41. Di Carli MF, Dorbala S, Hachamovitch R (2006) Integrated cardiac PET-CT for the diagnosis and management of CAD. J Nucl Cardiol 13:139–144

42. Klein I, Danzi S (2007) Thyroid disease and the heart. Circulation 116:1725–1735

43. Pingitore A, Landi P, Taddei MC et al (2005) Triiodothyronine levels for risk stratification of patients with chronic heart failure. Am J Med 118:132–136

44. Lowes BD, Minobe W, Abraham WT et al (1997) Changes in gene expression in the intact human heart. Downregulation of alpha-myosin heavy chain in hypertrophied, failing ventricular myocardium. J Clin Invest 100:2315–2324

45. Davis PJ, Davis FB (2002) Nongenomic actions of thyroid hormone on the heart. Thyroid 12:459–466

46. Fish SA, Mandel SJ (2005) The blood in thyrotoxicosis. In: Bravermann L, Utiger R (eds) Werner and Ingbar's The Thyroid. Lippincott Williams and Wilkins, Philadelphia, pp 595–598

47. Vargas F, Moreno JM, Rodríguez-Gómez I et al (2006) Vascular and renal function in experimental thyroid disorders. Eur J Endocrinol 154:197–212

48. Napoli R, Biondi B, Guardasole V et al (2001) Impact of hyperthyroidism and its correction on vascular reactivity in humans. Circulation 104:3076–3080

49. Kuzman JA, Gerdes AM, Kobayashi S, Liang Q (2005) Thyroid hormone activates Akt and prevents serum starvation-induced cell death in neonatal rat cardiomyocytes. J Mol Cell Cardiol 39:841–844

50. Laragh JH, Sealey JE (2003) Relevance of the plasma renin hormonal control system that regulates blood pressure and sodium balance for correctly treating hypertension and for evaluating ALLHAT. Am J Hypertens 16:407–415

51. Lewicki JA, Protter AA (1995) Physiological studies of the natriuretic peptide family. In: Laragh JH, Brenner BM (eds) Hypertension: pathophysiology, diagnosis and management. New York, Raven Press, pp 1029–1053

52. Klein I, Ojamaa K (2001) Thyroid hormone and the cardiovascular system. N Engl J Med 344:501–509

Neuroendocrine Control of the Cardiovascular System in Heart Failure

2

Claudio Ceconi and Roberto Ferrari

Abstract Neuroendocrine activation starts early in the natural history of left ventricular dysfunction, and the levels of circulating hormones increase in proportion to the severity of heart failure. The neurohormonal response evoked during congestive heart failure (CHF) is the same as that evolved to support the survival of the species under two main conditions that threaten life: hemorrhage and physical exercise. In these conditions, a short-term threat to blood pressure evokes a baroreceptor-mediated increase in sympathetic activity that causes venoconstriction, tachycardia, stimulation of the myocardium, and regional vasoconstriction. Augmented neuroendocrine activity in the syndrome of heart failure is initially beneficial, appears to be adaptive, and helps support blood pressure and cardiac output. Prolonged and excessive activation, however, has deleterious effects, with adverse consequences at both cardiac and vascular levels, which aggravate the clinical status of the syndrome and negatively affect its prognosis. Most studies suggest that high levels of neurohormones predict a poor prognosis, and antihormonal therapy is now the cornerstone of chronic heart failure treatment.

Keywords Neuroendocrine activation • Sympathetic system • Renin–angiotensin–aldosterone system • Natriuretic peptides • Adaptive mechanisms • Maladaptive mechanisms

2.1 Introduction

Heart failure is a clinical condition characterized by reduced cardiac function and impairment of the capacity of the heart to maintain output, reduced peripheral perfusion, and threatening of arterial pressure. As a consequence, a number of compensatory endocrine and paracrine mechanisms are activated to preserve circulatory homeostasis and maintain arterial pressure [1, 2]; these, however, ultimately result in a clinical syndrome characterized by vasoconstriction and water and fluid retention. Understanding of the events underlying this syndrome is complicated by the fact that heart failure is the end result of various diseases of multifactorial origin and usually develops after a chronic phase with several adaptation/de-adaptation processes occurring at the genetic, molecular, organ, or whole-organism level [1, 2]. The neuroendocrine response is indeed helpful for increasing or maintaining blood pressure under such conditions of short-term emergency as hypoglycemia, trauma, hemorrhage, and exercise. But heart failure is a chronic state in which, because of a primary abnormality in the cardiac pump, arterial pressure is continuously and chronically threatened. As a result, the body abnormally intensifies the neuroendocrine response by which arterial pressure should be main-

R. Ferrari (✉)
Department of Cardiology, University of Ferrara,
Cardiovascular Institute, Arcispedale S. Anna Hospital,
Ferrara, Italy

G. Iervasi, A. Pingitore (eds.), *Thyroid and Heart Failure*.
© Springer-Verlag Italia 2009

tained, and a vicious cycle is established. The existence of these vicious cycles both at the molecular level and at the level of the body is of paramount importance in the pathogenesis of heart failure syndrome.

2.2 Activation of Humoral Adaptive Responses in Heart Failure

Congestive heart failure (CHF) is a complex multiorgan syndrome that manifests itself by pump failure, cardiac dilation, intense systemic vasoconstriction, and avid sodium retention with edema formation [3]. Increasing evidence points to humoral substances that circulate and are also synthesized acting locally to mediate the terminal consequences of a failing heart. The principal humoral mechanisms activated in heart failure have opposing effects: vasoconstrictor hormones are antinatriuretic and antidiuretic and in general have growth-promoting properties, whereas vasodilator hormones are natriuretic and have antimitogenic effects [3–5]. Among

the former are, for example, norepinephrine (NE) and adrenaline, the components of the renin–angiotensin–aldosterone system (RAAS), and arginine vasopressin (AVP); among the latter are the natriuretic peptides, prostaglandins, kallikrein–kinin system, and calcitonin-gene-related peptide (CGRP). Indeed, this list is only partial as more than 100 humoral mediators have been well-investigated in CHF. Of these, NA. RAAS, and the atrial natriuretic peptides have been well-studied and in some circumstances used as a basis for making clinical and therapeutic decisions.

Despite the activation of these systems with their opposing actions, it is clear that in CHF the natriuretic and vasodilator effects of atrial natriuretic peptides are overwhelmed by baroreceptor-mediated influences that lead to vasoconstriction and salt and water retention through activation of the sympathetic system and the RAAS [3–5]. Thus, CHF sets in motion a complex and interacting network of events (Fig. 2.1). An extensive review of the hemodynamics and hormones in heart failure can be found in Schrier and Abraham [6].

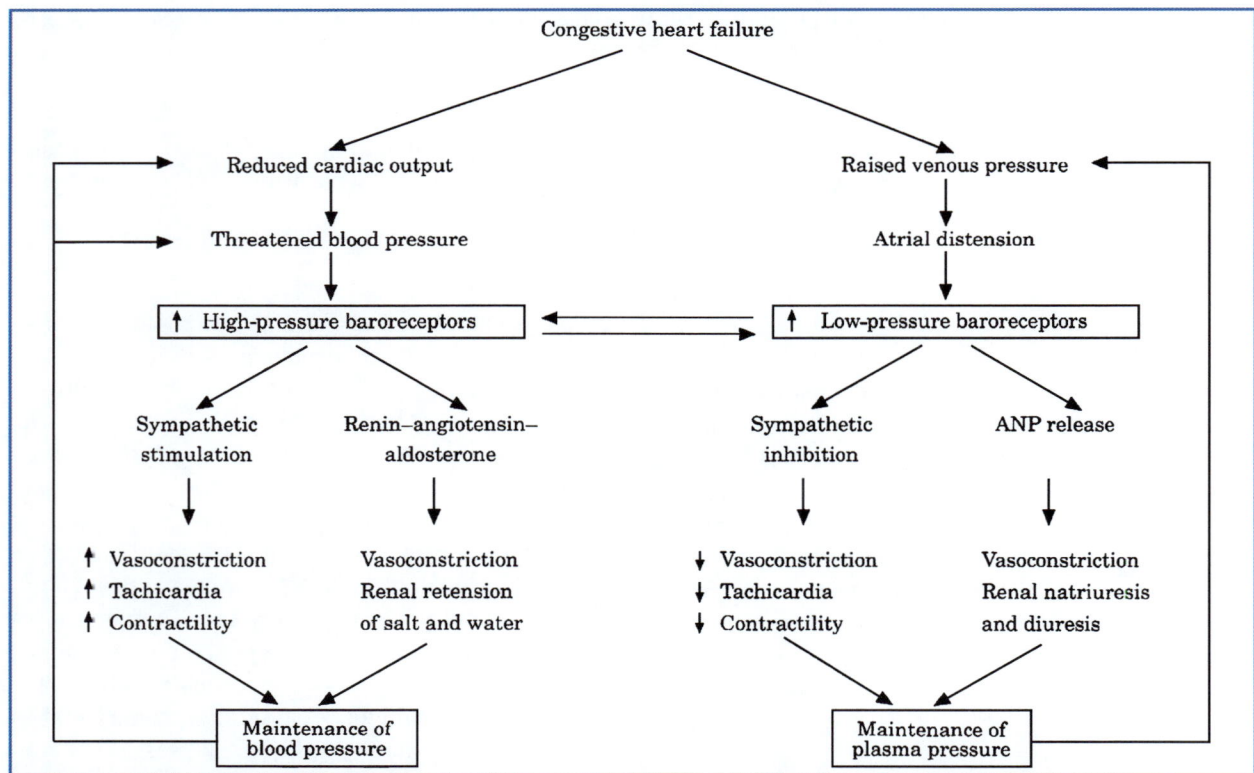

Fig. 2.1 Interplay between vasoconstrictor hormones (increased sympathetic and renin–angiotensin–aldosterone systems) and vasodilator substances (increased release of natriuretic peptides). *ANP* atrial natriuretic peptide

The majority of studies on the neuroendocrine response to CHF have been carried out in patients already treated with diuretics, digitalis, angiotensin-converting enzyme (ACE) inhibitors, and vasodilators [3, 7–9]. The data obtained are important as they provide a picture of the neuroendocrine activation in the treated patients who are referred to specific day hospitals and/or CHF clinics. From the physiopathological point of view, however, such data are misleading as the treatment itself may affect the mechanisms being studied. One unique small study has reported neurohormone measurements in untreated patients with water retention and reduced renal blood flow [10]. In these patients plasma levels of NA, renin activity, aldosterone, and atrial natriuretic peptide were increased even more than in the patients studied in the CONSENSUS I trial [7].

2.3 Underlying Mechanisms of the Neuroendocrine Response to CHF

The neurohormonal responses described above are seen in patients with heart disease and low-output CHF. However, an identical neurohormonal response and retention of salt and water also occur in a number of conditions in which the heart is entirely normal and cardiac output is even higher than normal. So-called high-output congestive heart failure is seen in a variety of conditions that include chronic severe anemia, chronic arteriovenous fistula, beriberi, Paget's disease, chronic obstructive pulmonary disease, and states with divergent hemodynamics [10]. The common factor in all forms of CHF appears to be a tendency towards low arterial blood pressure. Blood pressure is threatened in low-output states because of low cardiac output and in high-output states because of a decrease in systemic vascular resistance. However, the neurohormonal response of the body is similar. The neuroendocrine response has also been determined in untreated patients with constrictive pericarditis [11], chronic cor pulmonale [12], anemia [13], and arteriovenous fistula [14]. The data obtained are summarized in Figure 2.2.

Nor is this response unique to low- or high-output syndromes of CHF. The same neurohormonal response is also seen when blood pressure is

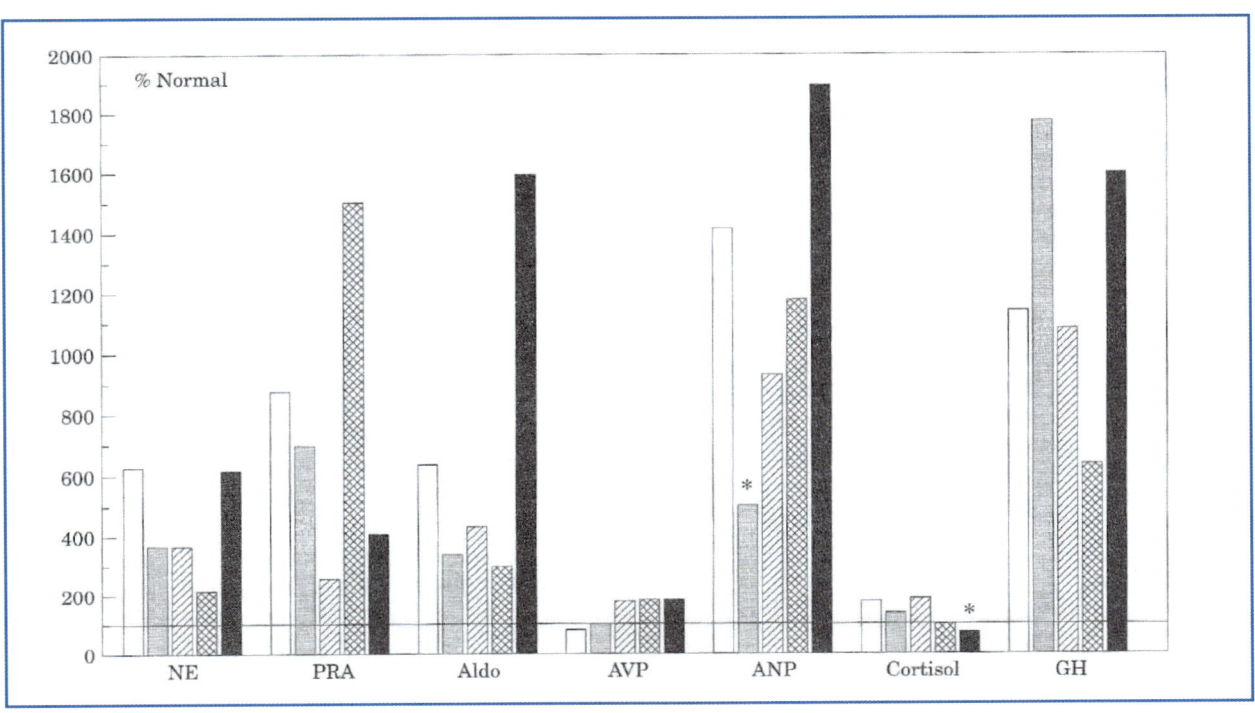

Fig. 2.2 Changes in a variety of neurohormones in untreated patients with low-output or high-output state and edema. The neurohormonal response is very similar. *NE* norepinephrine, *PRA* plasma renin activity, *Aldo* aldosterone, *AVP* arginine vasopressin, *ANP* atrial natriuretic peptide, *GH* growth hormone. (□) Dilated cardiomyopathy, (▨) chronic constrictive pericarditis, (▨) chronic obstructive pulmonary disease, (⊠) chronic severe anemia, (■) arteriovenous fistula. *P < 0.005 vs CHF. (Adapted from [48])

reduced for whatever reason; for example, during acute reduction of arterial pressure with nitroprusside [15], and during physical exercise [16, 17], when blood pressure is threatened by marked vasodilatation in exercising muscles. These findings, therefore, support the theory [1, 2] that the neurohormonal response evoked during CHF is the same as that evolved to support survival of the species under two main conditions that threaten life: hemorrhage and physical exercise. In these conditions, a short-term threat to blood pressure evokes a baroreceptor-mediated increase in sympathetic activity that causes venoconstriction, tachycardia, stimulation of the myocardium, and regional vasoconstriction. When blood pressure is threatened by reduced cardiac output due to left ventricular dysfunction, the body cannot distinguish whether the threat is from hemorrhage, exercise, or heart disease and therefore uses the same stereotyped response to which it is programmed. In heart disease (and other sustained vasodilated high-output states), however, blood pressure is threatened over a prolonged period and the effector mechanisms continue to operate for as long as the threat persists.

2.4 Activation of the Sympathetic System in Heart Failure: Adaptive or Maladaptive Process?

Many subsequent studies confirmed the original observation of Chidsey et al. [18] of an increased plasma concentration of norepinephrine in patients with CHF at rest [3, 7, 9]. In addition, the failing myocardium becomes depleted of norepinephrine (NE) [19, 20]. The reasons for this were debated, and a defect in the synthesis and uptake of NE was suggested [21]. It has been shown in experimental animals that the diminution in total myocardial norepinephrine content is specifically associated with CHF, whereas in the presence of ventricular hypertrophy without failure, the NE content remains unchanged. Its concentration, however, is decreased, simply because the volume of the myocytes is increased [22]. In untreated patients with cardiac edema, the plasma concentration of NE was consistently increased, the average being over six times that of the controls. In contrast, the plasma level of epinephrine was unchanged (Fig. 2.2) [10, 11, 17].

The magnification of the sympathetic outflow is likely to be mediated by the arterial stretch receptors [23]. These receptors normally send the central nervous system impulses that inhibit the activation of two vasoconstrictor mechanisms: the sympathetic nervous system and the release of vasopressin from the pituitary. When these inhibitory afferent impulses are reduced by a fall in systemic arterial pressure, central tonic inhibition is reduced, thereby triggering the activation of sympathetic activity and release of neurohormones (Fig. 2.1). An alternative hypothesis linking a diminished cardiac output with stimulation of the sympathetic system is that the low cardiac output causes underperfusion of the tissues, which in turn release a mediatory substance into the blood. There are, however, several observations against this hypothesis [23]. The increased sympathetic activity causes tachycardia, improves myocardial contractility, promotes venous constriction, and redistributes arterial resistance. All these mechanisms tend to maintain the systemic arterial pressure.

The effects of the sympathetic nervous system, although compensatory in their essence, as a whole are certainly not beneficial in the long run. Stimulation of mechanical performance with β-adrenergic agonists has proved an unsuccessful approach to the treatment of heart failure. β-Adrenergic blockers, on the other hand, have produced favorable effects in patients with chronic heart failure and are now a cornerstone of CHF treatment [3]. Consequently, the activation of this powerful system is not necessarily beneficial for patients in heart failure. Several factors must be considered in this regard.

Firstly, in heart failure there are abnormalities of the central neurohormonal regulation. Normally, feedback regulation exists between the sympathetic nervous system and blood pressure and intravascular volume. The increased sympathetic activity tends to enhance blood pressure and intravascular volume, which in turn, act on the high-pressure arterial and atrial baroreceptors, restoring the tonic inhibition of neurohormonal activity and thus suppressing sympathetic outflow. In CHF, however, the ability of atrial and arterial baroreceptors to suppress sympathetic activity is markedly impaired [24, 25]. Atrial receptors are no longer properly activated by the increase in atrial pressure. The desensitization of baroreceptors shifts the balance of circulatory homeostatic mechanisms to an equilibrium in which high circulating levels of NE and, therefore, vasoconstrictor force are continually dominant. This leads to an inability of the myocardium to respond to continuously high levels of endogenous or exogenous catecholamines [26]. β-Receptors are reduced in number, stimulation of adenylcyclase by isoprenaline is diminished, and the contractile response to catecholamines is lessened [27]. These findings have generated the concept that β-receptors are down-regulated in heart failure. As a consequence, patients with heart failure would be less responsive to adrenergic stimuli than healthy people, and the positive effects of sympathetic stimulation would diminish with time as the receptors are down-regulated [28].

It is important to emphasize here that the reduction in catecholamine responsiveness is relatively selective for the myocardium. Catecholamines do not become depleted in the kidney [21], where down-regulation does not take place. Furthermore, sympathetic neurotransmitter activity is augmented, rather than attenuated, in the peripheral blood vessels [29]. This explains why catecholamines in the long term are not beneficial for the patient with heart failure. Increased sympathetic activity will support excessive vasoconstriction with increased ventricular afterload and, through stimulation RAAS, water retention, thus leading to an increased ventricular preload. This will impose a greater workload on the myocardium, which cannot benefit from the positive inotropic effect mediated by catecholamines. This in turn will cause further deterioration of the cardiac pump, worsen heart failure, activate the neuroendocrine system, and further increase systemic resistance (Fig. 2.1). Overall, this represents a progressive spiral of heart failure [5, 30, 31].

2.5 Activation of the Renin–Angiotensin–Aldosterone System in Heart Failure: Adaptive or Maladaptive Process?

Early measurements of both aldosterone and renin activity in the plasma of patients with heart failure were confusing. Brown et al. [32] found plasma renin to be increased only in one-third of patients with untreated congestive cardiac failure of different causes.

Bayliss et al. [33] reported normal values for plasma renin activity in untreated patients with clinically mild heart failure. The same was true for aldosterone. This is quite in contrast with the common belief that the RAAS is stimulated in heart failure [34]. However, plasma renin activity and aldosterone concentrations are known to be influenced by diuretic therapy [35, 36]. In untreated patients with cardiac edema and excess accumulation of water, plasma renin activity and aldosterone levels varied considerably (Fig. 2.2). Some patients had normal values, whilst others had very high values. It seems, therefore, that both aldosterone and renin activity are increased in some patients independently of the administration of diuretic therapy, but are normal in others despite water retention.

An explanation of these results is provided by the pioneering experiments in dogs, carried out by Watkins et al. [37]. They showed that, after constriction of the pulmonary artery or inferior vena cava, the initial response was a reduction in blood pressure and a rise in plasma renin activity and aldosterone and in water intake. However, renin activity and aldosterone returned to normal levels in the following days, as soon as the plasma volume expanded and arterial blood pressure was restored. In those animals in which blood pressure was not restored, plasma renin activity and plasma aldosterone remained elevated throughout the period of constriction, suggesting the existence of a feedback mechanism between plasma volume and renin activity. Thus, activation of this system is likely to be transient rather than sustained, and is possibly related to the different phases of the development of heart failure. It has been suggested that plasma renin activity and angiotensin II are high in the initial stages of heart failure. With mild congestive chronic failure, they tend to fall toward normal as the condition is established. With severe heart failure they remain high.

The increased concentration of angiotensin II that will ultimately result from increased plasma renin activity has other important properties in heart failure in addition to stimulating aldosterone secretion. Angiotensin II acts on efferent arterioles to increase the glomerular hydraulic filtration pressure; it is the second most potent vasoconstrictor peptide after endothelin, enhances neuroeffector transmission, and is involved in the sensation of thirst. Metabolism and growth in nonmyocyte cells are also altered by circulating and locally generated angiotensin, which results in cardiac hypertrophy with both ventricular diastolic dysfunction and impaired systolic contractile activity [38].

Long-term treatment with ACE inhibitors has been shown in several trials to be beneficial for patients in heart failure [3]. The benefit is not simply due to a vasodilator action. These drugs also inhibit the facilitating action of angiotensin II on NE, enhance baroreceptor sensitivity, and prevent the consequences of this undesirable side effect of diuretics.

Thus, as in the case of catecholamines, it seems that every time we counteract the effects of the RAAS, the patient improves.

2.6 Activation of Natriuretic Peptides in Heart Failure: An Adaptive Compensatory Response

Microscopy studies have shown the presence of specific granules in atrial myocardium, the number of which varies with changes in water and electrolyte balance [39]. In addition, De Bold [40] demonstrated that an atrial extract has a natriuretic effect; the active principle has now been identified as a polypeptide and its amino acid sequence has been determined [41, 42]. Increased concentrations of natriuretic peptide were found in patients with treated CHF in the studies of Anand et al. ([10–13] and Fig. 2.2). In the untreated patient with cardiac edema, the plasma concentration of atrial natriuretic peptide was dramatically raised in every case, the average being 14 times the control valve.

The release of the peptide is stimulated by the stretching of atrial tissue [43] and by volume loading [44]; undoubtedly, increased concentrations in the blood of patients with CHF is due to excessive release from overstretched atria. Once released, natriuretic peptides exert a potent direct vasodilation by increasing intracellular cyclic GMP and natriuresis. Natriuretic peptide also suppresses the release of NE and renin, and counteracts the systemic vasoconstrictor actions of angiotensin II, as well as the ability of angiotensin II to stimulate thirst and to stimulate the secretion of aldosterone [45]. All these mechanisms, therefore, act together to lower systemic vascular resistances and to increase the sodium excretion (Fig. 2.1). This will unload the heart and reduce its energy consumption. Nonetheless, the natriuretic and vasodilator effects of the natriuretic peptides in patients with CHF are clearly outweighed by the sodium retention and vasoconstriction caused by the sympathetic stimulation and activation of the RAAS. As stated before, the atrial stretch receptors become impaired in chronic heart failure. Consequently, the ability of atrial distension to increase the release of atrial natriuretic peptide is blunted [25], and the slope of the curve of atrial pressure/atrial-natriuretic-peptide release is shifted so that circulating levels of atrial natriuretic peptide for a given atrial pressure are reduced [25]. In addition, it has been suggested that patients with heart failure may adapt to the physiological effects of atrial natriuretic peptide over time; in particular, the action of the peptide on the kidney is markedly attenuated [46].

2.7 Conclusions

Neuroendocrine response constitutes a mechanism of adaptation to the reduced capacity of the myocyte to support active contraction. Originally, the neuroendocrine response in CHF was viewed as a specific compensatory beneficial mechanism. However, we have learned that this view is too simplistic. All the changes in the peripheral autonomic and RAAS (among others) exacerbate the condition of heart failure, and the baroreflex responses as well as the natriuretic peptides system are outweighed in the chronic period. Consequently, pharmacological treatment aimed at reducing the effects of the neuroendocrine response has proven to be advantageous for patients with heart failure.

The problem is that the response of the body to heart failure is not specific [1, 2, 47]. It has been suggested that what is evoked is a stereotyped neuroendocrine response for which we have been programmed by natural selection in order to maintain arterial pressure, and therefore survival, in circumstances that threaten life directly, such as hypovolemia, trauma, hemorrhage, and exercise, on which daily life depends, and indeed the neuroendocrine response is very useful for these short-term conditions. Heart failure, however, is often a chronic state in which the arterial pressure is continuously and chronically threatened because of a primary abnormality in the cardiac pump. For this reason, the body abnormally intensifies the neuroendocrine responses, giving rise to series of deleterious vicious cycles.

Key Points

- Congestive heart failure is a complex multiorgan syndrome that manifests itself by pump failure, cardiac dilation, intense systemic vasoconstriction, and avid sodium retention with edema formation.

- This complex set of signs and symptoms is the direct consequence of activation of different neuroendocrine systems, including the sympathetic and renin–angiotensin–aldosterone systems.

- Neuroendocrine activation is not specific for heart failure, but seems to be a stereotyped response to support survival of the species in every acute condition in which arterial pressure and circulatory homeostasis are threatened.

- Heart failure, however, is often a chronic condition, and these mechanisms, initially compensatory, become maladaptive and cause disease progression.

- Measurement of the degree of neuroendocrine activation by means of various biomarkers (e.g., brain natriuretic peptide, noradrenaline) is an accepted method of estimating prognosis. Furthermore, treatment directed against neuroendocrine activation has dramatically improved the life expectancy of heart failure patients.

References

1. Harris P (1988) Role of arterial pressure in the edema of heart disease. Lancet 1(8593):1036–1038
2. Harris P (1983) Evolution and the cardiac patient. Cardiovasc Res 313:373–437
3. Task Force for Diagnosis and Treatment of Acute and Chronic Heart Failure 2008 et al (2008) ESC Guidelines for the diagnosis and treatment of acute and chronic heart failure 2008. Eur Heart J 29:2388–2442
4. Packer M, Lee WH, Kessler PD et al (1987) Role of neurohormonal mechanisms in determining survival in patients with severe chronic heart failure. Circulation 75(Suppl IV):IV–80
5. Packer M (1992) The neurohormonal hypothesis: a theory to explain the mechanism of disease progression in heart failure. J Am Coll Cardiol 20:248–254
6. Schrier RW, Abraham WT (1999) Hormones and hemodynamics in heart failure. N Engl J Med 341:577–585
7. Swedberg K, Eneroth P, Kjekshus J, Snapinn S (1990) Effects of enalapril and neuroendocrine activation on prognosis in severe congestive heart failure (follow-up of the CONSENSUS Trial Study Group). Am J Cardiol 66:40D–44D
8. Francis GS, Cohn IN, Johnson G et al (1993) Plasma norepinephrine, plasma renin activity and congestive heart failure. Relations to survival and the effects of therapy in V-HeFT II. The V-HeFT VA Cooperative Studies Group. Circulation 87:V140–148
9. Francis GS, Rector TS, Cohn IN (1988) Sequential neurohumoral measurements in patients with congestive heart failure. Am Heart J 116:1464–1468
10. Anand IS, Ferrari R, Kalra GS et al (1989) Edema of cardiac origin. Studies of body water and sodium, renal function, hemodynamic indexes, and plasma hormones in untreated congestive cardiac failure. Circulation 80:299–305
11. Anand IS, Ferrari R, Kalra GS et al (1991) Pathogenesis of edema in constrictive pericarditis. Circulation 83:1880–1887
12. Anand IS, Chandrashekhar Y, Ferrari R et al (1992) Pathogenesis of congestive state in chronic obstructive pulmonary disease. Circulation 86:12–21
13. Anand IS, Chandrashekhar Y, Ferrari R et al (1993) Pathogenesis of oedema in chronic severe anaemia: studies of body water and sodium, renal function, haemodynamic variables, and plasma hormones. Br Heart J 70:357–362
14. Anand IS (1997) Pathogenesis of salt and water retention in the congestive heart failure syndrome. In: Poole-Wilson PA, Colucci WS, Massie BM et al (eds) Heart failure. Churchill Livingstone, New York, pp 155–172
15. Ferrari R, Ceconi C, De Giuli F et al (1992) Temporal relations of the endocrine response to hypotension with sodium nitroprusside. Cardioscience 3:51–60
16. Ferrari R, Ceconi C, Rodella A et al (1991) Temporal relations of the endocrine response to exercise. Cardioscience 2:131–139
17. Ferrari R, Anand IS, Ceconi C et al (1996) Neuroendocrine response to standing and mild exercise in patients with untreated severe congestive heart failure and chronic constrictive pericarditis. Heart 76:50–5
18. Chidsey CA, Harrison DC, Braunwald E (1962) The augmentation of plasma norepinephrine response to exercise in patients with congestive heart failure. N Engl J Med 267:650–654
19. Chidsey CA, Braunwald E, Morrow AG (1965) Catecholamine excretion and cardiac stores of norepinephrine in congestive heart failure. Ann J Med 39:442–451
20. Chidsey CA, Sonnenblick EH, Morrow AG, Braunwald E (1966) Norepinephrine stores and contractile force of papillary muscle from the failing heart. Circulation 33:43–51

21. Spean JF, Chidsey CA, Pool PE, Braunwald E (1965) Mechanism of norepinephrine depletion in experimental heart failure produced by aortic constriction in the guinea pig. Circ Res 17:312–321

22. Ceconi C, Condorelli E, Quinzanini M et al (1989) Noradrenaline, atrial natriuretic peptide, bombesin and neurotensin in myocardium and blood of rats in congestive cardiac failure. Cardiovasc Res 23:674–682

23. Harris P (1987) Congestive cardiac failure: central role of the arterial blood pressure. Br Heart J 58:190–203

24. Hirsch AT, Dzau VJ, Creager MA (1987) Baroreceptor function in congestive heart failure: effect on neurohormonal activation and regional vascular resistance. Circulation 75(Suppl IV):IV-36

25. Tsutamoto T, Kanamori T, Morigami N et al (1993) Possibility of down regulation of atrial natriuretic peptide receptor coupled to guanylate cyclase in peripheral vascular beds of patients with chronic severe heart failure. Circulation 87:70–75

26. Fowler MB, Laser JA, Hopkins GL et al (1986) Assessment of beta-adrenergic receptor pathway in the intact failing human heart: progressive receptor down-regulation and sub sensitivity to agonist response. Circulation 74:1290–1299

27. Bristow MR, Ginsburg R, Minobe W (1982) Decreased catecholamine sensitivity and beta-adrenergic-receptor density in failing human hearts. N Engl J Med 307:205–211

28. Bristow MR, Minobe W, Rasmussen et al (1992) b-Adrenergic neuroeffector abnormalities in the failing human heart are produced by local rather than systemic mechanisms. J Clin Invest 89:803–815

29. Kramer PS, Mason DT, Braunwald E (1968) Augmented sympathetic neurotransmitter activity in the peripheral vascular bed of patients with congestive heart failure and cardiac norepinephrine depletion. Circulation 38:629–639

30. Cohn JN, Ferrari R, Sharpe N (2000) Cardiac remodeling – concepts and clinical implications: a consensus paper from an international forum on cardiac remodeling. J Am Coll Cardiol 35:569–582

31. Sutton MG, Sharpe N (2000) Left ventricular remodeling after myocardial infarction: pathophysiology and therapy. Circulation 101:2981–2988

32. Brown JJ, Davies DL, Johnson VW et al (1970) Renin relationships in congestive cardiac failure, treated and untreated. Am Heart J 80:329–342

33. Bayliss J, Norell M, Canepa Anson R et al (1987) Untreated heart failure: clinical and neuroendocrine effects of introducing diuretics. Br Heart J 57:17–22

34. Packer M (1992) The neurohumoral hypothesis: a theory to explain the mechanism of disease progression in heart failure. J Am Coll Cardiol 20:248–254

35. Skinner SL, McCubbin JW, Page JH (1964) Control of renin secretion. Circ Res 15:64–76

36. Ferrari R, Ceconi C, De Giuli F et al (1992) Temporal relations of the endocrine response to hypotension with sodium nitroprusside. Cardioscience 3:51–59

37. Watkins L Jr, Burton JA, Haber E et al (1976) The renin-aldosterone system in congestive failure on conscious dogs. J Clin Invest 57:1606–1607

38. Weber KT, Anversa P, Armostrong PW et al (1992) Remodeling and reparation of the cardiovascular system. J Am Coll Cardiol 20:3–16

39. Riegger GAJ, Liebau G, Kochsiek K (1982) Antidiuretic hormone in congestive heart failure. Am J Med 72:49–61

40. De Bold AJ (1979) Heart atria granularity. Effects of changes in water electrolyte balance. Proc Soc Exp Biol Med 161:508–511

41. Atlas SA, Kleinert HD, Camargo MJ (1984) Purification, sequencing and synthesis of natriuretic and vasoactive rat atrial peptide. Nature 309:717–719

42. De Bold AJ, Borenstein HB, Veress AT, Sonnenberg H (1981) A rapid and potent natriuretic response to intravenous injection of atrial myocardial extract in rats. Life Sci 28:89–94

43. Agnoletti G, Rodella A, Ferrari R, Harris P (1987) Release of atrial natriuretic peptide-like immunoreactive material during stretching of the rat atrium in vitro. J Mol Cell Cardiol 19:217–220

44. Agnoletti G, Curello S, Ceconi C et al (1992) Effects of isoproterenol (I) on the release of atrial natriuretic peptide (ANP) from isolated atria. Am J Cardiovasc Pathol 4:203–209

45. Laragh JH (1985) Atrial natriuretic hormone, the renin-angiotensin axis, and blood pressure-electrolyte homeostasis. N Engl J Med 313:1330–1343

46. Shaknovitch A, Pondolfino K, Clark M et al (1986) Atrial natriuretic factor in normal subjects and heart failure patients: plasma levels and renal, hormonal, and hemodynamic responses to peptide infusion. J Clin Invest 78:1362–1373

47. Harris P (1982) Biology of cardiac failure. Eur Heart J 3(Suppl D):5–10

48. Ferrari R, Ceconi C, Curello S, Visioli O (1998) The neuroendocrine and sympathetic nervous system in congestive heart failure. Eur Heart J 19(Suppl F):F45–51

Cardiac Morphology and Function in Mild Hypothyroidism

3

Bernadette Biondi

Abstract Subclinical hypothyroidism is an early and mild form of thyroid failure characterized by serum levels of thyroid hormones within their reference range but elevated serum TSH concentrations. The prevalence of subclinical hypothyroidism is 4–10% and this condition increases significantly with age. The management and treatment of subclinical hypothyroidism are controversial, and there is no consensus about the TSH concentration at which treatment should be started. The cardiovascular risk is increased in patients with overt hypothyroidism, with several potential cardiovascular risk factors similarly reported in patients with subclinical hypothyroidism. Identification of the potential cardiovascular risk factors could facilitate decision-making about the treatment of patients with subclinical hypothyroidism. Impaired left ventricular diastolic function, characterized by slowed myocardial relaxation and impaired early ventricular filling, is the most consistent cardiac abnormality identified in young and middle-aged patients with subclinical hypothyroidism. Moreover, vascular function is impaired in patients with mild and subclinical hypothyroidism, as documented by the increase in systemic vascular resistance and arterial stiffness and by the impaired endothelial function, increasing the risk of atherosclerosis and coronary artery disease. Epidemiological studies have investigated cardiovascular morbidity and mortality in patients with subclinical hypothyroidism; the results suggest that middle-aged individuals with mild thyroid hormone deficiency have a higher cardiovascular risk for coronary heart disease than the elderly with this condition. Moreover, cardiac death, particularly from ischemic heart disease, is significantly higher in cardiac patients with subclinical hypothyroidism. Replacement therapy with L-thyroxine (L-T$_4$) may reverse the cardiovascular risk associated with subclinical hypothyroidism. For this reason, L-T$_4$ replacement therapy should be considered in subclinically hypothyroid patients who have associated high cardiovascular risk factors.

Keywords Subclinical thyroid disease • Subclinical hypothyroidism • Thyrotropin • L-Thyroxine replacement therapy • Cardiovascular risk • Systolic function • Diastolic function • Cardiovascular mortality • Coronary heart disease • Heart failure

3.1 Causes, Prevalence, and Progression of Mild Subclinical Hypothyroidism

Subclinical hypothyroidism is an early and mild form of thyroid failure characterized by serum levels

B. Biondi (✉)
Department of Clinical and Molecular
Endocrinology and Oncology, University of Naples
Federico II, Naples, Italy

G. Iervasi, A. Pingitore (eds.), *Thyroid and Heart Failure*.
© Springer-Verlag Italia 2009

of thyroid hormones within their reference range but elevated serum TSH concentrations [1, 2]. Most patients with subclinical hypothyroidism have chronic autoimmune thyroiditis, with positive tests for serum antithyroid peroxidase (anti-TPO) antibodies. Poor compliance with L-T$_4$ therapy or suboptimal treatment of overt disease may also result in subclinical hypothyroidism [1, 2]. Moreover, some medications (lithium, iodine, interferon, etc.), ^{131}I therapy, or thyroidectomy and external irradiation of the neck are other important causes of transient or persistent subclinical hypothyroidism [1]. Only persistent subclinical hypothyroidism should be considered an early stage of thyroid disease [1].

The epidemiological data provided by three large population-based screening studies (the Whickham Survey, the Colorado Thyroid Disease Prevalence Study, and the National Health and Nutrition Examination Survey III) [3–5] showed that the prevalence of subclinical hypothyroidism is 4–10% and that this condition increases significantly with age, so that by the ninth decade of life the prevalence may be 15–20%. Progression to overt hypothyroidism occurs at a rate of 2–5% and is increased in patients with TSH concentrations above 6 mIU/L and positive thyroid antibodies [6]. The management and treatment of subclinical hypothyroidism are controversial and there is no consensus about the TSH concentration at which treatment should be started [7, 8]. According to recent consensus guidelines, treatment with L-T$_4$ should be considered in patients with increased serum TSH levels (>10 mIU/L), whereas it is controversial in patients with only mildly increased serum TSH levels (4.5–10 mIU/L) [8]. In the Colorado study, 75% of individuals with subclinical hypothyroidism had serum TSH levels between 5 and 10 mIU/L [4]. Given this high prevalence of mild hypothyroidism in the general population, it is important to establish whether mild thyroid dysfunction is associated with an increased cardiovascular risk, in order to establish the necessity of treatment with replacement therapy.

3.2 Cardiac Morphology and Function in Subclinical Hypothyroidism

Identification of the potential cardiovascular risk in subclinical hypothyroidism could facilitate decision-making about the treatment of these patients [1, 9–11]. Systolic and diastolic functions have been assessed in patients with subclinical hypothyroidism during the last 10–15 years by a variety of techniques. At-rest systolic function, as assessed using Weissler's method (simultaneous recording electrocardiography, carotid tracing, and phonocardiogram), showed no difference in early studies of patients with subclinical hypothyroidism compared to healthy subjects [12–14]. In contrast, more sensitive echocardiographic studies showed that left ventricular function at rest was impaired, as indicated by a longer pre-ejection period (PEP) and increased ratio of pre-ejection period to left ventricular ejection time (PEP/ET) in patients as compared with healthy subjects [15–17]. These alterations in systolic time intervals were similar to those reported in patients with overt disease. Moreover, a mild (albeit significant) decrease in mean aortic acceleration was reported in patients with mild thyroid hormone deficiency [18].

Doppler echocardiography was first used in 1999 to evaluate left ventricular diastolic function in subjects with mild thyroid hormone deficiency [18]. Doppler-derived indices of left ventricular diastolic filling revealed abnormalities of myocardial relaxation. Impaired left ventricular diastolic function, characterized by slowed myocardial relaxation and impaired early ventricular filling, was the most consistent cardiac abnormality identified in young and middle-aged patients with Hashimoto thyroiditis and a mild but persistent increase in TSH compared to controls [18]. Isovolumic relaxation time (IRT) was significantly prolonged in all studies performed in patients with mild hypothyroidism [15–19]. Moreover, the ratio of early to late diastolic mitral flow velocity (E/A ratio) was significantly reduced [17–19], mainly because of an increased A wave [17–19]. Interestingly, diastolic function improved in all studies in which patients were evaluated after replacement therapy [16–18]; two such studies were double-blind placebo-controlled investigations [16, 17].

Impaired left ventricular diastolic function at rest may be an important cause of systolic dysfunction on effort in patients with thyroid hormone deficiency [9]. The slowed rate of left ventricular relaxation could critically impair ventricular filling during exercise, leading to left ventricular systolic dysfunction. Impaired left ventricular systolic [20] and diastolic [21] function on effort were documented by Doppler echocardiography and cardiopulmonary exercise testing in patients with subclinical hypothyroidism compared with euthyroid controls. Moreover, systolic and diastolic function on effort improved after L-T₄ replacement therapy in patients with subclinical hypothyroidism in studies performed with radionuclide ventriculography, Doppler echocardiography, and cardiopulmonary exercise testing [20–23].

Ultrasonic video densitometry was used to evaluate young and middle-aged patients affected by Hashimoto thyroiditis and subclinical hypothyroidism [24]. Video densitometric analysis revealed a lower cyclic variation index (CVI) in these patients than in controls at both the septum and posterior wall, resulting in an inverse relationship between CVI and the PEP/ET ratio [24]. Pulsed tissue Doppler imaging, which is minimally affected by alterations of afterload and heart rate, was used to provide, for the first time, information about myocardial systolic and diastolic properties in the various regional segments of the left ventricle, thereby permitting quantitative analysis of myocardial wall motion in subclinical hypothyroidism [15]. The results of tissue Doppler imaging analysis revealed that patients with mild hypothyroidism had changes in myocardial time intervals in several left ventricular segments similar to those reported in overt disease [15, 19]. Myocardial time intervals, evaluated as precontraction time (PTCm), the PTCm/myocardial contraction time ratio, and myocardial relaxation time (RTm), were prolonged at the level of both the posterior septum and the mitral annulus in patients with autoimmune subclinical hypothyroidism compared to controls [15].

More sophisticated techniques have recently been used to assess systolic and diastolic function in patients with subclinical hypothyroidism. Cardiac magnetic resonance imaging is currently the most accurate and reproducible noninvasive technique, providing an excellent evaluation of cardiac volumes and function. Cardiac volumes and systolic performance were significantly altered in patients with subclinical hypothyroidism. Moreover, preload (end-diastolic volume) was significantly decreased and afterload (systemic vascular resistance, SVR) significantly increased, leading to impaired cardiac performance in patients with mild thyroid failure [25]. The end-diastolic volume, stroke volume, ejection fraction, and cardiac index increased and SVR decreased after L-T₄ therapy [25].

All these studies, performed in young and middle-aged subjects with mild thyroid hormone deficiency, support the hypothesis that long-term subclinical hypothyroidism can affect cardiac morphology and function, depressing systolic function at rest, inducing left ventricular diastolic dysfunction at rest and during exercise, and impairing left ventricular systolic function on exercise (Table 3.1).

All the cardiovascular alterations reported in patients with subclinical hypothyroidism are similar to those observed in patients with overt hypothyroidism, suggesting that there is a continuum in the cardiac changes that occur: through mild, subclinical disease into overt hypothyroidism [26, 27]. Only one study was performed in elderly subjects (mean age 61 years) with a mean serum TSH level of 5.4 mIU/L [28]. In that study, using tissue Doppler imaging, subclinical hypothyroidism was not associated with significant differences in diastolic or systolic function compared with euthyroid controls. However, these elderly subjects were recruited from an epidemiological study and not from clinical practice [29]; thus, it is not possible to rule out that these patients were affected by transient subclinical hypothyroidism.

Many patients with subclinical hypothyroidism are elderly, and the onset or progression of the disease in these vulnerable subjects may precipitate cardiac decompensation and promote congestive heart failure [26]. Only one study evaluated the risk of heart failure in patients with subclinical hypothyroidism and stratified the risk according to TSH levels (4.5–6.9, 7.0–9.9, and ≥ 10 mIU/L) (30). This study reported an increased risk of congestive heart failure among adults aged 70–79 years with a TSH level of 7.0 mIU/L or greater [30].

Table 3.1 Long-term cardiovascular consequences of persistent mild thyroid hormone deficiency

Cardiac morphology and function:
- Depressed systolic function at rest
- Left ventricular diastolic dysfunction at rest and during exercise
- Impaired left ventricular systolic function on exercise

Vascular abnormalities:
- Increased systemic vascular resistance
- Increased prevalence of diastolic hypertension
- Increased arterial stiffness
- Endothelial dysfunction
- Increased carotid artery intima–media thickness

3.3 Effects of Mild Hypothyroidism on the Vascular System

Overt hypothyroidism is associated with premature atherosclerosis and coronary artery disease [31]. The mechanisms potentially responsible for atherosclerosis and coronary artery disease in patients with subclinical hypothyroidism remain unknown. Subclinical hypothyroidism could impair vascular function by inducing an increase in systemic vascular resistance and arterial stiffness and by altering endothelial function, increasing the risk of atherosclerosis and coronary artery disease [1] (Table 3.1).

In various studies, diastolic blood pressure was found to be significantly higher in normotensive subjects with mild hypothyroidism than in euthyroid subjects [11]. Moreover, an increase in systemic vascular resistance and in mean arterial pressure was reported in normotensive patients with subclinical hypothyroidism compared with euthyroid subjects [18, 32]. Furthermore, using cardiac magnetic resonance imaging, a significant increase in SVR was reported in patients with subclinical hypothyroidism compared to euthyroid controls [25]. These data suggest that even mild thyroid hormone deficiency, like overt hypothyroidism, affect vascular tone [1, 11, 26].

Increased central arterial stiffness is an important risk factor for cardiovascular disease. Changes in arterial wall elasticity may occur before and during the early stages of atherosclerosis and may have detrimental effects on left ventricular function and coronary perfusion. Increased arterial stiffness, identified from an increased augmentation gradient, augmentation index, and corrected augmentation index, was reported in patients with subclinical hypothyroidism compared to controls [33]. Furthermore, brachial-ankle pulse wave velocity (baPWV), a parameter of arterial stiffening, was significantly higher in patients with subclinical hypothyroidism [34, 35]. Central and peripheral PWV were reported to be significantly higher in these patients than in normal subjects [34, 35]. Finally, like overt hypothyroidism, subclinical hypothyroidism was associated with endothelial dysfunction [36, 37] due to impaired availability of nitric oxide. Moreover, higher carotid artery intima-media thickness (CIMT) was reported in patients with subclinical hypothyroidism that in age-and sex-matched controls; mean CIMT was positively related to age and to TSH and low-density lipoprotein cholesterol (LDL-C) concentrations [38].

In uncontrolled clinical trials, appropriate replacement therapy with L-T_4 induced a significant decrease in systemic vascular resistance [25, 32], mean arterial pressure [32], and central arterial stiffness [33] in normotensive, subclinically hypothyroid patients. Moreover, L-T_4 treatment improved endothelium-dependent vasodilation in a randomized double-blind crossover study of L-T_4 versus placebo [37]. In a double-blind placebo-controlled study of individuals aged 55 years, replacement therapy with L-T_4 significantly decreased CIMT [38]. The reduction was directly related to the decrease of both total cholesterol and TSH [38].

3.4 Epidemiological Evidence on the Risk of Atherosclerosis and Coronary Disease in Subclinical Hypothyroidism

Although some important cardiovascular risk factors are associated with mild and subclinical hypothyroidism, conflicting results have been reported in epidemiological studies assessing the risk of atherosclerosis and coronary disease (Table 3.2). In the Whickham survey, autoimmune thyroid disease (defined as treated hypothyroidism, positive antibodies, or elevated serum TSH) was not associated with coronary disease [39]. In the large cross-sectional Rotterdam study of 1149 women aged 55 years or older, subclinical hypothyroidism (defined as TSH >4.0 mIU/L) was associated with atherosclerosis and myocardial infarction only in cross-sectional analysis [40]. However, the risk of myocardial infarction was not significantly increased during an average follow-up of 4.6 years. In another study, from England and Wales, subclinical hypothyroidism (defined as TSH >5.0 mIU/L with a prevalence of 10.8%) was not associated with death from circulatory disease during the 10-year follow-up [41], but 40% of individuals with subclinical hypothyroidism developed overt hypothyroidism during follow-up and began thyroxine replacement therapy [41]. Furthermore, subclinical hypothyroidism (defined as TSH >4.50 mIU/L) was not associated with an increased incidence of coronary heart disease, cerebrovascular disease, cardiovascular disease, or all-cause death in the cross-sectional and longitudinal components of the Cardiovascular Health Study, a population-based longitudinal study of risk factors for the develop-

Table 3.2 Epidemiological evidence for an association between subclinical hypothyroidism and coronary heart disease

Study	No. of patients	Sex	TSH (mIU/L)	Age (years)	Follow-up (years)	Cardiovascular risk
Vanderpump et al. [39]	2779	Both	ATD	≥ 18	20	No association of autoimmune thyroid disease with coronary disease
Hak et al. [40]	1149, 124 subclinically hypothyroid	F only	> 4.0	≥ 55	4 .6	Risk of atherosclerosis; risk of myocardial infarction only in cross-sectional analysis
Imaizumi et al. [43]	2550, 257 subclinically hypothyroid	Both	> 5.0	≥ 40	10	Increased risk of ischemic heart disease only in the baseline cross-sectional analysis in men
Walsh et al. [44]	2108, 119 subclinically hypothyroid	Both	0.4–2 2.0–4 < 10 > 10	17–89	20	Risk of coronary events in subjects with serum TSH levels of 10 mIU/L or less and >10 mIU/L
Rodondi et al. [30]	2730, 338 subclinically hypothyroid	Both	4.5–6.9 7–9.9 ≥ 10	70–79	4	Subclinical hypothyroidism was not associated with coronary heart disease
Cappola et al. [42]	5888, 496 subclinically hypothyroid	Both	≥ 4.5	≥ 65	13	Subclinical hypothyroidism was not associated with coronary heart disease
Iervasi et al. [49]	3121 cardiac patients, 208 subclinically hypothyroid	32.6% F	> 4.5	60.7–61.5	2.7	Significantly higher cardiac death rate, particularly from ischemic heart disease, in subclinically hypothyroid subjects compared to euthyroid subjects

TSH thyroid-stimulating hormone
ATD patients had autoimmune thyroid disease

ment of cardiovascular disease in US community dwellers aged 65 years or older [42].

In contrast, subclinical hypothyroidism (defined as TSH >5.0 mIU/L) was associated with ischemic heart disease and increased all-cause mortality in the cross-sectional analysis of a cohort of atomic bomb survivors from the Nagasaki Adult Health Study [43]. Moreover, subclinical hypothyroidism was an independent predictor of coronary heart disease in middle-aged subjects (mean age of 50 years) in the cross-sectional and longitudinal analyses of the community-based study carried out in Busselton, Western Australia [44]. The increased risk of coronary events associated with subclinical hypothyroidism was found in this study in subjects with a serum TSH level of 10 mIU/L or less as well as in those with a serum TSH >10 mIU/L. The risk remained significant after adjustment for standard cardiovascular risk factors.

The discrepancies in epidemiological data about the risk of coronary heart disease in subclinical hypothyroidism are probably related to differences in the populations studied in terms of age, sex, race/ethnicity, life style, the TSH range used to define subclinical hypothyroidism, methods of evaluation of cardiovascular disease, differences in adjustments for known risk factors for cardiovascular disease, and the duration of follow-up [1, 45] (Table 3.2). Few studies stratified the analysis by TSH levels [1]. Furthermore, not all epidemiological studies included follow-up data on thyroid function, and in other studies some patients were treated with thyroid hormone during follow-up [1, 45]. Moreover, associated atherosclerotic risk factors were evaluated in only a few studies [45]. For this reason, the meta-analysis by Völzke et al. [46], assessing the risk of coronary heart disease and cardiovascular mortality, concluded that not all possible relevant confounders of the association between subclinical hypothyroidism and mortality were considered in each of the prospective cohort studies. Consequently, the authors concluded that the current evidence for a causal relation between subclinical hypothyroidism and mortality is weak and should not be used to decide whether or not to treat patients with subclinical hypothyroidism [46].

The cardiovascular risk factors potentially responsible for coronary heart disease in subclinical hypothyroidism remain unknown. In the Whickham Survey, subclinical hypothyroidism was not related to hyperlipidemia [39]. In the Rotterdam Study, total cholesterol was lower in women with subclinical hypothyroidism than in euthyroid women [40]. In the Nagasaki study, the prevalence of ischemic heart disease was independent of such coronary risk factors as blood pressure, body mass index, total cholesterol level, smoking status, and the presence of diabetes mellitus [43]. Moreover, in the Cardiovascular Heath Study, there were no differences in serum cholesterol concentration, lipoprotein (a), C-reactive protein, or fasting insulin and glucose concentrations between individuals with subclinical hypothyroidism and those with normal thyroid function [42]. Contrary to this, in the study by Rodondi et al. [30], participants had no increase in coronary heart disease despite significantly higher cholesterol levels, and cholesterol itself was not associated with an increased risk of atherosclerotic events. Only in the Busselton study was serum total cholesterol significantly higher in subjects with subclinical hypothyroidism than in euthyroid subjects, but the difference was barely significant after adjustment for age and sex [44]. Moreover, LDL-C was significantly increased in subjects with mild subclinical hypothyroidism and TSH ≥ 10 mIU/L [44].

There is a need to clarify the role of "nontraditional" blood markers for atherosclerosis risk, such as homocysteine, C-reactive protein, and alterations in coagulation parameters in patients with subclinical hypothyroidism compared with euthyroid age-matched controls [1]. However, data about the potential association of subclinical hypothyroidism with such "nontraditional" cardiovascular risk factors are not consistent [1].

3.5 Cardiovascular Mortality in Subclinical Hypothyroidism

Cardiovascular mortality was assessed in seven studies in subclinical hypothyroidism [30, 39, 41–44, 47]. It was increased in only two studies [43, 47]. In the longitudinal follow-up study of a cohort of atomic bomb survivors in the Nagasaki Adult Health Study, all-cause mortality was increased at

6 years only in men, although the specific causes of death were not determined [43]. However, mortality was not increased at a 10-year follow-up [43]. In the Leiden prospective cohort study of subjects aged 85 years, subclinical hypothyroidism was associated with greater longevity and a reduced risk of death from cardiovascular disease during the 4-year follow-up; this was attributed to a lower metabolic rate [47]. Individuals with overt and subclinical hypothyroidism had lower all-cause and cardiovascular mortality than clinically euthyroid individuals, although serum cholesterol levels were higher [47]. These two studies involved selected populations of subclinically hypothyroidism individuals (atomic bomb survivors in the Nagasaki study and 85-year-olds in the Leiden study), which limits conclusions based on these findings.

3.6 Association between Subclinical Hypothyroidism and Cardiovascular Risk in Elderly Subjects and Those with Comorbid Conditions: Epidemiological Evidence

In a recent meta-analysis by Ochs et al. [48], ten population-based cohort studies were evaluated to establish the risk of coronary heart disease and mortality. In a random-effects model, the relative risk (RR) for coronary heart disease in subclinical hypothyroidism was 1.2. Risk estimates were lower when high-quality studies were pooled and were higher among participants younger than 65 years. The RR was 1.18 for cardiovascular mortality and 1.12 for total mortality. The RR of all-cause mortality was increased only in patients with co-morbid conditions. In fact, cardiac death, particularly as regards ischemic heart disease, was significantly higher in cardiac patients with subclinical hypothyroidism than in those who were euthyroid [49]. Moreover, patients with type 2 diabetes who were subclinically hypothyroid had an increased risk of nephropathy and cardiovascular events [50].

Fifteen studies were included in a recent meta-analysis by Razvi et al. [51], in which subclinical hypothyroidism was associated with increased ischemic heart disease (both prevalence and incidence) and cardiovascular mortality only in subjects from younger populations (subjects less than 65 years old); moreover, it was statistically significant only in women [51]. In fact, in epidemiological studies, the risk of coronary heart disease was increased in young and middle-aged patients but not in elderly and very elderly patients with subclinical hypothyroidism.

These results suggest that middle-aged individuals with mild thyroid hormone deficiency have a higher cardiovascular risk for coronary heart disease than the elderly with this condition, and that subclinical hypothyroidism may have a protective effect in subjects older than 85 years [1, 45].

3.7 Conclusions

Whether to treat subclinical hypothyroidism remains a controversial issue. Replacement therapy with L-T$_4$ may reverse the systolic and diastolic dysfunction, arterial hypertension, increased central arterial stiffness, endothelial dysfunction, and other cardiovascular risk factors associated with this condition [1, 11, 26]. However, there are no data showing that thyroxine therapy improves outcomes such as cardiac morbidity or mortality. Additional randomized controlled trials and longitudinal studies are necessary to evaluate whether replacement therapy with thyroxine reduces the risk of coronary heart disease and congestive heart failure in subjects with subclinical hypothyroidism. In the meantime, it could be useful to identify patients with subclinical hypothyroidism who have associated high cardiovascular risk factors and to consider L-T$_4$ replacement treatment in them, with the aim of reducing cardiovascular risk. Current data suggest that middle-aged individuals benefit more from treatment than the elderly [1]. On this basis, treatment of subclinical hypothyroidism should be individualized, taking into account the age of the patient and the presence of associated comorbid conditions [1, 45].

Key Points

- Subclinical hypothyroidism is an early and mild form of thyroid failure characterized by serum levels of thyroid hormones within their reference range but elevated serum TSH concentrations.

- The prevalence of subclinical hypothyroidism is 4–10% and this condition increases significantly with age.

- The management and treatment of subclinical hypothyroidism are controversial; there is no consensus about the TSH concentration at which treatment should be started.

- Identification of the potential cardiovascular risk could facilitate decision-making about the treatment of patients with subclinical hypothyroidism.

- Impaired left ventricular diastolic function, characterized by slowed myocardial relaxation and impaired early ventricular filling, is the most consistent cardiac abnormality identified in young and middle-aged patients with subclinical hypothyroidism.

- Subclinical hypothyroidism could impair vascular function by inducing an increase in systemic vascular resistance and arterial stiffness and by altering endothelial function, increasing the risk of atherosclerosis and coronary artery disease.

- Replacement therapy with L-T$_4$ may reverse the cardiovascular risk associated with subclinical hypothyroidism.

- Middle-aged individuals with mild thyroid hormone deficiency have a higher cardiovascular risk for coronary heart disease than the elderly with this condition.

- Cardiac death, particularly as regards ischemic heart disease, is significantly higher in cardiac patients with subclinical hypothyroidism.

- L-T$_4$ replacement should be considered in patients with subclinical hypothyroidism who have associated high cardiovascular risk factors, with the aim of reducing cardiovascular risk.

References

1. Biondi B, Cooper DS (2008) The clinical significance of subclinical thyroid dysfunction. Endocr Rev 229:76–131
2. Cooper DS (2001) Clinical practice. Subclinical hypothyroidism. N Engl J Med 345:260–265
3. Vanderpump MP, Tunbridge WM, French JM et al (1995) The incidence of thyroid disease in the community: a twenty-year follow-up of the Whickham Survey. Clin Endocrinol 43:55–68
4. Canaris GJ, Manowitz NR, Mayor G, Ridgway EC (2000) The Colorado thyroid disease prevalence study. Arch Intern Med 160:526–534
5. Hollowell JG, Staehling NW, Flanders WD et al (2002) Serum TSH, T(4), and thyroid antibodies in the United States population (1988 to 1994): National Health and Nutrition Examination Survey (NHANES III). J Clin Endocrinol Metab 87:489–499
6. Huber G, Staub JJ, Meier C et al (2002) Prospective study of the spontaneous course of subclinical hypothyroidism: prognostic value of thyrotropin, thyroid reserve, and thyroid antibodies. J Clin Endocrinol Metab 87:3221–3226
7. Gharib H, Tuttle RM, Baskin HJ et al (2005) Subclinical thyroid dysfunction: a joint statement on management from the American Association of Clinical Endocrinologists, the American Thyroid Association, and The Endocrine Society. J Clin Endocrinol Metab 90:581–585
8. Surks MI, Ortiz E, Daniels GH et al (2004) Subclinical thyroid disease: scientific review and guidelines for diagnosis and management. JAMA 291:228–238
9. Biondi B, Palmieri EA, Lombardi G, Fazio S (2002) Effects of subclinical thyroid dysfunction on the heart. Ann Intern Med 137:904–914
10. Biondi B, Palmieri EA, Lombardi G, Fazio S (2002) Subclinical hypothyroidism and cardiac function. Thyroid 12:505–510
11. Biondi B (2007) Cardiovascular effects of mild hypothyroidism. Thyroid 17:625–630
12. Bough EW, Crowley WF, Ridgway EC et al (1978) Myocardial function in hypothyroidism: relation to disease severity and response to treatment. Arch Intern Med 138:1476–1480
13. Cooper DS, Halpern R, Wood LC, et al (1984) Thyroxine therapy in subclinical hypothyroidism. A double-blind, placebo-controlled trial. Ann Intern Med 101:18–24
14. Staub JJ, Althaus BU, Engler H et al (1992) Spectrum of subclinical and overt hypothyroidism: effect on thyrotropin, prolactin, and thyroid reserve, and metabolic impact on peripheral target tissues. Am J Med 92:631–642
15. Vitale G, Galderisi M, Lupoli, GA et al (2002) Left ventricular myocardial impairment in subclinical hypothyroidism assessed by a new ultrasound tool: pulsed tissue Doppler. J Clin Endocrinol Metab 87:4350–4355
16. Monzani F, Di Bello V, Caraccio N et al (2001) Effect of levothyroxine on cardiac function and structure in subclinical hypothyroidism: a double blind, placebo-controlled study. J Clin Endocrinol Metab 86:1110–1115
17. Yazici M, Gorgulu S, Sertbas Y et al (2004) Effects of thyroxin therapy on cardiac function in patients with subclinical hypothyroidism: index of myocardial performance in the evaluation of left ventricular function. Int J Cardiol 95:135–143
18. Biondi B, Fazio S, Palmieri EA et al (1999) Left ventricular diastolic dysfunction in patients with subclinical hypothyroidism. J Clin Endocrinol Metab 84:2064–2067
19. Aghini-Lombardi F, Di Bello V, Talini E et al (2006) Early textural and functional alterations of left ventricular myocardium in mild hypothyroidism. Eur J Endocrinol 155:3–9
20. Kahaly GJ (2000) Cardiovascular and atherogenic aspects of subclinical hypothyroidism. Thyroid 10:665–679
21. Brenta G, Mutti LA, Schnitman M et al (2003) Assessment of left ventricular diastolic function by radionuclide ventriculography at rest and exercise in subclinical hypothyroidism, and its response to L-thyroxine therapy. Am J Cardiol 91:1327–1330
22. Bell GM, Todd WT, Forfar JC et al (1985) End-organ responses to thyroxine therapy in subclinical hypothyroidism. Clin Endocrinol 22:83–89
23. Forfar JC, Wathen CG, Todd WT et al (1985) Left ventricular performance in subclinical hypothyroidism. Q J Med 57:857–865
24. Di Bello V, Monzani F, Giorgi D et al (2000) J Am Soc Echocardiogr 13:832–840
25. Ripoli A, Pingitore A, Favilli B et al (2005) Does subclinical hypothyroidism affect cardiac pump performance? Evidence from a magnetic resonance imaging study. J Am Coll Cardiol 45:439–445
26. Biondi B, Klein I (2004) Hypothyroidism as a risk factor for cardiovascular disease. Endocrine 24:1–13
27. Galderisi M, Vitale G, D'Errico A et al (2004) Usefulness of pulsed tissue Doppler for the assessment of left ventricular myocardial function in overt hypothyroidism. Ital Heart J 5:257–264
28. Iqbal A, Schirmer H, Lunde P et al (2007) Thyroid stimulating hormone and left ventricular function. J Clin Endocrinol Metab 92:3504–3510
29. Cappola AR (2007) Subclinical thyroid dysfunction and the heart. J Clin Endocrinol Metab 92:3404–3405
30. Rodondi N, Newman AB, Vittinghoff E et al (2005) Subclinical hypothyroidism and the risk of heart failure, other cardiovascular events, and death. Arch Intern Med 165:2460–2466
31. Cappola AR, Ladenson PW (2003) Hypothyroidism and atherosclerosis. J Clin Endocrinol Metab 88:2438–2444
32. Faber J, Petersen L, Wiinberg N et al (2002) Hemodynamic changes after levothyroxine treatment in subclinical hypothyroidism. Thyroid 12:319–324
33. Owen PJD, Rajiv C, Vinereanu D et al (2006) Subclinical hypothyroidism, arterial stiffness and myocardial reserve. J Clin Endocrinol Metab 9:2126–2132
34. Nagasaki T, Inaba M, Kumeda Y et al (2006) Increased pulse wave velocity in subclinical hypothyroidism. J Clin Endocrinol Metab 91:154–158
35. Nagasaki T, Inaba M, Kumeda Y et al (2007) Central pulse wave velocity is responsible for increased brachial–ankle pulse wave velocity in subclinical hypothyroidism. Clin Endocrinol (Oxf) 66:304–308
36. Taddei S, Caraccio N, Virdis A et al (2003) Impaired endothelium-dependent vasodilatation in subclinical hypothyroidism: beneficial effect of levothyroxine therapy. J Clin Endocrinol Metab 88:3731–3737
37. Razvi S, Ingoe L, Keeka G et al (2007) The beneficial effect of L-thyroxine on cardiovascular risk factors, endothe-

lial function and quality of life in subclinical hypothyroidism: randomised, crossover trial. J Clin Endocrinol Metab 92:1715–1723

38. Monzani F, Caraccio N, Kozakowa M et al (2004) Effect of levothyroxine replacement on lipid profile and intima-media thickness in subclinical hypothyroidism: a double-blind, placebo-controlled study. J Clin Endocrinol Metab 89:2099–2106

39. Vanderpump MP, Tunbridge WM, French JM et al (1996) The development of ischemic heart disease in relation to autoimmune thyroid disease in a 20-year follow-up study of an English community. Thyroid 6:155–1560

40. Hak AE, Pols HA, Visser TJ et al (2000) Subclinical hypothyroidism is an independent risk factor for atherosclerosis and myocardial infarction in elderly women: the Rotterdam Study. Ann Intern Med 132:270–278

41. Parle JV, Maisonneuve P, Sheppard MC et al (2001) Prediction of all-cause and cardiovascular mortality in elderly people from one low serum thyrotropin result: a 10-year cohort study. Lancet 358:861–865

42. Cappola AR, Fried LP, Arnold AM et al (2006) Thyroid status, cardiovascular risk, and mortality in older adults. JAMA 295:1033–1041

43. Imaizumi M, Akahoshi M, Ichimaru S et al (2004) Risk for ischemic heart disease and all-cause mortality in subclinical hypothyroidism. J Clin Endocrinol Metab 89:3365–3370

44. Walsh JP, Bremner AP, Bulsara MK et al (2005) Thyroid dysfunction and serum lipids: a community-based study. Clin Endocrinol (Oxf) 63:670–675

45. Biondi B (2008) Should we treat all subjects with subclinical thyroid disease the same way? Eur J Endocrinol 159:343–345

46. Völzke H, Schwahn C, Wallaschofski H, Dörr M (2007) The association of thyroid dysfunction with all-cause and circulatory mortality: is there a causal relationship? J Clin Endocrinol Metab 92:2421–2429

47. Gussekloo J, van Exel E, de Craen AJ et al (2004) Thyroid status, disability and cognitive function, and survival in old age. JAMA 292:2591–2599

48. Ochs N, Auer R, Bauer DC et al (2008) Meta-analysis: subclinical thyroid dysfunction and the risk for coronary heart disease and mortality. Ann Intern Med 148:832–845

49. Iervasi G, Molinaro S, Landi P et al (2007) Association between increased mortality and mild thyroid dysfunction in cardiac patients. Arch Intern Med 167:1526–1532

50. Chen HS, Wu TE, Jap TS et al (2007) Subclinical hypothyroidism is a risk factor for nephropathy and cardiovascular diseases in type 2 diabetic patients. Diabet Med 24:1336–1344

51. Razvi S, Shakoor A, Vanderpump M et al (2008) The influence of age on the relationship between subclinical hypothyroidism and ischemic heart disease: a meta-analysis. J Clin Endocrinol Metab 93:2998–3007

Cardiovascular Hemodynamics and Work Capacity in Thyroid Dysfunction

4

George J. Kahaly

Abstract Thyroid dysfunction strongly involves the cardiovascular system, especially systemic vascular resistance and the cardiac ejection fraction. The observed increase in cardiac output results from the interactions of several factors: preload, afterload, myocardial contractility, and heart rate. In thyrotoxicosis, cardiac output is enhanced due to the increase in heart rate and stroke volume. Stroke volume is also enhanced due to a decreased afterload and increased myocardial contractility and preload. The latter is explained by the increase in blood volume, the reduction in venous compliance, and the improvement in ventricular diastolic filling. Although cardiac function at rest is enhanced, an abnormal response of the cardiac ejection fraction to physical exercise has been reported in thyrotoxic patients without underlying heart disease. Dyspnea and reduced exercise tolerance in patients with thyroid dysfunction are due to a reduction of the cardiac functional reserve. Cardiac output cannot adequately increase in response to physical exercise because all the mechanisms involved in the hemodynamic response to exercise are already activated at rest, depending on the degree of thyroid hormone excess. A further aspect is the cardiac hypertrophy that develops in long-term thyrotoxicosis due to the direct effect of thyroid hormone on myocardiocyte protein synthesis, thus indirectly leading to an increased cardiac workload. Also, left ventricular mass frequently increases in patients with long-term subclinical hyperthyroidism and may counteract the beneficial effect of thyroid hormone on diastolic performance, thereby impairing diastolic ventricular filling and systolic performance on effort. Cardiac hypertrophy may be prevented or partially reversed by β-blockade in individuals with long-term exposure to thyroid hormone excess.

Keywords Cardiovascular hemodynamics • Cardiovascular exercise capacity • Pulmonary exercise capacity • Mild subclinical thyroid disease • Overt thyroid dysfunction • Hyperthyroidism • Thyrotoxicosis • Myxedema • Hypothyroidism

4.1 Hemodynamics in Hyperthyroidism

The hemodynamic consequences of excess thyroid hormones result from a direct effect of thyroid hormones on the heart and vasculature. Heart rate, blood volume, left ventricular stroke volume, ejection fraction, and cardiac output increase (Table 4.1). Peripheral vasodilation occurs as a result of rapid utilization of oxygen, increased metabolic end products, and induction of arterial smooth muscle cell relaxation by thyroid hormones. Vasodilation results in a marked decrease in systemic vascular resistance, which plays a central role in the hemodynam-

G.J. Kahaly (✉)
Department of Medicine I, Gutenberg University Hospital, Mainz, Germany

G. Iervasi, A. Pingitore (eds.), *Thyroid and Heart Failure*.

Table 4.1 Cardiovascular hemodynamic changes in thyroid dysfunction

	Hyper-	Hypothyroidism
Systemic vascular resistance	↓↓	↑
Circulation time	↓↓	↑
Diastolic blood pressure	↓	↑
Arterial resistance	↓	↑
Venous resistance	↑	–
Systolic blood pressure	↑	↓
Cardiac output	↑	↓
Cardiac index	↑	↓
LV stroke volume	↑	↓
LV systolic function	↑	↓
Pulse pressure	Widened	Narrow

LV left ventricular

ic changes that accompany thyrotoxicosis, resulting in an increase in heart rate, a selective increase in blood flow to certain organs such as skin, skeletal muscles, and heart, and a drop in diastolic blood pressure with widening of the pulse pressure. Vasodilation and the lack of rise in renal blood flow cause a decrease in renal perfusion pressure and an activation of the renin–angiotensin system, thus increasing sodium reabsorption and blood volume. The combination of expanded blood volume and improvement in diastolic relaxation of the heart contribute to increased left ventricular end-diastolic volume or preload. Similarly, the drop in systemic vascular resistance and the improved myocardial contractility result in a smaller left ventricular end-systolic volume or afterload. The net effect of an increased preload and a decreased afterload translates into a significant increased in left ventricular stroke volume. In turn, the rise in heart rate and the increased stroke volume combine to cause a two- to threefold increase in cardiac output, greater than accounted for by the changes in the body metabolic rate. Of all contributing factors, the increase in preload accounts for most of the increase in cardiac output. In addition to the improvement in systolic contractile parameters, echocardiographic data indicate that newly diagnosed thyrotoxicosis is accompanied by an improvement in left ventricular diastolic function as manifested by an enhancement in left ventricular relaxation, diastolic flow velocities, and isovolumic relaxation time. All diastolic parameters normalize when thyrotoxic patients are ren-

dered euthyroid. This has led to the suggestion that the dyspnea on exertion and exercise intolerance that accompany thyrotoxicosis may not be of cardiac origin. Findings of improvement in diastolic function have not been confirmed invasively and should be accepted with caution since the increase in contractility and in preload that accompany hyperthyroidism may also affect echocardiographic indices of diastolic function [1–7].

4.2 Experimental Findings

Thyrotoxicosis may be associated with as much as a 50% decline in systemic vascular resistance, and free T_3 (fT_3) is capable of causing rapid relaxation of vascular smooth muscle cells in culture. Since the vascular smooth muscle of resistance arterioles primarily determines systemic vascular resistance, fT_3 may directly regulate systemic vascular resistance, which in turn causes alterations in blood pressure and cardiac output. A significant decrease in cardiac output after administration of phenylephrine to thyrotoxic but not to normal subjects has been noted. The ability to block the elevated cardiac output by pharmacologically reversing the changes in systemic vascular resistance of thyrotoxicosis reinforces the possibility that many of the cardiovascular changes of hyperthyroidism occur in response to changes in peripheral tissues. Thyrotoxicosis markedly increases oxygen consumption in the periphery and increases metabolic demands, which require increased blood supply and pumping action of the heart. Arterial resistance decreases and venous tone increases in thyrotoxic animals, leading to an augmented return of blood to the heart. The effects of fT_3 on venous compliance and blood volume displayed in thyrotoxic calves include an increase in mean circulatory filling pressure, no change in blood volume, and a decrease in venous compliance, whereas hypothyroid animals showed a decrease in mean circulatory filling pressure and blood volume but no change in venous compliance. This hemodynamic effect of fT_3 in the periphery markedly contributes to the increased cardiac contraction. Studies using heterotopic cardiac isographs have shown that fT_3-induced changes in protein synthesis and cardiac growth primarily result from secondary changes in cardiac work. In contrast, T_3-induced changes in myosin isoenzyme predominance occur to the same extent in the heart in situ and in the heterotopic isograft. Thus, T_3-induced hemodynamic effects originating in the periphery may influence increases in total protein synthesis and cardiac hypertrophy [1–5].

4.3 Hemodynamics in Hypothyroidism

The pathophysiological basis of the hemodynamic cardiovascular changes in hypothyroidism is the opposite of those discussed for the thyrotoxic heart. In addition to decreased direct effects of thyroid hormones in cardiac myocytes, indirect effects occur through decreases in peripheral oxygen consumption and changes in hemodynamic parameters (e.g., increased arterial resistance). In addition, it is possible but not proven that decreased sensitivity of the sympathoadrenal system also plays a role in hypothyroid patients. Cardiac papillary muscle obtained from animals with hypothyroidism shows a depression of the force–velocity curve and a reduced rate of tension development, indicating significant contractile abnormalities. After administration of thyroid hormones, all of these abnormalities revert to normal. Myxedema is characterized by a low cardiac index, decreased stroke volume, decreased vascular volume, and increased systemic vascular resistance. Total blood volume is decreased in myxedema and varies directly as a function of basal metabolic rate. Renal perfusion, when measured by glomerular filtration, is also decreased. Although sodium excretion is normal, free water clearance is impaired and can lead to hyponatremia. Total-body albumin distribution is expanded in myxedema, in keeping with the development of high-protein-content effusions in many body cavities [8–11].

Thyroid dysfunction alters blood pressure. Thyrotoxicosis has only minor effects on mean arterial blood pressure, because increases in systolic blood pressure caused by increased stroke volume are offset by decreases in diastolic blood pressure due to peripheral vasodilatation. Estimates of the occurrence of hypertension in the hypothyroid population have varied widely. However, a true increased incidence of hypertension has been found in most studies. Therefore, it is important to wait with definitive treatment of hypertension until thyroid hormone values have been normalized. Hypertension of hypothyroidism appears to be hypertension of a low-renin state, and the main pathophysiological reason for the development of hypertension is an increased peripheral systemic vascular resistance. Conversely, myxedema is associated with increases in diastolic blood pressure. Overtreatment of thyrotoxic patients that resulted in myxedema was associated with an increase in diastolic blood pressure which was reversible when thyroid function returned to normal. Hypothyroidism was found in 3.6% of 688 consecutive hypertensive patients, and in this subset diastolic blood pressure fell significantly after adequate T_4 replacement, suggesting a cause-and-effect relation. Renin, angiotensin, and aldosterone play minor roles in this form of hypertension. Finally, very recently, the expression of cardiac angiotensin II type 1 and 2 receptors was enhanced in rats subjected to experimental hypothyroidism [8, 12].

4.4 Interactions with the Sympathoadrenal System

Sympathomimetic agents and thyroid hormones lead to similar cardiac symptoms, especially inducing tachycardia and increasing the force and velocity of cardiac contraction. Treatment of thyrotoxic patients with sympatholytic agents ameliorates rate-related cardiac changes. These observations have resulted in the hypothesis that some effects of T_3 are mediated by an increased activity of the sympathoadrenal system or an increased responsiveness and sensitivity of cardiac tissue to normal sympathomimetic stimuli. Since plasma and urine levels of catecholamines are normal in thyrotoxicosis, the hypothesis that thyroid status leads to increased sensitivity of the sympathoadrenal system has been favored. The enhanced sympathetic sensitivity of the thyrotoxic heart may be mediated by an increased number of β-adrenergic receptors. In humans, short-term hyperthyroidism is associated with an increase in the sensitivity of heart rate and left ventricular shortening velocity to isoproterenol stimulation. In addition, the levels of other components of the sympathetic transmission system increase. Specifically, investigations in thyrotoxic pigs show that fT_3 markedly increases the amount of stimulatory guanine nucleotide regulatory protein. Studies of the various components of the adrenergic-receptor complex in plasma membranes have also shown that β-adrenergic receptors, guanine-nucleotide regulatory proteins, and adenylyl cyclase types V and VI all are altered by changes in thyroid status [13–21].

Cardiac tissue contains both β_1- and β_2-adrenergic receptor subtypes. In most species studied, β_1-receptors account for 70% of all β-adrenergic receptors. Furthermore, the level of β-adrenoceptors in the sinoatrial node are approximately twice those in surrounding myocytes. The β-adrenoceptors in the sinoatrial node comprise predominantly β_1-receptors (75%). In contrast, β_2-receptors are the predominant species in nonmyocyte vascular cells (75%). Thus, β_1-receptors are the predominant β-adrenoceptors in cells of myocyte origin and might be responsive to T_3 regulation. Indeed, there appears to be a differential induction of cardiac β_1- and β_2-adrenergic receptor mRNA in rat myocytes by T_3. T_3 causes a fourfold induction of cardiac β_1-adrenoceptor mRNA, but no significant change in β_2-receptor mRNA. The effects of T_3 on β_1-adrenergic gene transcription occur within 30 min, with elevations lasting for 72 h. Following the rise in β_1-mRNA, there is a threefold increase in the density of cardiac β_1-receptors, which persists for 48 h. In contrast, β_2-receptors are not significantly increased following T_3 administration. These studies suggest that in cardiac tissue the β_1-adrenoreceptor gene is sensitive to T_3, whereas the β_2-receptor gene is minimally influenced. Extrapolation of these animal and in vitro studies to the human heart is premature since cardiac β_1-receptor gene regulation by T_3 in hypothyroid humans has not been studied. However, the cardiac β_2-adrenoreceptor in myxedema may be refractory to T_4 therapy, as determined by polymerase chain reaction amplification of the β_2-mRNA in cardiac tissue from a hypothyroid subject before and after therapy [19–21].

4.5 Metabolic Involvement

Thyroid hormone controls the expression of myocyte-specific genes coding for the myosin isoforms of the Na^+, K^+-ATPase pumps and the Ca^{2+}-ATPase canals of the sarcoplasmic reticulum. This explains the increase in contractility and relaxation of skeletal muscles observed in thyrotoxicosis as opposed to myxedema. Control of key enzymes of the main energetic pathways accounts for inhibition of oxidative metabolism in hypothyroidism and excessive glycolysis recruitment in hyperthy-

roidism. In both cases, muscle performance is reduced, with accumulation of lactic acid on exercise. This is due to defective pyruvate oxidation and proton expulsion in hypothyroidism, and to the acceleration of glycolysis in hyperthyroidism. Muscle glycolysis exceeds mitochondrial oxidation of pyruvate, enhancing the shunting of pyruvate to lactate via lactic dehydrogenase activity and thus leading to an increased lactate/pyruvate ratio. This mitochondrial oxidative dysfunction during exercise in thyroid dysfunction mostly causes intracellular acidosis. These abnormalities partly explain why people with dysthyroidism are intolerant of exertion. Regarding other possible metabolic causes of the impaired inotropic and chronotropic response to incremental exercise in patients with thyroid dysfunction, thyrotoxicosis increases fast-myosin and fast-twitch fibers in skeletal muscle, which are less economic in oxygen utilization during contraction than are slow-twitch muscle fibers. Reduced exercise efficiency may also be induced by excessive heat production in hyperthyroidism. Effort tolerance is also impaired in thyrotoxicosis, because of decreased skeletal muscle mass and oxidative capacity related to accelerated protein catabolism. Thyroid hormone affects mitochondrial mass and enzyme activities, and clinical symptoms of exercise intolerance in hyperthyroidism may be due to decreased rather than increased muscle oxidative capacity.

In myxedema, inadequate cardiovascular support appears to be one of the principal factors involved. Insufficient skeletal muscle blood flow compromises both exercise capacity, via reduced oxygen delivery, and endurance, through decreased delivery of blood-borne substrates. The latter effect results in increased dependence on intramuscular glycogen. In addition, decreased mobilization of free fatty acids from adipose tissue and, consequently, lower plasma levels of free fatty acids compound the problem of reduced lipid delivery to active skeletal muscle in the hypothyroid state. In contrast, cardiovascular support is enhanced in thyrotoxicosis, implicating other factors in exercise tolerance. Greater reliance on muscle glycogen appears to be one of the primary reasons for decreased endurance. Biochemical changes with hyperthyroidism that would favor enhanced flux through glycolysis may account for this dependence on glycogen [22–28].

Patients with myxedema often complain of muscular weakness, cramps, and excessive fatigability. Hypothyroidism induces a metabolic myopathy, with a fall in energy production and, especially, in mitochondrial metabolism. This is due to a global inhibition of the main oxidative pathways (substrate incorporation, substrate oxidation) and of the respiratory chain. Diminished energy consumption is partly related to a transition to myosin isoforms that express a slower ATPase, and to partly impairment of the trans-sarcolemmic transport. Exercise intolerance could be due to abnormal recruitment of several metabolic pathways, such as glycolysis, related to the mitochondrial metabolism impairment and including an abnormal accumulation of protons and monovalent phosphate ions, which are involved in the alteration of the actin–myosin interaction, and also by an abnormal calcium metabolism. The decreased number of Na^+,K^+-ATPase-dependent pumps could imply an abnormal intracellular sodium level and explain the frequent disorders of membrane excitability. Studies of rats performing treadmill running have shown that blood flows during exercise to high-oxidative, extensor-type muscles are lower in hypothyroid rats than in euthyroid rats. Abnormal cardiac and vascular functions appear to contribute to this hypoperfusion. Experiments involving isolated segments of arterial vessels have demonstrated that potential for constriction is normal in vessels from hypothyroid animals; however, reduced vasodilator potential is associated with myxedema. Dysfunction of both endothelium and vascular smooth muscle appears to contribute to blunt the potential for vasodilation. An altered ability to generate vasodilator substances and/or changes in responses to these vasodilators—e.g., markedly decreased acetylcholine-induced vasorelaxation—may account for vascular dysfunction. It appears that impaired vascular function interacts with other factors, such as poor myocardial function and changes in energy metabolism, to compromise exercise tolerance [28–34].

4.6 Experimental Thyroid Dysfunction and Work Capacity

To study the role of thyroid hormones in exercise-induced muscle growth and protein synthesis, skeletal and cardiac muscle protein synthesis as well as myosin heavy chain (MHC) gene expression were measured in hypothyroid rats allowed to exercise voluntarily. The ratios of heart weight to body weight in hypothyroid (thyroidectomized) and hypothyroid + overfed rat groups were indicative of marked cardiac atrophy over a 28-day period. However, running-wheel exercise in a hypothyroid rat subgroup prevented heart, gastrocnemius, and soleus muscle atrophy over the same time period. Heart, gastrocnemius, and soleus muscle showed markedly suppressed protein synthesis rates in the hypothyroid and hypothyroid + overfed groups versus the euthyroid control rats. However, exercise increased the protein synthesis rate by 50% compared with hypothyroidism alone in all three muscle groups. Exercise did not modify hypothyroidism-induced alterations of cardiac myosin isoform expression. Thus, exercise-mediated effects on skeletal and cardiac muscle growth but not on cardiac MHC gene expression appear to be independent of thyroid hormones [35–42].

Compared with a normal control group, hypothyroid female rats subjected to an 8-week physical training (running) program showed reductions in maximum oxygen uptake (−32%), skeletal muscle homogenate respiratory capacity (−50%), cardiac myosin ATPase (−58%), and in-situ-derived left ventricular pressure (−58%). The training program restored skeletal muscle oxidative capacity and maximum oxygen uptake to within normal limits, but it did not improve cardiac myosin ATPase or calcium regulation of myofibril ATPase. However, the heart-weight-to-body-weight ratio was highest in the hypothyroid trained group. These findings suggest that the maximum oxygen utilization capacity of hypothyroid rats can be normalized by physical training, even though the intrinsic contractile capacity of the heart can not. The effects of hypo- and hyperthyroidism on in vivo cardiovascular functional capacity were ascertained in the context of phosphorylation of cardiac myosin light chain 2, a proposed modulator of myocardial function at rest and during exercise. Compared with normal controls, calcium-regulated myofibril ATPase was reduced by 39% in rats with myxedema and increased by 9% in thyrotoxic rats. This response was associated with a 20-fold increase in the V_3 isoform and an 11% increase in the V_1 isoform in hypothyroid and hyperthyroid rats, respectively. Submaximum treadmill exercise elicited significant elevations in all myocardial functional indices examined in thyrotoxic rats compared with the control group, whereas the opposite occurred in the hypothyroid group. Despite the marked contrast in cardiac function among the three groups, intrinsic levels of myosin light chain 2 were similar among the groups when at rest and were significantly reduced in both the hypothyroid and the hyperthyroid group relative to controls during exercise. These data suggest that, although thyroid state exerts a profound impact on intrinsic myocardial functional state, it exerts little control over cellular processes regulating myosin light chain 2 during rest and exercise.

Muscle glycogen, glycolytic intermediate, and high-energy phosphate contents were compared in five intact (control) and five hypothyroid (thyroidectomized) dogs after 30 min of treadmill exercise of low (40 W) and high (70 W) intensity [40]. Although after the low-intensity exercise the rate of glycogenolysis and muscle lactate accumulation in hypothyroid dogs exceeded those in controls, the diminished oxidative capacity in the former was inadequately compensated, resulting in lowering of the ATP contents. Thus, inadequate fuel utilization may be considered as a factor limiting the ability for heavy exercise in myxedema.

To investigate the mechanism of reduced exercise capacity in thyrotoxicosis, the effects of excess thyroid hormone administration (daily ingestion of 0.1 mg T_3 for 2 weeks) on cardiac and metabolic responses to graded-dose isoproterenol infusion, skeletal muscle β-adrenergic receptor density, and physiological determinants of exercise capacity in young healthy subjects were characterized. The slope of the heart rate response to isoproterenol was 36% greater after T_3 administration. In addition, β-adrenergic receptor density was increased in all types of skeletal muscle fibers. Maximum oxygen uptake during treadmill exercise declined 5% after T_3 administration because of a decrease in the arteriovenous oxygen difference. The plasma lactate response to submaximum exercise was 25% greater in the thyrotoxic state. These effects were paralleled by a decrease in skeletal muscle oxidative capacity (21–37% decline in activities of oxidative and glycolytic enzymes in skeletal muscle) and a 15% decrease in cross-sectional area of type 2a skeletal myocytes. Lean body mass was reduced and the rates of whole-body leucine oxidation and protein breakdown were enhanced. Thus, work or exercise capacity was impaired in short-duration experimental thyrotoxicosis because of decreased skeletal muscle mass (type 2a fiber atrophy) and oxidative

capacity related to accelerated protein catabolism, but cardiac pump function was not reduced [40–42]. Thyroid hormone excess enhanced cardiac β-adrenergic sensitivity under in vivo conditions in human subjects. In contrast, no change in adrenergic sensitivity was found in other primates.

4.7 Cardiovascular and Pulmonary Work Capacity

Stress echocardiography compares two-dimensional echocardiographic images obtained before, during, and after exercise. It is an accurate technique for the evaluation and follow-up of global and regional left ventricular function as well as of exercise capacity. In the normal subject, when cardiac performance is monitored during exercise, the most striking physiological changes are the increase in left ventricular contractility and the decrease in end-systolic volume. These alterations can be detected by analysis of left ventricular wall motion and measurement of the ejection fraction response to stress. Failure of these changes to occur during exercise is abnormal. Possible causes include cardiomyopathy, reduced exercise capacity, medications such as β-blockers, and ischemia. Based on the linear relationship between cardiac output and oxygen uptake, direct breath-to-breath gas exchange measurements during exercise allow accurate determinations of cardiorespiratory function. The advantage of gas exchange analysis is that it gives an objective determination of maximum oxygen uptake and ventilator anaerobic threshold (the reflection point at which there is a disproportionate increase in carbon dioxide production compared with oxygen uptake). The term "anaerobic threshold" has also been used to define the peak work rate or oxygen uptake at which aerobic metabolic processes can no longer meet the skeletal muscle requirements for ATP. As work is increased above the anaerobic threshold, progressive increases in anaerobic glycolysis must accompany aerobic metabolism to sustain adequate levels of ATP regeneration. The acceleration in glycolysis leads to an elevated muscular concentration of lactic acid and a consequent metabolic acidosis. Therefore, the anaerobic threshold obtained by respiratory gas analysis on a ramp-loading cycle ergometer is an objective measure of work or exercise capacity [43–48].

Abnormal left ventricular function has been

observed in thyrotoxicosis, independent of β-adrenoceptor activation, suggesting a reversible functional cardiomyopathy due to a direct effect on the myocardium of excessive circulating T_3. Left ventricular ejection fraction was also decreased in patients with myxedema and increased after levothyroxine (LT_4) therapy. Furthermore, thyrotoxicosis has been implicated as a primary cause of reduced cardiorespiratory exercise tolerance. Although cardiac function is enhanced at rest, an abnormal response of the left ventricular ejection fraction to physical exercise has been reported in subjects with thyrotoxicosis without underlying heart disease. Dyspnea and reduced exercise capacity in thyrotoxicosis are most probably due to reduction of the cardiac functional reserve. Cardiac output cannot adequately increase in response to physical work because all the mechanisms involved in the hemodynamic response to exercise are potentially already maximally activated at rest (enhanced heart rate, myocardial contractility, and preload, together with reduced afterload) in relation to the degree of hyperthyroidism. Furthermore, subjects with long-standing thyrotoxicosis may have developed cardiac hypertrophy, caused directly by the effect of thyroid hormones on myocardial protein synthesis and indirectly by the increase in cardiac workload. An increase in left ventricular mass has also been reported in long-term overt hyperthyroidism and may counteract the beneficial effect of thyroid hormones on diastolic performance, impairing diastolic ventricular filling and the systolic performance of the thyrotoxic individual on effort [1–3].

4.8 Long-Term Experience at the Gutenberg University Joint Cardiac–Thyroid Laboratory

To analyze alterations of cardiovascular function and work capacity thought to occur in patients with thyroid disease, stress echocardiography, spiroergometry, and spirometry were performed at our institution in more than 300 people with untreated mild or subclinical thyroid disease or with overt thyroid dysfunction and again after restoration of euthyroidism in these patients [43–48]. The results were compared to those obtained in a group of 50 age- and sex-matched healthy controls. At rest, the majority of cardiorespiratory parameters were similar in the patients with thyroid dysfunction and in

the control group. During exercise, however, cardiac indices were significantly different, and the Doppler parameters were markedly modified, all of which reverted to normal when euthyroidism was reinstated. At rest, systemic vascular resistance was 36% lower in hyperthyroid patients than in the control group, but no further decline was noted at maximum exercise. The change in end-systolic volume index between rest and maximum exercise was lower in the hyperthyroid than in the control group. At rest, left ventricular ejection fraction, stroke volume, and cardiac indices were significantly increased in thyrotoxicosis but exhibited a blunted response to exercise, which normalized after restoration of a euthyroid state. Even in subjects with mild or subclinical hyperthyroidism vs. controls, the changes in minute ventilation (Δ_{MV}: respiratory rate Δ tidal volume), oxygen pulse (Δ_{OP}: oxygen uptake per heart beat, a measure of effective cardiorespiratory function), and workload were significantly smaller than in controls both at the anaerobic threshold (Fig. 4.1) and at maximum exercise. In subjects with a fT_3 concentration above 20 pg/ml, Δ_{OP} and the changes in left ventricular ejection fraction (Δ_{LVEF}) (Fig. 4.2), cardiac index (Δ_{CI}), and systemic vascular resistance (Δ_{SVR}) were markedly smaller than in controls. Negative correlations between fT_3 concentration and diastolic blood pressure, maximum workload, changes in heart rate, and Δ_{LVEF} were noted. Normal left ventricular wall motion was observed, and no wall motion abnormalities devel-

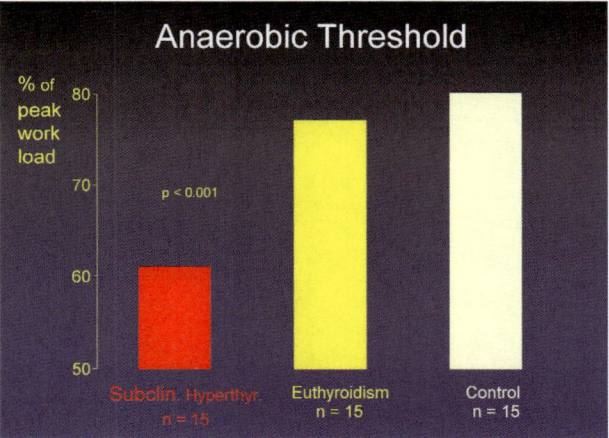

Fig. 4.1 Compared to controls, the anaerobic threshold is reached earlier and peak workload is markedly lower in patients with subclinical hyperthyroidism. These changes are reversible when biochemical euthyroidism is achieved

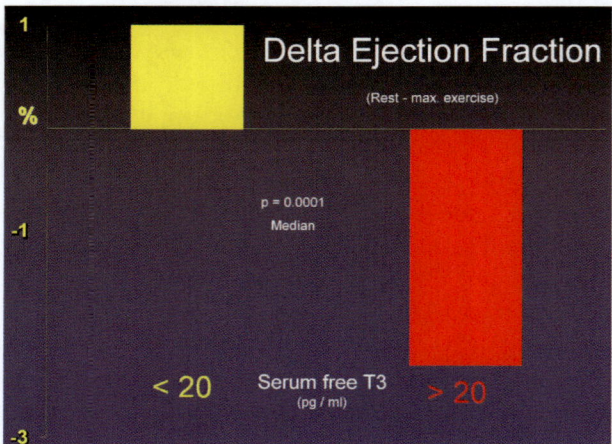

Fig. 4.2 Severe hyperthyroidism markedly impairs left ventricular ejection fraction during exercise

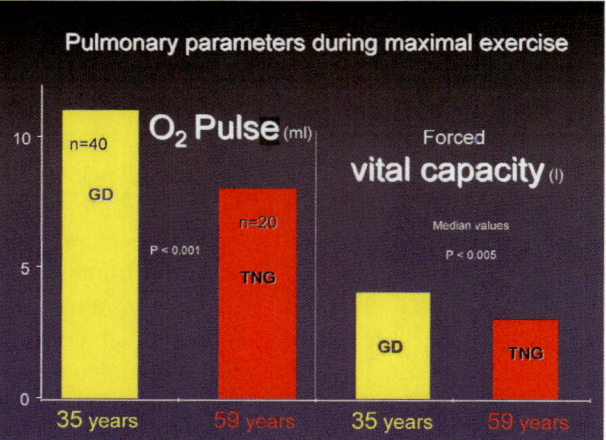

Fig. 4.3 Patients with thyrotoxic nodular goiter (*TNG*) were, on average, older than those with Graves' disease (*GD*) and showed markedly impaired cardiorespiratory parameters during exercise

oped with exercise. It two groups of patients with thyrotoxicity of different etiologies and with different mean ages, marked but reversible alterations of cardiopulmonary function were noted in the older group (Figs. 4.3 and 4.4).

In patients with myxedema, reduced forced vital capacity and tidal volume at the anaerobic threshold compared were observed to the euthyroid state. In those with subclinical or mild hypothyroidism, the oxygen uptake per heart beat (also defined as oxygen pulse) was markedly impaired (Fig. 4.5). This key cardiorespiratory parameter reverted to near normal after LT$_4$ substitution.

In contrast to healthy controls and to patients in the euthyroid state, heart rate did not increase significantly during exercise in thyrotoxic patients, a sign of impaired chronotropic reserve. The results are consistent with a described depression of the efferent activity of the vagal component of the autonomic nervous system during exercise in hyperthyroid individuals. Furthermore, although the rate–pressure product was significantly higher in hyperthyroidism than in euthyroidism, workload was markedly lower in hyperthyroidism. This product is an index of cardiac work that correlates with myocardial oxygen consumption. During exercise, the smaller increase in rate–pressure product in thyrotoxic patients was most likely due both to the higher resting heart rate

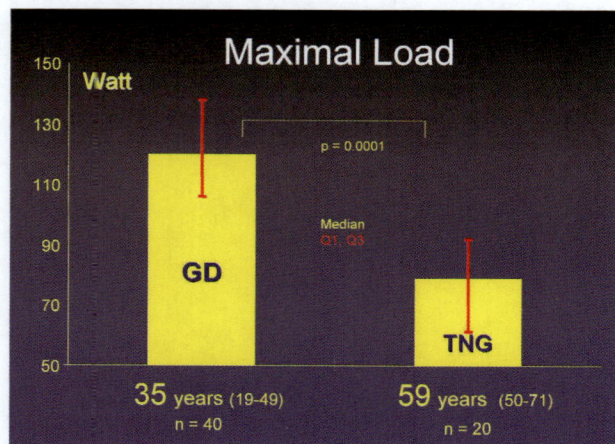

Fig. 4.4 Work capacity during maximum exercise was markedly lower in the older subjects with thyrotoxic nodular goiter. *Q*1, 25%; *Q*3, 75%

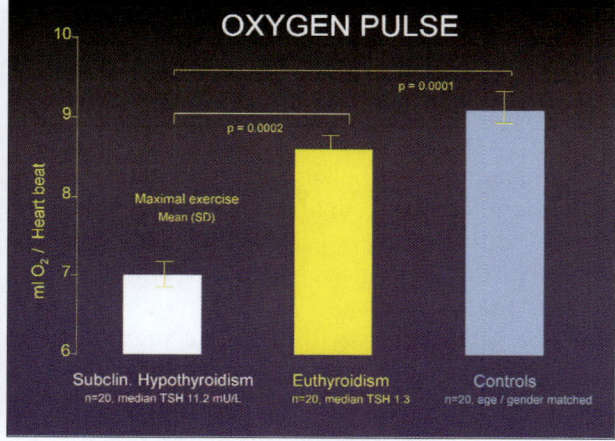

Fig. 4.5 In contrast to euthyroidism and controls, the oxygen uptake per heart beat was markedly lower in patients with subclinical hypothyroidism; after levothyroxine substitution it became nearly normal

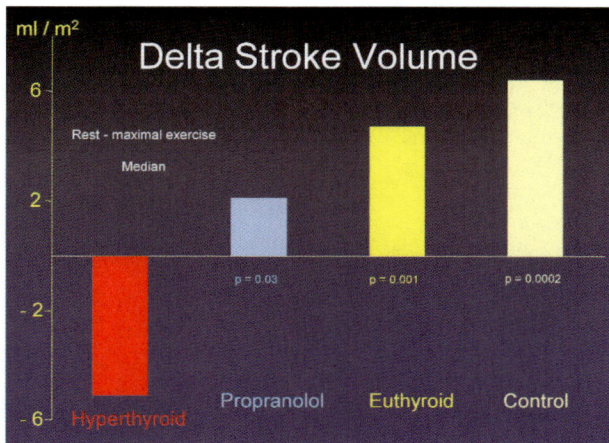

Fig. 4.6 In contrast to controls, left ventricular stroke volume was markedly reduced in overt hyperthyroidism. It was improved after propranolol administration and nearly normal after biochemical euthyroidism was achieved

and systolic blood pressure and to the lower systemic vascular resistance seen in hyperthyroidism, consistent with decreased contractile cardiac reserve. Propranolol treatment led to a significant increase in the change in stroke volume index (Δ_{SVI}) between resting and maximum exercise (Fig. 4.6). The action of thyroid hormones may be mediated by adrenergic receptor stimuli that can be blocked by β-antagonists. This effect is plausible since there is a high cardiac sensitivity to β-adrenergic stimulation in thyrotoxicosis. In contrast to the effects of β-blockade in controls, propranolol partially improved skeletal muscle weakness in hyperthyroid patients and reversed T_4-induced cardiac hypertrophy in both animals and humans. Thyroid hormones and catecholamines in concert appear to mediate the muscle dysfunction in thyrotoxicosis. Although older patients with hyperthyroidism lack an appropriate peripheral circulatory response, propranolol therapy may enhance workload and reduce the response of heart rate to exercise. Thus, β-blockade leads to more economical work and higher efficiency of cardiovascular function. This may explain the clinical amelioration of symptoms in thyrotoxic patients during propranolol therapy [49, 50].

4.9 Conclusions

The heart is an organ that is sensitive to the action of thyroid hormones, and measurable changes in cardiovascular performance are detected with small variations in serum concentrations of thyroid hormones. Most patients with thyroid dysfunction experience cardiovascular manifestations, and the most serious complications of thyroid disease are a result of cardiac involvement. To meet the increased metabolic state and oxygen consumption that occur in thyrotoxic patients, an increased supply of oxygen and the removal of metabolic products from the periphery are required. This is accomplished by increasing the cardiac output to meet the needs of the periphery. Circulation time is decreased in hyperthyroid patients, and a lowered arterial resistance and increased venous resistance promote the return of blood to the heart. Thyroid hormones may significantly decrease the strength of both respiratory and skeletal muscles and affect regulatory mechanisms of adaptation to incremental effort. In thyrotoxicosis, cardiovascular exercise testing and analysis of respiratory gas exchange demonstrate a low efficiency of cardiopulmonary function and impaired chronotropic, contractile, and vasodilatatory reserves, which are reversible when euthyroidism is restored. During exercise, the increases in minute ventilation and oxygen pulse are significantly lower in thyroid dysfunction than in euthyroidism. Especially in older patients with thyroid disease, markedly reduced workload is observed both at the anaerobic threshold and at maximum exercise. In hyperthyroidism, mitochondrial oxidative dysfunction during exercise mostly causes intracellular acidosis, whereas in hypothyroidism the inadequate cardiovascular support appears to be one of the principal factors involved. These abnormalities partly explain why people with dysthyroidism are intolerant of exertion: in thyroid dysfunction, both cardiac structures and cardiac function may remain normal at rest, but exercise unmasks impaired cardiovascular and respiratory adaptability to effort.

Key Points

- The cardiovascular system is deeply involved in thyroid dysfunction.

- Marked changes in systemic vascular resistance mainly explain the modified clinical cardiovascular signs in thyroid dysfunction.

- Even subclinical thyroid dysfunction involves the cardiovascular and respiratory systems significantly.

- The close interaction between thyroid hormones and the sympathoadrenal system enhances the arrhythmic effect in both subclinical and overt hyperthyroidism.

- β-Blockade markedly improves cardiovascular work capacity and significantly decreases the risk of atrial arrhythmias in both subclinical and overt hyperthyroidism.

References

1. Kahaly GJ, Dillmann WH (2005) Thyroid hormone action in the heart. Endocr Rev 26:704–728

2. Dillmann WH (1996) Thyroid hormones and the heart: basic mechanistic and clinical issues. Thyroid Today 19:1–11

3. Klein I, Danzi S (2007) Thyroid disease and the heart. Circulation 116:1725–1735

4. Klein I, Ojamaa K (2001) Thyroid hormone and the cardiovascular system. N Engl J Med 344:501–509

5. Klein I, Levey GS (2000) The cardiovascular system in thyrotoxicosis. In: Braverman LE, Utiger RD (eds) Werner & Ingbar's The thyroid: a fundamental and clinical text, 8th edn. Lippincott Williams & Wilkins, Philadelphia, pp 596–604

6. Kahaly GJ, Matthews CH, Mohr Kahaly S et al (2002) Cardiac involvement in thyroid hormone resistance. J Clin Endocrinol Metab 87:204–212

7. Kahaly GJ, Nieswandt J, Mohr-Kahaly S (1998) Cardiac risks of hyperthyroidism in the elderly. Thyroid 8:1165–1169

8. Klein I, Ojamaa K (2000) The cardiovascular system in hypothyroidism. In: Braverman LE, Utiger RD, eds. Werner & Ingbar's The thyroid: a fundamental and clinical text, 8th edn. Lippincott Williams & Wilkins, Philadelphia, pp 777–782

9. Kahaly GJ (2000) Cardiovascular and atherogenic aspects of subclinical hypothyroidism. Thyroid 10:665–679

10. Kahaly GJ, Mohr-Kahaly S, Beyer J, Meyer J (1995) Left ventricular function analyzed by Doppler and echocardiographic methods in short-term hypothyroidism. Am J Cardiol 75:645–648

11. Wieshammer S, Keck FS, Waitzinger J (1989) Acute hypothyroidism slows the rate of left ventricular diastolic relaxation. Can J Physiol Pharmacol 67:1007–1010

12. Carneiro-Ramos MS, Diniz GP, Almeida J et al (2008) Cardiac angiotensin II type I and type II receptors are increased in rats submitted to experimental hypothyroidism. J Physiol 583.1:213–223

13. Ransnas L, Hammond HK, Insel PA (1988) Increased Gs in myocardial membranes from hyperthyroid pigs. Clin Res 36:552A

14. Hammond HK, White FC, Buxton IL et al (1987) Increased myocardial b-receptors and adrenergic responses in hyperthyroid pigs. Am J Physiol 252:H283–H290

15. Hoit BD, Khoury SF, Shao Y et al (1997) Effects of thyroid hormone on cardiac beta-adrenergic responsiveness in conscious baboons. Circulation 96:592–598

16. Ojamaa K, Klein I, Sabet A, Steinberg SF (2000) Changes in adenylyl cyclase isoforms as a mechanism for thyroid hormone modulation of cardiac beta-adrenergic receptor responsiveness. Metabolism 49:275–279

17. Carvalho-Bianco SD, Kim BW, Zhang JX et al (2004) Chronic cardiac-specific thyrotoxicosis increases myocardial beta-adrenergic responsiveness. Mol Endocrinol 18:1840–1849

18. Bachman ES, Hampton TG, Dhillon H et al (2004) The metabolic and cardiovascular effects of hyperthyroidism are largely independent of beta-adrenergic stimulation. Endocrinology 145:2767–2774

19. Brodde OE (1991) b1- and b2-adrenoreceptors in the human heart: properties, function, and alterations in chronic heart failure. Pharmacol Rev 43:203–242

20. Bahouth SW (1991) Thyroid hormones transcriptionally regulate the b1-adrenergic receptor gene in cultured ventricular myocytes. J Biol Chem 266:15863–15869

21. Bahouth SW, Cui X, Beauchamp MJ, Park EA (1997) Thyroid hormone induces ?1-adrenergic receptor gene transcription through a direct repeat separated by five nucleotides. J Mol Cell Cardiol 29:3223–3237

22. Ianuzzo CD, Patel P, Chen V (1977) Thyroidal trophic influence on skeletal muscle myosin. Nature 270:74–76

23. Caiozzo VJ, Herrick RE, Baldwin KM (1991) Influence of hyperthyroidism on maximal shortening velocity and myosin isoform distribution in skeletal muscles. Am J Physiol 261:C285–295

24. Crow MT, Kushmerik MJ (1982) Chemical energetics of slow- and fast-twitch muscles of the mouse. J Gen Physiol 79:147–166

25. Nazar K, Chwalbinska-Moneta J, Machalla J (1978) Meta-

bolic and body temperature changes during exercise in hyperthyroid patients. Clin Sci 54:323–327

26. Winder WW, Holloszy JO (1977) Response of mitochondria of different types of muscle to thyrotoxicosis. Am J Physiol 232:C180–184

27. Sestoft L, Saltin B (1985) Working capacity and mitochondrial enzyme activities in muscle of hyperthyroid patients before and after 3 months of treatment. Biochem Soc Trans 13:733–734

28. Bengel FM, Nekolla SG, Ibrahim T et al (2000) Effect of thyroid hormones on cardiac function, geometry, and oxidative metabolism assessed noninvasively by positron emission tomography and magnetic resonance imaging. J Clin Endocrinol Metab 85:1822–1827

29. Weiss RE, Murata Y, Cua K et al (1998) Thyroid hormone action on liver, heart and energy expenditure in thyroid hormone receptor b deficient mice. Endocrinology 139:4945–4952

30. Wikstrom L, Johansson C, Salto C et al (1998) Abnormal heart rate and body temperature in mice lacking thyroid hormone receptor a1. EMBO J 17:455–461

31. Swanson EA, Gloss B, Belke DD et al (2003) Cardiac expression and function of thyroid hormone receptor beta and its PV mutant. Endocrinology 144:4820–4825

32. Morkin E, Pennock GD, Spooner PH et al (2002) Clinical and experimental studies on the use of 3,5-diiodothyropropionic acid, a thyroid hormone analogue, in heart failure. Thyroid 12:527–533

33. Trost SU, Swanson EA, Gloss B et al (2000) The thyroid hormone receptor-b-selective agonist GC-1 differentially affects plasma lipids and cardiac activity. Endocrinology 141:3057–3064

34. Grover GJ, Mellström, Ye L et al (2003) Selective thyroid hormone receptor-? activation: a strategy for reduction of weight, cholesterol, and lipoprotein (a) with reduced cardiovascular liability. Proc Natl Acad Sci U S A 100:10067–10072

35. McAllister RM, Sansone JC, Laughlin JR (1995) Effect of hyperthyroidism on muscle blood flow during exercise in rats. Am J Physiol 268:H330–335

36. McAllister RM, Luther Kl, Pfeifer PC (2000) Thyroid status and response to endothelin-1 in rat arterial vessels. Am J Physiol 279:E252–258

37. Katzeff HL, Ojamaa KM, Klein I (1994) Effects of exercise on protein synthesis and myosin heavy chain gene expression in hypothyroid rats. Am J Physiol 267:E63–67

38. Baldwin KM, Ernst SB, Herrick RE et al (1980) Exercise capacity and cardiac function in trained and untrained thyroid-deficient rats. J Appl Physiol 49:1022–1026

39. Fitzsimons DP, Bodell PW, Herrick RE, Baldwin KM (1990) Effect of thyroid state on cardiac myosin P-light chain phosphorylation during exercise. J Appl Physiol 69:313–320

40. Martin WH III, Spina RJ, Korte E et al (1991) Mechanisms of impaired exercise capacity in short duration experimental hyperthyroidism. J Clin Invest 88:2047–2053

41. Martin WH III, Korte E, Tolley TK, Saffitz JE (1992) Skeletal muscle b-adrenoreceptor distribution and responses to isoproterenol in hyperthyroidism. Am J Physiol 262:E504–510

42. Martin WH III, Spina RJ, Korte E (1992) Effect of hyperthyroidism of short duration on cardiac sensitivity to beta-adrenergic stimulation. J Am Coll Cardiol 19:1185–1191

43. Kahaly GJ, Wagner S, Nieswandt J et al (1999) Stress echocardiography in hyperthyroidism. J Clin Endocrinol Metab 84:2308–2313

44. Wassermann K (1997 Diagnosing cardiovascular and lung pathophysiology from exercise gas exchange. Chest 112:1091–1101

45. Forfar JC, Muir AL, Sawers SA, Toft AD (1982) Abnormal left ventricular function in hyperthyroidism. Evidence for a possible reversible cardiomyopathy. N Engl J Med 307:1165–1170

46. Forfar JC, Muir AL, Toft AD (1982) Left ventricular function in hypothyroidism. Responses to exercise and beta adrenoceptor blockade. Br Heart J 48:278–284

47. Kahaly GJ, Hellermann J, Mohr-Kahaly S, Treese N (1996) Impaired cardiopulmonary exercise capacity in hyperthyroidism. Chest 109:57–61

48. Kahaly GJ, Nieswandt J, Wagner S et al (1998) Ineffective cardiorespiratory function in hyperthyroidism. J Clin Endocrinol Metab 83:4075–4078

49. Kollai B, Kollai M (1988) Reduced cardiac vagal excitability in hyperthyroidism. Brain Res Bull 20:785–790

50. Biondi B, Fazio S, Carella C et al (1994) Control of adrenergic overactivity by beta-blockade improves quality of life in patients on long-term suppressive therapy with levothyroxine. J Clin Endocrinol Metab 78:1028–1033

Mechanism of Action of Thyroid Hormone on the Cardiac Vascular System

5

Wolfgang H. Dillmann

Abstract The influences of thyroid hormone action on cardiovascular function present a complex mix of beneficial adaptive and maladaptive effects. Increased thyroid hormone action mediates an increased speed of diastolic relaxation and an increased speed and force of systolic contraction. Beneficial thyroid hormone effects are caused in part by alterations in calcium handling, which are based on changes in the expression of important proteins involved in this process. These include increases in the level of calcium ATPase of the sarcoplasmic reticulum (SERCa2) and decreases in phospholamban levels. Increased thyroid hormone action also has marked electrophysiological effects resulting in increased heart rate and an increased propensity for cardiac arrhythmias, especially atrial fibrillation. In addition, thyroid hormone exerts marked effects, on the vascular system, decreasing arterial resistance and thus diminishing cardiac afterload. Hyperthyroidism of some duration results in cardiac hypertrophy. Recently, thyroid hormone analogues have been developed that target the thyroid hormone receptor-β in the liver, mediating the lowering of lipid levels without significant other cardiac effects, especially without an increase in heart rate or cardiac arrhythmias. Severe heart failure of different causes can lead to the nonthyroidal illness syndrome, resulting in decreased thyroid hormone levels. Studies in human beings and animal models have also shown that the levels of thyroid hormone receptor-α and -β are decreased in the failing heart. Alternatively, the syndrome may lead to a cardiac status compatible with a "hypothyroid heart." It is currently unclear whether the nonthyroidal illness syndrome presents an adaptive or a maladaptive phenomenon whit respect to cardiac function. In some clinical trials, administration of thyroid hormone to patients with heart-failure-induced nonthyroidal illness syndromes has had beneficial effects; however, other trials did not show improvements in cardiac function.

Keywords Thyroid hormone action • Cardiovascular system • Contractile effects of thyroid hormone • Vascular function • Angiogenesis • Gene expression • Cardiac myocyte • Calcium flux • Heart failure • Nonthyroidal illness syndrome • Thyroid hormone receptor isoforms • Ion channels • Thyroid hormone analogues • Viral vectors • Calcium ATPase of the sarcoplasmic reticulum

5.1 Introduction

In one of the earliest description of hyperthyroidism, in 1785, the British physician C.H. Parry alluded to the close correlation between alterations

W.H. Dillmann (✉)
Department of Medicine, University of California,
San Diego, CA, United States

G. Iervasi, A. Pingitore (eds.), *Thyroid and Heart Failure.*
© Springer-Verlag Italia 2009

in thyroid and cardiac function. Parry noted that the coincidence of thyroid enlargement, a rapid heartbeat, and cardiac enlargement occurred in several of his patients [1]. About 50 years later the Irish physician R.J. Graves, after whom autoimmune-based hyperthyroidism, or Graves' disease, is named, reported that he had observed continued palpitation in four of his hyperthyroid patients [2]. A similar connection between thyroid disease and cardiac disease was noted in 1840 by C.A. von Basedow, who described goiter, palpitation, and exophthalmos in several of his patients [3]. The cardiac manifestations of hypothyroidism were identified much later. In 1918, the physician H. Zondek, in Munich, described cardiac manifestations in his patients with severe hypothyroidism [4]. He termed this condition "das Myxoedemherz," which can be translated as "the myxedemic heart."

In subsequent years, the marked influence of thyroid hormone action on cardiac function was elaborated in further detail [5–8]. The contractile function changes, including increased speed and force of systolic contraction, or the inotropic activity, and increased speed of diastolic relaxation, or lusitropic activity. In addition, electrophysiological influences of hyperthyroidism, especially those leading to tachycardia and a propensity to atrial arrhythmias due to alterations in specific ion channels, have been described [9, 10]. Furthermore, thyroid hormone has significant vascular effects, leading to arterial vasodilation and increased vascular density in the heart [11, 12]. Very recent studies have demonstrated that the thyroid hormone receptor (TR) isoforms TR-α and TR-β exert differential effects on cardiac function [13, 14]. Novel thyroid hormone analogues under development attempt to target the TR-β in the liver, leading to lipid lowering without exerting adverse cardiovascular effects such as increases in heart rate [15, 16]. In addition, interesting questions are being asked about the heart-failure-induced nonthyroidal illness syndrome, specifically that it may be of a maladaptive nature for cardiac function [17, 18].

5.2 Mechanism of Thyroid Hormone Action

Significant influences on cardiac function are exerted by the binding of thyroid hormone, especially T_3, to specific nuclear-based TRs, leading to altered transcription of specific genes [19, 20]. In addition, rapid nongenomic effects of T_4 and T_3 have been described which occur within minutes and include binding to integrins and effects on signaling cascade members, cardiac ion channels, and specific proteins [21]. These effects have been well-established in ex vivo and cell culture systems.

We will first describe the mechanisms of TR action. It was demonstrated in 1986 that the cellular homologue of the *erb* proto-oncogene, which binds T_3 with high affinity and limited capacity, has binding characteristics identical to those of nuclear T_3 receptors [13, 14]. Two separate genes, *TRα* and *TRβ*, were identified that encode several mRNA splice variants [20]. The *TRα* gene codes for the T_3-binding TRα1 isoform and nonligand splice variants including TRα2 [20]. In addition, several internal transcription start sites leading to δ isoforms, which do not bind T_3, have been identified [20]. Furthermore, a specific splice variant of the *TRα* gene with preferential mitochondrial localization has been described [20]. For the *TRβ* gene several splice variants lead to the widely distributed TRβ1 mRNA [20]. TRβ2 mRNA is preferentially concentrated in the pituitary and the central nervous system, and an additional isoform, TRβ3, is more ubiquitously distributed [20]. In the mouse heart, TRα1 accounts for 70% of total cardiac thyroid hormone receptor mRNA, and TRβ1 for the remaining 30% [14]. TRα1 and TRβ1 have different N-terminal regions and more limited amino acid differences in other regions [19]. TRs reside primarily in the nucleus, with some cytosolic accumulation [21]. The TR protein can be divided into protein domains exhibiting different functions related to gene expression. The T_3-mediated transcriptional activity of TRs on positive thyroid hormone response elements (TRE) occurs by recruitment of co-activator proteins which bind to specific regions in the C-terminal area of the THs. These co-activator proteins include SRC1, GRIP-1, and others; are involved in local promoter chromatin remodeling; and communicate with the basal transcription machinery to increase transcription [22]. In contrast, TRs not occupied by T_3 associate with co-repressors like SMRT1 or NCor. These co-repressors form a multiprotein complex with other factors, including histone deacetylases, leading to decreased acetylation of histones. A more compact chromatin structure results in inhibitory interaction with the basal transcriptional machinery, leading to gene repression or silencing [23]. Different isoforms of SMRT occur, and SMRTα exhibits preferential interaction with T_3 receptor isoforms [24]. On negative TREs T_3-occupied TRs suppress gene expression [23]. Stimulatory TR action is a complex process influenced by receptor isoform levels, occupancy of the receptors by T_3, and interactions with co-activators and communication with the basal transcriptional machinery. Levels of TRs and T_3 are key determinants and their interaction is governed by the law of mass action [25]. Decreases in T_3 can be partially compensated by increases in TRs. In addition, cell-type-specific transcriptional factors can interact with the T_3 receptor complex and T_3 action can be modified by interactions with other signaling systems. For example, β-adrenergic sympathetic stimulation leads to an increased heart rate and thyroid hormone action has similar effects [26, 27].

5.3 Thyroid Hormone Receptors and Thyroid-Hormone-Responsive Cardiac Genes

The heart is primarily composed of cardiac myocytes, fibroblasts, endothelial cells, and vascular smooth muscle cells, with cardiac myocytes contributing the majority of protein and mRNA. In the heart of mice, TRα1 is predominant, and the predominance of isoforms is reflected in the phenotype of mice with TR deletions thyroid hormone receptors. Mice with ubiquitous deletion of TRα exhibit a significant cardiac phenotype, with a heart rate that is significantly lower than that of wild-type mice [13, 14]. In addition, the contractile performance of the heart is abnormal. The speed of diastolic relaxation is markedly decreased and the speed and force of systolic relaxation are delayed [14]. The contractile phenotype of the TRα knockout mice mimics that of the hypothyroid heart. In contrast, in mice with ubiquitous deletion of TRβ, thyroid hormone levels are elevated and the mice have a corresponding increase in heart rate. If thyroid hormone levels are normalized by treating the mice with a low-iodine/6-propyl-2-thiouracil (PTU)-containing diet and a physiological dose of replacement thyroid hormone, they have a normal heart rate and a completely normal contractile phenotype [14]. Corresponding to the decreased contractile phenotype, mRNAs coding for proteins involved in cardiac contraction, such as MHCα or SERCa2A, are markedly diminished and the mRNA coding for myosin heavy chain β is increased [6]. In contrast, the levels of SERCa2 and

MHCs are normal in mice with a knockout of TRβ. The diminished heart rate in mice with a knockout of TRα can be increased towards the normal range by T_3 administration [13]. These findings indicate that, although TRα is more predominant in the heart and in the sinus node (SN), a significant contribution is made by TRβ to SN pacemaker regulation. In very interesting and recent studies, it was determined that a cardiac-specific microRNA (miRNA208) is encoded by an intron of the MHCα gene [28]. The miRNA208 plays a role in mediating cardiac hypertrophy and fibrosis, and it also regulates MHCβ expression and cardiac remodeling. These studies therefore demonstrate that the MHCα gene encodes a major cardiac contractile protein, but in addition plays a role in regulating cardiac growth and gene expression in response to stress and thyroid hormone signaling through miRNA208.

In addition to the influence of thyroid hormone on the expression of SERCa2 and MHC genes, it should be noted that thyroid hormone influences the expression of a large number of additional genes that play a role in electrophysiological effects. Thyroid-status-induced changes in the expression of some of these genes are shown in Table 5.1. For example, genes coding for the I_f current HCN2 and HCN4 are thyroid hormone responsive. In addition, various potassium channel genes, such as Kv4.2 and Kv1.5, show marked thyroid hormone responsiveness [29–31]. Acting through to proteins involved in calcium handling and a positively influencing the transcription of the SERCa2 gene, thyroid hormone likewise regulates in a positive fashion the mRNA coding for the calcium channel of the sarcoplasmic reticulum, the ryanodine channel [32]. In hypothyroidism, phospholamban levels are increased [33]. Unphosphorylated phospholamban inhibits SERCa2 activity, and the hypothyroidism-mediated delay in diastolic relaxation most likely results from a combination of decreases in SERCa2 expression and further inhibition of SERCa2 activity by elevated phospholamban levels.

5.4 Thyroid Hormone Effects on Cardiac Vascular Function

Thyroid hormone's influences on vascular function in human beings and animal models have been less well-appreciated than its effects on cardiac contractile and electrophysiological function, but such

Table 5.1 Effects of thyroid hormone on gene expression in the heart

Gene	Transcription	TRE	mRNA	Protein	Activity
Myocytes – myofibrils					
MHCα	—	Yes	—	—	Speed contraction
MHCβ	—	Yes	—	—	Speed contraction
C-actin	n.d.	n.d.	—	n.d.	Thin filament contractile protein
S-actin	n.d.	n.d.	—	n.d.	Thin filament contractile protein
Troponin I	n.d.	n.d.	—	n.d.	Thin filament regulatory protein
Myocytes – sarcoplasmic reticulum					
SERCA2	—	Yes	—	—	Ca sequestration
Phospholamban	n.d.	n.d.	T_3/T_x	n.d.	SERCA2 inhibition
Ryanodine channel	n.d.	n.d.	—	n.d.	Ca efflux
Myocytes – sarcolemma					
Na,K-ATPase					
α1			$T_x\,E$	$T_x\,E$	Na efflux
α2			$T_x\,E$	$T_x\,E$	
β			$T_x\,E$	$T_x\,E$	
βi Receptor	—	n.d.	—	—	Adrenergic
Giα	n.d.	n.d.	—	—	Adrenergic
Giβ	n.d.	n.d.	—	—	Adrenergic
Gs	n.d.	n.d.	n.d.	—	Adrenergic
Myocytes – atrium					
Ion channel					
Kv1.5	n.d.	n.d.	—	—	Delayed rectifier K channel
Kv2.1	n.d.	n.d.	—	—	Delayed rectifier K channel
Kv1.4	n.d.	n.d.	$T_x\,E$	n.d.	Voltage gated K channel
Kv1.2	n.d.	n.d.	$T_x\,E$	n.d.	Voltage gated K channel
minK	n.d.	n.d.	—	n.d.	K channel β-subunit
Myocytes – ventricle					
HCN2	n.d.	n.d.	—	n.d.	I_f current
HCN4	n.d.	n.d.	—	n.d.	I_f current
Kv4.2	n.d.	n.d.	—	n.d.	Voltage gated K channel
Kv1.1	n.d.	n.d.	—	n.d.	Delayed rectifier K channel
Kv1.5	n.d.	n.d.	—	n.d.	Delayed rectifier K channel

TRE thyroid hormone response elements, an increase of parameter after TH administration, a decrease in the hypothyroid state. *n.d.* not determined, *E* extranuclear effect
Modified from [65]

effects have been well documented in the literature. For example, hypothyroidism leads to increased vascular resistance, with hypertension occurring in 20–40% of hypothyroid patients [34]. In contrast, hyperthyroidism has the opposite effects, leading to vascular relaxation. Furthermore, influences of thyroid status on cardiac blood flow have been demonstrated. In animal models of hypothyroidism, cardiac perfusion is decreased and cardiac blood flow is returned to normal when a euthyroid status is achieved [35]. In hyperthyroid animals, cardiac blood flow is increased above the normal level. Mechanisms mediating these changes have only been explored in a limited fashion. Increasing thyroid hormone action enhances endothelial-based nitric oxide (NO) generation, and such effects have been noted in smooth muscle of mesenteric arteries [36]. In addition, direct thyroid hormone effects on aortic vascular smooth muscle relaxation have been described, but without identification of a clear underlying mechanism [37]. Earlier reports indicated that in isolated vascular smooth muscle cells obtained from mesenteric arteries thyroid hormone inhibited myosin light chain kinase activity, which is linked to increased vascular tone [38]. Only one study has focused on thyroid hormone receptor isoform effects. In aortic rings from mice with an ubiquitous knock-in of a thyroid hormone receptor mutant, the TRβ PV mutant, which similarly occurs in patients with the thyroid hormone resistance syndrome, a decrease in endothelial-based relaxation in response to acetylation was noted [39]. The predominance of thyroid hormone receptor isoforms in the cells of the vascular system is also unclear. In vascular smooth muscle, a strong TRα1 and TRα2 mRNA predominance was reported as was weak expression of TRβ1 and TRβ2 but without precise quantitation [40]. Our recent preliminary data indicate that in endothelial cells as well as vascular smooth muscle cells over 90% of total TR isoform mRNA is represented by TRα.

In addition to its effects on vascular tone, thyroid hormone stimulates angiogenesis. Angiogenesis in this context is defined as the formation of new capillaries from postcapillary venules. Hyperthyroidism mediates increases in cardiac vascular density, with opposite effects to those of hypothyroidism described [12, 35]. In addition, thyroxin administration was accompanied by elevated basic fibroblast growth factor mRNA and protein levels [41]. Furthermore, very interesting recent studies have demonstrated that the T_3 analogue DITPA stimulates coronary vascular growth [42, 43]. Similarly, proangiogenic effects of T_3 analogues, which appear to be initiated at the cell surface and by integrins, representing nongenomic effects, have also been noted [44]. Hyperthyroidism in general leads to a cardiac hypertrophy compatible with a physiological type of hypertrophy in contrast to a pathological hypertrophy. Studies in other areas indicate that the difference between physiological and pathological hypertrophy may in part be linked to capillary formation [45]. It is therefore interesting to note that thyroid hormone not only stimulates protein synthesis in cardiac myocytes, leading to cardiac hypertrophy, but simultaneously provides for an increased blood supply by increasing vascular relaxation and mediating an enhancement of angiogenesis.

5.5 Thyroid Hormone Analogues and Cardiovascular Effects

The $TR\alpha$ and $TR\beta$ genes code for different TR isoforms with different tissue distributions. These findings have provided an impetus to develop novel thyroid hormone analogues which have differential

potencies in different tissues and on different pathophysiological mechanisms. As mentioned above, TRα predominates in the heart; in contrast, in the liver TRβ1 is the predominant thyroid hormone receptor isoform. The liver is one of the major sites for lipoprotein and cholesterol production, and attempts to develop novel thyroid hormone analogues with preferred liver accumulation and binding to TRβ1 have recently been actively pursued. A TRβ1-specific analogue may lead to significant lipid lowering without exerting unwanted cardiac effects. Several years ago, a TRβ-preferred agonist termed GC1 was synthesized in the laboratory of T. Scanlan [46, 47]. In GC1, iodine atoms on the inner ring are replaced by methyl groups and an isopropyl group replaces the iodine atom on the outer ring. In addition, the linkage of the two six-carbon rings occurs through a carbon bond rather than an ether bridge. The alanine site chain is markedly modified as well. The binding affinity of GC1 for the TRβ1 isoform is 10 times higher than binding for the TRα1 isoform. Influences of GC1 on cardiac and hepatic action were compared to those of T_3 in hypothyroid mice [47]. In rats placed on a hypercholesterolemic diet and treated with equimolar concentrations of T_3 and GC1, GC1 had better triglyceride-lowering and similar cholesterol-lowering effects to T_3. In T_3-treated animals, but not in GC1-treated animals, an increased heart rate was accompanied by an elevated mRNA coding for the I_f channel HCN2 cardiac-pacemaker-related protein. It was also observed that GC1 had preferential accumulation in the liver versus the heart, which probably contributed to its marked lipid-lowering effects in the absence of effects on heart rate [47]. Overall, these data indicate that GC1 presents a prototype for new drugs for the treatment of high lipid levels.

In subsequent studies, a cytochrome P_{450}-activated prodrug of a phosphonate-containing TR agonist was evaluated [16]. This prodrug showed preferential accumulation in hepatic tissue. After first-pass hepatic extraction and cleavage, the prodrug generates a negatively charged TR agonist that distributes poorly in other tissues and has TRβ-preferred binding activities. This compound, MB07811, significantly reduces cholesterol and both serum and hepatic triglyceride levels at doses devoid of influences on body weight, glycemia, or heart rate. Similar beneficial effects of the TRβ-preferred agonists KB2115 and KB141, with marked lowering of cholesterol and lipoprotein levels without significant effects on heart rate, have been reported [15, 48]. In prior studies thyroid hormone analogues like triiodothyroacetic acid appeared to have more potent hepatic than cardiac actions [49], but not at the level of the liver-preferred effects observed with the newer analogues. It should also be noted that D-thyroxine was previously claimed to have preferred cholesterol-lowering effects. However, more detailed studies showed that D-thyroxine was as active in stimulating cardiac action as L-thyroxine, which may have been in part due to contamination with LT_4 [50].

5.6 Thyroid Hormone Action, Cardiac Hypertrophy, and Heart Failure

Several reports indicate that hypothyroidism, including subclinical hypothyroidism, presents an increased risk to develop heart failure [51–53]. One report describes a patient with severe hypothyroidism who had significant heart failure [54]. Myocardial biopsies were undertaken and indicated that, during the time the patient was hypothyroid, MHCα mRNA was of markedly lower predominance with opposite changes occurring for MHCβ. Furthermore, the mRNA coding for atrial natriuretic factor was markedly elevated in the hypothyroid heart. In addition, phospholamban, which in its non-phosphorylated state inhibits the SERCa2 pump, was 10-fold higher in the hypothyroid than in the euthyroid heart. With thyroid hormone replacement and the achievment of a euthyroid status, those changes reverted to normal and normal cardiac function resumed [54]. Results in animal models of hypothyroidism indicate that the level and activity of the SERCa2 protein markedly decrease and contribute in a significant way to the delayed diastolic relaxation of the heart. For example, if transgenic mice in which a promoter driving a SERCa2 transgene that does not contain thyroid hormone response elements are made hypothyroid, and their SERCa2 level remains in the normal range, no decrease in diastolic function occurs [55]. These findings indicate the important role that normal SERCa2 activity and calcium handling play in the manifestation of abnormal diastolic function in hypothyroidism. Other proteins related to calcium handling, such as the ryanodine receptor, are also markedly decreased with hypothyroidism [56].

In earlier investigations cross-talk between sig-naling cascades mediated by thyroid hormone and by cytokines, which are elevated in the failing heart, were noticed [52]. For example, when neonatal myocytes are incubated with a SERCa2 promoter driving a β-galactosidase reporter gene, addition of thyroid hormone to the cell culture increases SERCa2 expression twofold [57]. In contrast, when the cytokines LIF and IL-6 are added to the cell culture in addition to T_3, the T_3-mediated increase in SERCa2 gene expression is completely abolished. One could therefore speculate that the elevated cytokine levels occurring with heart failure contribute to the down-regulation of SERCa2 by preventing thyroid-hormone-mediated stimulation of SERCa2 gene expression.

5.7 The Nonthyroidal Illness Syndrome, Heart Failure, and Thyroid Hormone Signaling

Severe illness, including heart failure, leads to a down-regulation of the thyroid hormone axis. The detailed mechanisms responsible are not completely clear, but with heart failure and in many severe systemic illnesses cytokines increase that are known to decrease thyroid hormone secretion and divert the metabolism of thyroxine to the biologically inactive reverse T_3 instead of T_3. A decrease in T_4 to T_3 conversion occurs initially, followed by decreased secretion of thyroid stimulating hormone (TSH) and diminished thyroid hormone release from the thyroid gland [58]. Characteristic laboratory findings of nonthyroidal illness syndrome are increases in reverse T_3 accompanied by decreases in T_3 and followed by decreases in T_4 and TSH. With recovery from the severe illness, a rebound happens and thyroid hormone levels return to the normal range. In several recent reports it was clearly demonstrated that a strong correlation exists between the decrease in T_3 levels induced by congestive heart failure and survival [17, 18]. These findings therefore raise the question of whether the heart-failure-induced nonthyroidal illness is of a beneficial, adaptive or a maladaptive nature. Studies in human beings have demonstrated that hearts obtained from patients undergoing cardiac transplantation have decreased levels of thyroid hormone receptors [17]. In addition, in the serum of these patients T_3 is markedly decreased. Similarly, in animal models in which constriction of the ascending aorta induces cardiac hypertrophy and heart failure, marked decrease of TRα and TRβ in cardiac myocytes occurs [59]. To determine whether the decreased T_3 action in heart failure is maladaptive, animal studies were carried out in which heart failure was induced by ascending aortic constriction. TRα or TRβ was cloned into adeno-associated viruses (AAV), that were then injected into the left ventricular wall of the heart. The AAV-based TR expression led to an increased TR level in about 50% of cardiac myocytes. In addition, some of the mice received a physiological replacement dose of 3.5 ngT_3 per gram body weight per day. Cardiac function, especially diastolic relaxation, was determined 2 weeks after viral-vector-based TR administration. In mice with ascending aortic constriction treated with AAV expressing the TR versus empty adenovirus, a significant improvement in cardiac function, especially diastolic relaxation, occurred. In other investigations, a tetracycline-system-based increase in the expression of the deiodinase type II, which converts T_4 to T_3, was used. These studies also showed significant improvement in contractile function in mice with pressure-overload-induced cardiac hypertrophy [54]. It could therefore be speculated that the failing heart represents a hypothyroid heart because of decreased TR levels and decreased levels of the ligand T_3.

5.8 Heart Failure, the Nonthyroidal Illness Syndrome, and Decreased Thyroid Hormone Action: To Treat or Not To Treat

Several studies have been undertaken exploring the results of thyroid hormone administration to patients after cardiac surgery, or in heart failure. In one of these reports, when T_3 was administered to patients after cardiac surgery a beneficial effect was realized from lowering the incidence of atrial fibrillation [60]. In a very recent study, patients with ischemic and nonischemic dilated cardiomyopathy received T_3 infusion for 3 days or underwent a placebo infusion [18]. The patients were followed by clinical examination, echocardiography, and cardiac magnetic resonance determination of cardiac function, and the biohormonal profile was established, including thyroid hormone values, norepinephrine, brain natriuretic peptide, and IL-6. In the group receiving T_3, the neuroendocrine profile and ventricular performance had improved. It should, however, also be noted that in other studies using a randomized double-blind placebo-controlled trial design, intravenous administration of T_3 to patients undergoing coronary bypass graft surgery did not show significant cardiac improvement [61]. It was discussed above that in animal models TR levels are significantly decreased in patients with heart failure. It may therefore not be possible for thyroid hormone administration to exert its maximum beneficial effects in cardiac myocytes. In recent clinical trials, the administration of AAV-encoded SERCa2 was undertaken in patients with heart failure [62]. Trials in large animal models of heart failure have shown that with this approach viral-vector-encoded transgenes can be efficiently delivered to the cardiac myocyte [63, 64]. Although these early results await further confirmation and expansion, novel treatment modalities are being developed for the treatment of heart failure involving components of the thyroid hormone signaling system.

Key Points

- Thyroid hormone action in the cardiovascular system is predominantly mediated by the actions of thyroid hormone receptor α1 and thyroid hormone receptor β1 (TRα1 and TRβ1).

- TRα1 action predominates in cardiac myocytes.

- TRα1 action increases cardiac diastolic relaxation and systolic contraction.

- Thyroid hormone receptor effects increasing SERCa2 expression make an important contribution to calcium handling and diastolic relaxation.

(Cont. →)

(cont.)

- Thyroid hormone receptor action can result in largely beneficial contractile effects and some maladaptive electrophysiological effects, such as resting tachycardia and atrial fibrillation.

- Thyroid hormone receptor action has beneficial cardiac vascular effects, such as arterial relaxation and increased angiogenesis.

- Novel thyroid hormone analogues that result in lipid lowering without significant heart rate effects are being developed.

- Heart failure results in a nonthyroidal illness syndrome with decreased serum thyroid hormone levels and diminished cardiac thyroid hormone receptor levels. Animal experiments indicate that these changes may be maladaptive.

References

1. Parry CH (1825) Collections from the unpublished papers of the late Caleb Hilliel Parry, vol 2. London, p 111
2. Graves RJ (1835) Clinical lectures. Lond Med Surg J 7:516
3. von Basedow CA (1840) Exophthalmos durch Hypertrophie des Zellgewebes in der Augenhöhle. Wochenschr Heilkd 6:197
4. Zondek H (1918) Das Myxoedemherz. Munch Med Wochenschr 65:1180
5. Klein I, Ojamaa K (2001) Thyroid hormone and the cardiovascular system. N Engl J Med 344:5011–5019
6. Kahaly GJ, Dillmann WH (2005) Thyroid hormone action in the heart. Endocr Rev 26:704–728
7. Fazio S, Palmieri EA, Lombardi G, Biondi B (2004) Effects of thyroid hormone on the cardiovascular system. Recent Prog Horm Res 59:31–50
8. Boelaert K, Franklyn JA (2005) Thyroid hormone in health and disease. J Endocrinol 187:1–15
9. Shimizu T, Koide S, Noh JY et al (2002) Hyperthyroidism and the management of atrial fibrillation. Thyroid 12:489–493
10. Le Bouter S, Demolombe S, Chambellan A et al (2003) Microarray analysis reveals complex remodeling of cardiac ion channel expression with altered thyroid status: relation to cellular and integrated electrophysiology. Circ Res 92:234–242
11. Owen PJ, Sabit R, Lazarus JH (2007) Thyroid disease and vascular function. Thyroid 17:519–524
12. Tomanek RJ, Busch TL (1998) Coordinated capillary and myocardial growth in response to thyroxine treatment. Anat Rec 251:44–49
13. Johansson C, Göthe S, Forrest D et al (1999) Cardiovascular phenotype and temperature control in mice lacking thyroid hormone receptor beta or alpha1 and beta. Am J Physiol 276(6 Pt 2):H2006–2012
14. Gloss B, Trost S, Bluhm W et al (2001) Cardiac ion channel expression and contractile function in mice with deletion of thyroid hormone receptor alpha or beta. Endocrinology 142:544–550
15. Berkenstam A, Kristensen J, Mellström K et al (2008) The thyroid hormone mimetic compound KB2115 lowers plasma LDL cholesterol and stimulates bile acid synthesis without cardiac effects in humans. Proc Natl Acad Sci U S A 105:663–667
16. Erion MD, Cable EE, Ito BR et al (2007) Targeting thyroid hormone receptor-beta agonists to the liver reduces cholesterol and triglycerides and improves the therapeutic index. Proc Natl Acad Sci U S A 104:15490–15495
17. Kinugawa K, Minobe WA, Wood WM et al (2001) Signaling pathways responsible for fetal gene induction in the failing human heart: evidence for altered thyroid hormone receptor gene expression. Circulation 103:1089–1094
18. Pingitore A, Galli E, Barison A et al (2008) Acute effects of triiodothyronine (T3) replacement therapy in patients with chronic heart failure and low-T3 syndrome: a randomized, placebo-controlled study. J Clin Endocrinol Metab 93:1351–1358
19. Yen PM, Ando S, Feng X et al (2006) Thyroid hormone action at the cellular, genomic and target gene levels. Mol Cell Endocrinol 246(1–2):121–127
20. Bassett JH, Harvey CB, Williams GR (2003) Mechanisms of thyroid hormone receptor-specific nuclear and extra nuclear actions. Mol Cell Endocrinol 213:1–11
21. Davis PJ, Leonard JL, Davis FB (2008) Mechanisms of nongenomic actions of thyroid hormone. Front Neuroendocrinol 29:211–218
21. Kenessey A, Ojamaa K (2006) Thyroid hormone stimulates protein synthesis in the cardiomyocyte by activating the Akt-mTOR and p70S6K pathways. J Biol Chem 281:20666–20672
22. McKenna NJ, O'Malley BW (2002) Minireview: nuclear receptor coactivators – an update. Endocrinology 143:2461–2465
23. Shupnik MA (2000) Thyroid hormone suppression of pituitary hormone gene expression. Rev Endocr Metab Disord 1(1–2):35–42
24. Goodson ML, Jonas BA, Privalsky ML (2005) Alternative mRNA splicing of SMRT creates functional diversity by generating corepressor isoforms with different affinities for different nuclear receptors. J Biol Chem 280:7493–7503
25. Oppenheimer JH, Schwartz HL, Koerner D, Surks MI (1974) Limited binding capacity sites for L-triiodothyronine in rat liver nuclei. Nuclear-cytoplasmic interrelation, binding constants, and cross-relativity with L-thyroxine. J Clin Invest 53:768–777

26. Carvalho-Bianco SD, Kim BW, Zhang JX et al (2004) Chronic cardiac-specific thyrotoxicosis increases myocardial b-adrenergic responsiveness. Mol Endocrinol 18:1840–1849

27. Bachman ES, Hampton TG, Dhillon H et al (2004) The metabolic and cardiovascular effects of hyperthyroidism are largely independent of b-adrenergic stimulation. Endocrinology 145:2767–2774

28. van Rooij E, Sutherland LB, Qi X et al (2007) Control of stress-dependent cardiac growth and gene expression by a microRNA. Science 316(5824):575–579

29. Shimoni Y, Fiset C, Clark RB et al (1997) Thyroid hormone regulates postnatal expression of transient K+ channel isoforms in rat ventricle. J Physiol 500(Pt 1):65–73

30. Ojamaa K, Sabet A, Kenessey A et al (1999) Regulation of rat cardiac Kv1.5 gene expression by thyroid hormone is rapid and chamber specific. Endocrinology 140:3170–3176

31. Le Bouter S, Demolombe S, Chambellan A et al (2003) Microarray analysis reveals complex remodeling of cardiac ion channel expression with altered thyroid status: relation to cellular and integrated electrophysiology. Circ Res 92:234–242

32. Jiang M, Xu A, Tokmakejian S, Narayanan N (2000) Thyroid hormone-induced overexpression of functional ryanodine receptors in the rabbit heart. Am J Physiol Heart Circ Physiol 278:H1429–1438

33. Shenoy R, Klein I, Ojamaa K (2000) Differential regulation of SR calcium transporters by thyroid hormone in rat atria and ventricles. Am J Physiol Heart Circ Physiol 281:H1690–1696

34. Danzi S, Klein I (2003) Thyroid hormone and blood pressure regulation. Curr Hypertens Rep 5:513–520

35. Khalife WI, Tang YD, Kuzman JA et al (2005) Treatment of subclinical hypothyroidism reverses ischemia and prevents myocyte loss and progressive LV dysfunction in hamsters with dilated cardiomyopathy. Am J Physiol Heart Circ Physiol 289:H2409–2415

36. Zwaveling J, Pfaffendorf M, van Zwieten PA (1997) The direct effects of thyroid hormones on rat mesenteric resistance arteries. Fundam Clin Pharmacol 11:41–46

37. Ojamaa K, Klemperer JD, Klein I (1996) Acute effects of thyroid hormone on vascular smooth muscle. Thyroid 6:502–512

38. Mamiya S, Hagiwara M, Inoue S, Hidaka H (1989) Thyroid hormones inhibit platelet function and myosin light chain kinase. J Biol Chem 264:8575–8579

39. Owen PJ, Ying H, Lang D et al (2007) Endothelial dysfunction in a murine model of thyroid hormone resistance. Eur J Clin Invest 37:390–395

40. Mizuma H, Murakami M, Mori M (2001) Thyroid hormone activation in human vascular smooth muscle cells: expression of type II iodothyronine deidinase. Circ Res 88:313–318

41. Tomanek RJ, Doty MK, Sandra A (1998) Early coronary angiogenesis in response to thyroxine: growth characteristics and upregulation of basic fibroblast growth factor. Circ Res 82:587–593

42. Wang X, Zheng W, Christensen LP, Tomanek RJ (2003) DITPA stimulates bFGF, VEGF, angiopoietin, and Tie-2 and facilitates coronary arteriolar growth. Am J Physiol Heart Circ Physiol 284:H613–618

43. Tomanek RJ, Zimmerman MB, Suvarna PR et al (1998) A thyroid hormone analogue stimulates angiogenesis in the post-infarcted rat heart. J Mol Cell Cardiol 30:923–932

44. Mousa SA, O'Connor L, Davis FB, Davis PJ (2006) Proangiogenesis action of the thyroid hormone analogue 3,5-diiodothyropropionic acid (DITPA) is initiated at the cell surface and is integrin mediated. Endocrinology 147:1602–1607

45. Shiojima I, Sato K, Izumiya Y et al (2005) Distribution of coordinated cardiac hypertrophy and angiogenesis contributes to the transition of heart failure. J Clin Invest 115:2108–2118

46. Chiellini G, Apriletti JW, Yoshihara HA et al (1998) A high-affinity subtype-selective agonist ligand for the thyroid hormone receptor. Chem Biol 5:299–306

47. Trost SU, Swanson E, Gloss B et al (2000) The thyroid hormone receptor-beta-selective agonist GC-1 differentially affects plasma lipids and cardiac activity. Endocrinology 141:3057–3064

48. Bryzgalova G, Effendic S, Khan A et al (2008) Anti-obesity, anti-diabetic, and lipid lowering effects of the thyroid receptor beta subtype selective agonist KB-141. J Steroid Biochem Mol Biol 111:262–267

49. Sherman SI, Ringel MD, Smith MJ et al (1997) Augmented hepatic and skeletal thyromimetic effects of tiratricol in comparison with levothyroxine. J Clin Endocrinol Metab 82:2153–2158

50. Young WF Jr, Gorman CA, Jiang NS et al (1984) L-thyroxine contamination of pharmaceutical D-thyroxine; probable cause of therapeutic effect. Clin Pharmacol Ther 36:781–787

51. Shuvy M, Shifman OE, Nusair S et al (2008) Hypothyroidism-induced myocardial damage and heart failure: an overlooked entity. Cardiovasc Pathol Feb 21 (Epub ahead of print). doi:10.1016/j.carpath.2007.12.015

52. Schmidt-Ott UM, Ascheim DD (2006) Thyroid hormone and heart failure. Curr Heart Fail Resp 3:114–119

53. Rodondi N, Bauer DC, Cappola AR et al (2008) Subclinical thyroid dysfunction, cardiac function, and the risk of heart failure. The Cardiovascular Health study. J Am Coll Cardiol 52:1152–1159

54. Ladenson PW, Sherman SI, Baughman KL et al (1992) Reversible alterations in myocardial gene expression in a young man with dilated cardiomyopathy and hypothyroidism. Proc Natl Acad Sci U S A 89:5251–5255

55. Blumh WF, Meyer M, Sayen MR et al (1999) Overexpression of sarcoplasmic reticulum Ca(2+)-ATPase improves cardiac contractile function in hypothyroid mice. Cardiovasc Res 43:382–388

56. Arai M, Otsu K, MacLennan DH et al (1991) Effect of thyroid hormone on the expression of mRNA encoding sarcoplasmic reticulum proteins. Circ Res 69:266–273

57. Gloss B, Villegas S, Villarreal FJ et al (2000) Thyroid hormone-induced stimulation of the sarcoplasmic reticulum Ca(2+) ATPase gene is inhibited by LIF and IL-6. Am J Physiol Endocrinol Metab 278:E738–743

58. Adler SM, Wartofsky L (2007) The nonthyroidal illness syndrome. Endocrinol Metab Clin North Am 36:657–672

59. Belke DD, Gloss B, Swanson EA, Dillmann WH (2007) Adeno-associated virus-mediated expression of thyroid hormone receptor isoforms-alpha1 and -beta1 improves contractile function in pressure overload-induced cardiac hypertrophy. Endocrinology 148:2670–2677

60. Klemperer JD, Klein IL, Ojamaa K et al (1996) Triiodothyronine therapy lowers the incidence of atrial fibrillation after cardiac operations. Ann Thorac Surg 61:1323–1327

61. Bennett-Guerrero E, Jimenez JL, White WD et al (1996) Cardiovascular effects of intravenous triiodothyronine in patients undergoing coronary artery bypass graft surgery. A randomized, double-blind, placebo-controlled trial. Duke T3 study group. JAMA 275:687–692

62. Hajjar RJ, Zsebo K, Deckelbam L et al (2008) Design of a phase 1/2 trial of intracoronary administration of AAV1/SERCA2a in patients with heart failure. J Card Fail 14:355–367

63. Byrne MJ, Power JM, Preovolos A et al (2008) Recirculating cardiac delivery of AAV2/1SERCA2a improves myocardial function in an experimental model of heart failure in large animals. Gene Ther 15:1550-1557

64. Vinge LE, Raake PW, Koch WJ (2008) Gene therapy in heart failure. Circ Res 102:1458–1470

65. Kahaly GJ, Dillman WH (2005) Thyroid hormone action in the heart. Endocrine Rev 26:704–728

Cardiac Functional Effects of 3-Iodothyronamine, a New Endogenous Thyroid Hormone Derivative

6

Riccardo Zucchi, Sandra Ghelardoni and Grazia Chiellini

Abstract   Thyronamines are decarboxylated derivatives of thyroid hormone. 3-Iodothyronamine (T_1AM) has been detected in blood and in several tissues, where it is likely produced from thyroid hormone by the consequent action of aromatic amino acid decarboxylase and deiodinases. In vitro, high-affinity interaction has been observed between T_1AM and a novel G-protein-coupled receptor known as trace-amine-associated receptor 1 (TAAR1). TAAR1 and other receptors of this family are expressed in several tissues, including the heart. Functional effects have been observed after administration of exogenous T_1AM: in the isolated heart, a negative inotropic and chronotropic action was produced, and the resistance to ischemic injury was increased, possibly as a consequence of an action on intracellular calcium homeostasis. Extracardiac effects include reduction of body temperature, increased lipid versus carbohydrate metabolism, modulation of insulin secretion, and inhibition of neuronal catecholamine reuptake. T_1AM may play an important physiological or pathophysiological role, and this signaling system might allow the development of new therapeutic agents.

Keywords   Heart • Thyroid • Thyroid hormone • G-protein-coupled receptors • Trace-amine-associated receptors • Signaling • Contraction • Calcium • Ischemia • Metabolism

6.1 Introduction

The term "thyroid hormone" refers to two different molecules (Fig. 6.1): thyroxine (T_4) and 3,5,3'-tri-iodothyronine (T_3). T_4 is the main product of the thyroid gland, and in the human circulation total T_4 exceeds total T_3 content by about two orders of magnitude [1, 2]. T_3 is produced by T_4 deiodination mostly in target tissues (liver, kidney, adipose tissue, heart, brain), and it is the most effective agonist of thyroid hormone receptors. For this rea-son, T_3 is regarded as the active form of thyroid hormone, while T_4 is regarded as a prohormone. Thyroid hormone receptors two subtypes comprise TRα (or NR1A1) and TRβ (or NR1A2), which act as activators of transcription, as detailed in other chapters of this book. The corresponding function-al effects therefore occur on a relatively slow time scale. However, there are many rapid effects asso-ciated with thyroid hormone, occuring within a matter of seconds to minutes and insensitive to inhibitors of protein synthesis such as cyclohex-imide [3]. The effects relate to calcium uptake, oxygen consumption, ion channel activation, and cardiac function. They are referred to as nonge-nomic effects and are thought to be mediated by membrane receptors.

R. Zucchi (✉)
Professor of Biochemistry, University of Pisa, Pisa, Italy

G. Iervasi, A. Pingitore (eds.), *Thyroid and Heart Failure.*
© Springer-Verlag Italia 2009

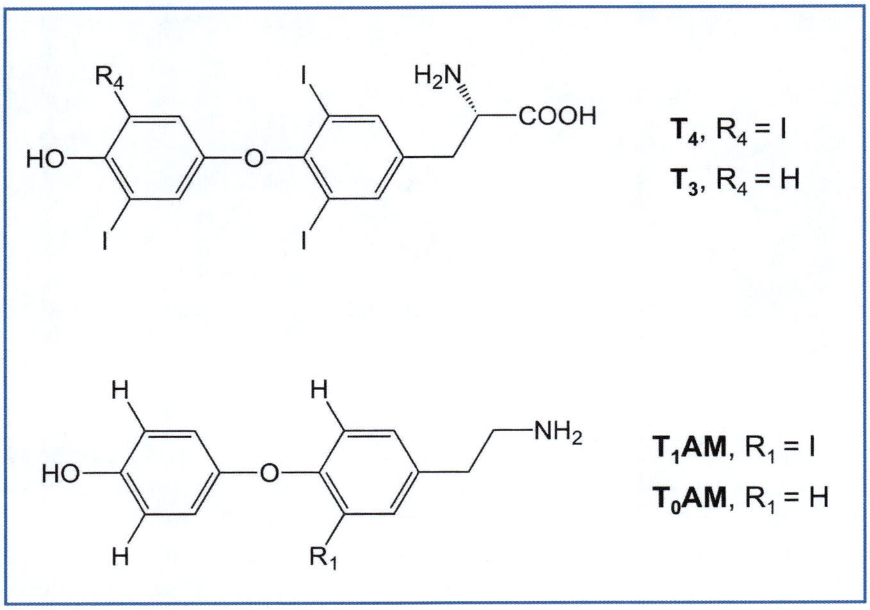

Fig. 6.1 Thyroid hormones and the endogenous derivatives thyronamine (T_0AM) and 3-iodothyronamine (T_1AM)

In the last 5 years it has been observed that some iodothyronamines, endogenous thyroid hormone derivatives, are able to interfere with G-protein-coupled receptors [4]. While it was initially believed that iodothyronamines might to be responsible for the nongenomic effects of thyroid hormone, it was soon recognized that their functional effects often antagonize classical thyroid hormone responses. This discovery has shown that the picture of thyroid hormone signaling is more complex than previously thought, opening a new line of research.

6.2 Chemical Structure and Metabolism

With respect to the structure of T_4, the common characteristic of all iodothyronamines is the absence of the carboxylate group within the β-alanine side chain. In addition, one or more iodine atoms may be substituted by hydrogen atoms (Fig. 6.2). The nomenclature used for iodothyronamines follows the rules applied for thyronines, and the different compounds are usually abbreviated as T_xAM, with "x" indicating the number of iodine atoms per molecule. In the past, several compounds of this class have been synthesized in vitro, and a few studies have evaluated the biological effects of thyronamine (the totally deiodinated molecule, usually indicated as T_0AM), 3,5,3'-triiodothyronamine (T_3AM, also

called "triam"), 3,5-diiodothyronamine (T_2AM) and 3,5,3', 5'-tetraiodothyronamine (T_4AM, also called "thyroxamine") [5–12]. Recently, the discovery of a novel group of mammalian orphan G-protein-coupled receptors [13, 14], now called the trace-amine-associated receptors (TAARs) [15], has renewed the interest in iodothyronamines, and particularly in 3-iodothyronamine (T_1AM), which is a novel compound since it had never been synthesized or evaluated before 2004 [4].

So far, no pathway for de novo iodothyronamine synthesis has been described. However, some well-known enzymes might yield iodothyronamines from thyroid hormone. Aromatic amino acid decarboxylase has been proposed as the candidate enzyme for thyronine decarboxylation, due to its relatively broad substrate specificity, which includes L-3,4-dihydroxyphenylalanine (L-dopa) and 5-hydroxytryptophane [16, 17]. Three deiodinase isozymes (D1, D2, and D3) catalyze the sequential reductive removal of iodide from iodothyronines and various iodothyronine metabolites (Fig. 6.3), thus controlling the bioavailability of thyroid hormone [18]. Deiodinases are a family of homologous selenoproteins, consisting of 250–280 amino acids and containing an essential selenocysteine residue in the active center. D1 has a low affinity for T_3 and T_4 (in the order of 0.1–1 μM) and can remove iodide from both the phenolic (i.e., the outer) and the tyrosyl (i.e., the inner) ring. D2 and D3 have much higher

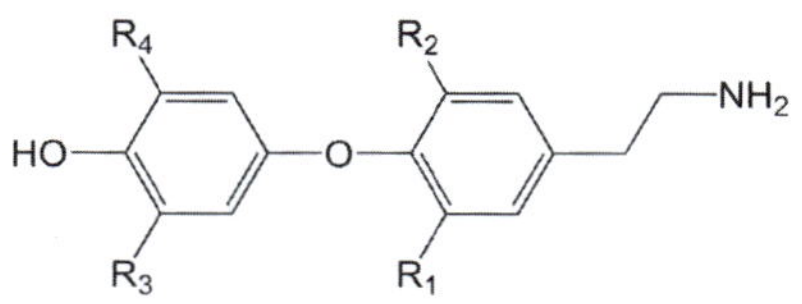

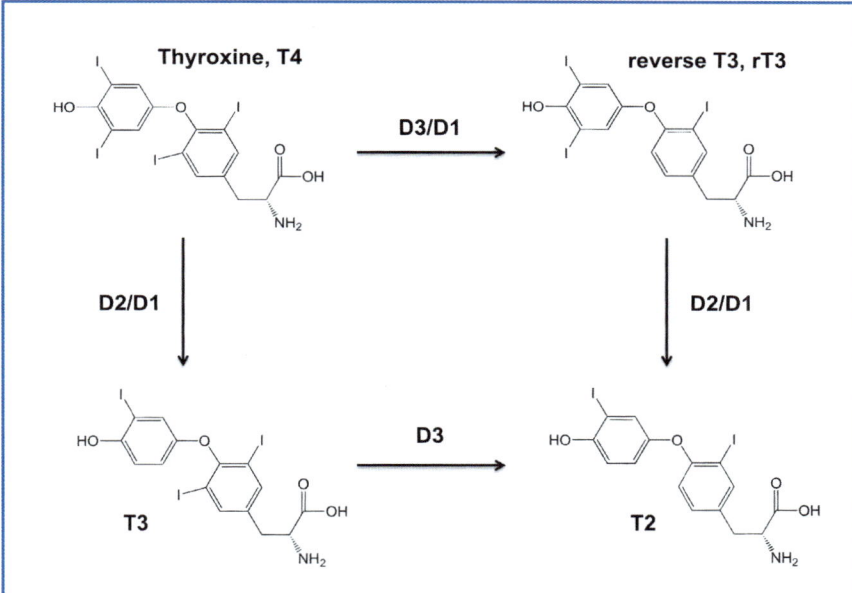

Thyronamine	R_1	R_2	R_3	R_4
T_1AM	I	H	H	H
$3,3'-T_2AM$	I	H	I	H
T_2AM	I	I	H	H
T_3AM	I	I	I	H
T_0AM	H	H	H	H
$3'-T_1AM$	H	H	I	H
$3',5'-T_2AM$	H	H	I	I
rT_3AM	H	I	I	I
T_4AM	I	I	I	I

Fig. 6.2 Natural and synthetic iodothyronamines

Fig. 6.3 Basic deiodinase reactions. The reactions catalyzed by the deiodinases remove iodine moieties from the phenolic (outer) or tyrosyl (inner) rings of the iodothyronines. These pathways can activate T_4 by transforming it into T_3 (via D1 or D2) or prevent it from being activated by converting it to the metabolically inactive form, reverse T_3 (via D1 or D3). T_2 is an inactive product common to both pathways that is rapidly metabolized by further deiodination

affinities (in the order of 1 nM) and are more specific since they act exclusively on the phenolic ring and on the tyrosyl ring, respectively.

Decarboxylation and deiodination are known to play a major role in thyroid hormone catabolism [17], as detailed elsewhere in this volume (Chap. 7). Decarboxylation is usually thought to occur after the amino group has been removed by amino oxidases or amino transferases, yielding thyroacetic or thyropyruvic acid derivatives. However, it cannot be ruled out that decarboxylation precedes deamination, as occurs in the biosynthesis of catecholamines, so that T_4, T_3, or their lower-iodination-state metabolites, are converted to the corresponding iodothyronamines. Notably, both deiodinases and aromatic amino acid decarboxylase are expressed in many tissues.

Iodothyronamines can be further metabolized by

different pathways. First of all, iodothyronamines themselves are deiodinase substrates [19]. D1 and D2 can only deiodinate rT_3AM and 3',5'-diiodothyronamine at their phenolic rings, while they are inactive on the other iodothyronamines. In contrast, D3 can deiodinate all iodothyronamines with iodine atoms in the tyrosyl ring, with an apparent Michaelis constant (K_M) of about 1 μM. So, deiodinases might potentially convert all iodothyronamines to T_0AM.

By analogy to thyroid hormone metabolism, it is assumed that alternative inactivation pathways include amine group oxidation by amine oxidases, glucuronidation, or sulfation. In particular, T_0AM, T_1AM, and T_3AM have been shown to be substrates for human liver sulfotransferases, especially for $SULT_1A3$ [20]. The K_M for T_1AM is about 32 μM, and significant sulfotransferase activity is also present in brain and heart.

6.3 Endogenous Concentration

So far, it has been impossible to assay iodothyronamines by immunological methods or by conventional high-performance liquid chromatography (HPLC) techniques. The only reliable assay is liquid chromatography coupled with tandem mass spectrometry. With this technique, T_0AM and T_1AM were detected in blood and in tissue homogenates, showing that they must be considered as endogenous compounds. Quantitative estimates of T_1AM concentrations using deuterated standards have been reported. In rat brain homogenate, T_1AM was present at subpicomole per gram quantities, corresponding to an average concentration close to 1 nM [4]; in rat heart homogenate T_1AM levels averaged 68 pmol/g, corresponding to a concentration of 70 nM [21]; in Djungarian hamster blood, T_1AM assays yielded 5.9 ± 1.7 nM [22]. However, different procedures have been followed for tissue preparation and extraction in these investigations, and their yield is uncertain. In particular, the extent of T_1AM binding to proteins is unknown, although it is likely to be relevant. Given the structural similarity between T_1AM and biogenic amines, the existence of membrane transporters has been hypothesized, but none of the candidate transporters tested so far appears to transport T_1AM. Thus, the subcellular distribution of T_1AM has not been determined and its concentration in specific compartments might be

significantly different from the average concentration. In spite of these uncertainties, it should be pointed out that T_1AM content appears to be of the same order of magnitude as T_4 content, and definitely higher than T_3 content, at least in brain and heart.

6.4 Receptors for Iodothyronamines: From Adrenergic Receptors to TAARs

Decarboxylated derivatives of thyroid hormone have been classically regarded as inactive metabolites, since they do not bind to the nuclear thyroid hormone receptors. The hypothesis that iodothyronamines may bind to G-protein-coupled receptors was first proposed by Meyer and Hesch [11], who determined the influence of some iodothyronamines on the binding of [^{3}H]-dihydroalprenolol, a specific β_2-adrenergic ligand, in turkey erythrocytes. T_3AM displaced dihydroalprenolol with a K_i in the order of 5 μM, while T_2AM and T_0AM showed lower affinities. However, in HEK293 cells stably expressing either the dopamine D_1 receptor or the β_2-adrenergic receptor, no change in cAMP was produced by T_0AM or T_1AM at concentrations as high as 10 μM [4]. More recently, it has been reported that T_1AM displaced [^{3}H]-RX821002, an α_{2A}-adrenergic ligand, in Cos7 cells transiently transfected with the human or mouse α_{2A}-adrenergic receptor gene [23]. The K_i was again in the micromolar range.

While these results suggest that some iodothyronamines interact with some adrenergic receptors, a crucial discovery was the observation that T_1AM can interact with a novel G-protein-coupled receptor, known as trace-amine-associated receptor 1 (TAAR1) and that biochemical effects are produced at nanomolar concentrations.

As reviewed by Grandy [24], the discovery of TAAR1 was based on a degenerate polymerase chain reaction (PCR) approach, using complex mixtures of oligonucleotides whose sequences were chosen based on the G-protein-coupled receptors for serotonin [13] or dopamine [14]. Several novel sequences were identified; these predicted a 332-amino-acid protein that showed the biochemical features of an aminergic G-protein-coupled receptor. After expression of the novel receptor in heterologous cell models, cAMP production was observed upon exposure to *p*-tyramine or β-phenylethylamine, but not to the classical biogenic amines, i.e., dopamine, norepinephrine, epinephrine, serotonin, and histamine. The new receptor was therefore called trace-amine receptor (the term "trace amines" applies to *p*-tyramine, β-phenylethylamine, octopamine, and tryptamine). Additional degenerate PCR experiments and extensive genomic analysis allowed the identification of several putative trace-amine receptors [15, 25]. They all share a polypeptide sequence that is 100% specific when used to query all current Swiss-Prot entries. This sequence, defined as NSXXNPXX[YH]XXX[YF]XWF, is therefore considered as a hallmark of the new receptor family. It has been very difficult to express these genes in heterologous models to identify their properties. However, a clear response to trace amines has been reported only for TAAR1 and possibly for a few other members of the family (e.g., TAAR4), whose name has therefore been modified to trace-amine-associated receptors, or TAARs.

The human and chimpanzee genomes contain nine TAAR genes, TAAR1–TAAR9. The rat and mouse genomes contain additional genes, which are called paralogue genes since on the basis of sequence homologies they appear to have been generated by duplication events within the lineage of each species. Together, 19 TAARs have been identified in rat and 16 in mouse. Paralogue genes are designated by a letter suffix (e.g., TAAR7a, TAAR7b). Some TAARs do not contain an open reading frame and are therefore classified as pseudogenes. In particular, there are three pseudogenes in human, six in chimpanzee, two in rat, and one in mouse [15, 26]. A summary of TAAR classification is given in Table 6.1. In invertebrate species, genomic analysis did not reveal any TAAR sequence. Instead, the effects of trace amines appear to be mediated by a different class of receptors, more similar to serotonin receptors [25].

Table 6.1 TAAR classification and nomenclature: TAAR genes in human, chimpanzee, rat, and mouse[a]

Human	Chimpanzee	Rat	Mouse
TAAR1	TAAR1	TAAR1	TAAR1
TAAR2	(TAAR2)	TAAR2	TAAR2
(TAAR3)	(TAAR3)	TAAR3	TAAR3
(TAAR4)	(TAAR4)	TAAR4	TAAR4
TAAR 5	TAAR5	TAAR5	TAAR5
TAAR6	TAAR6	TAAR6	TAAR6
(TAAR7)	(TAAR7)	TAAR7a	TAAR7a
		TAAR7b	(TAAR7b)
		TAAR7c	TAAR7c
		TAAR7d	TAAR7d
		TAAR7e	TAAR7e
		(TAAR7f)	TAAR7f
		TAAR7g	
		TAAR7h	
		(TAAR7i)	
TAAR8	(TAAR8)	TAAR8a	TAAR8a
		TAAR8b	TAAR8b
		TAAR8c	TAAR8c
TAAR9	(TAAR9)	TAAR9	TAAR9

[a] The rat and mouse genomes contain several genes that on the basis of sequence homologies appear to have been generated by duplication events within the lineage of each species. Such genes are called paralogue genes and are identified by a letter suffix, while genes with the same number, which were likely generated by speciation events, are called orthologous genes. Pseudogenes are shown in parentheses

Quantitative reverse-transcription (RT-)PCR has allowed the identification of TAAR transcripts in many tissues, including brain, stomach, amygdala, kidney, lung, small intestine, heart, liver, pancreas, prostate, skeletal muscle, spleen, pituitary, and leukocytes (reviewed in [26]). Expression levels were usually low and reliable antibodies for Western blot experiments are not available, so the actual receptor concentration is unknown.

Since it is likely that several, and possibly most, TAARs do not respond to trace amines, it was hypothesized that different physiological ligands should exist. Liberles and Buck [27] reported that all TAAR subtypes except for TAAR1 are expressed at very high levels in the mouse olfactory epithelium. They also provided evidence that specific TAARs when expressed in heterologous cell models, could be activated by volatile amines, suggesting a role for TAARs in olfaction.

Another potential class of endogenous ligands is represented by iodothyronamines. The structural similarity between iodothyronamines and trace amines prompted testing of their effects on TAAR1 [4]. In HEK293 cells expressing the rat TAAR1, several different iodothyronamines induced a concentration-dependent increase in cAMP concentration. T_1AM was the most effective compound, with EC_{50} = 14 nM, followed by T_2AM, T_3AM, and T_0AM (EC_{50} = 41, 56, 87, and 131 nM, respectively). Similar results were obtained with cells expressing the mouse TAAR1, although in this case only T_1AM and T_2AM were effective at submicromolar concentrations (EC_{50} = 112 and 371 nM, respectively). In this model some synthetic thyronamine derivatives turned out to be more active than T_1AM. They included 3-methyl-thyronamine, N-methyl-O-(p-trifluoromethyl)benzyl-tyramine, O-phenyl-3-iodotyramine, and O-(p-fluoro)phenyl-3-iodotyramine [28]. With regard to the structure–activity relationship, these studies suggested that a basic amino group at $C\alpha$ is required for activity and that an iodide or methyl substituent at the 3-position of the thyronamine scaffold is optimal for activity, while modifying the outer ring of the phenoxyphenylamine core can improve potency. It has also been observed that incorporating unsaturated hydrocarbon substituents and hydrogen-bond-accepting groups in the ethylamine portion increases activity of rat and mouse TAAR1, respectively [29]. These results have been used to develop theoretical models of receptor–agonist interaction, based on the so-called rotamer toggle switch model [30].

While extensive data have been reported with TAAR1, there is still no direct evidence about the interaction of T_1AM or other iodothyronamines with different TAAR subtypes, as a consequence of the difficulty in obtaining their stable expression in heterologous cell models.

6.5 Effects on Body Temperature

The observation that T_1AM is an endogenous compound able to interact with a specific receptor prompted an investigation of its functional effects. The first interesting finding was the observation that intraperitoneal injection of T_1AM in mouse (20–50 mg/kg) induced within 30 min profound hypothermia which lasted for 6–10 h and was not associated with any compensatory homeostatic response such as shivering or piloerection [4]. T_0AM produced similar effects, although it had about one-tenth of the potency of T_1AM. The doses of T_1AM and T_0AM required for half maximal stimulation were 59 and 178 µmol/kg, respectively. So their relative potency was similar to the potency shown in TAAR1 activation.

6.6 Metabolic and Endocrine Effects

In some small mammals, hypothermia may be associated with depressed metabolism, producing a state known as torpor. It therefore seemed interesting to investigate the metabolic effects of T_1AM [22]. Both in mouse and in Djungarian hamster, T_1AM (50 mg/kg) produced within minutes a substantial drop in body temperature, which lasted for 6–12 h. This was associated with decreased oxygen consumption and a decreased respiratory quotient. The latter represents the ratio between CO_2 produced and O_2 consumed and reflects the balance between glucose utilization and lipid utilization, since the respiratory quotient is close to 0.9 for glucose oxidation, and to 0.7 for fatty acid oxidation. Therefore T_1AM apparently produced a shift from carbohydrate to fatty acids as the preferred metabolic fuel. Consistent with this conclusion, treatment with T_1AM also caused ketonuria and a significant loss of body fat. The metabolic effects were more prolonged than the hypothermic effect since the respiratory quotient was still depressed after 24 h.

T_1AM has recently been reported to modulate insulin secretion [23]. In mice, intraperitoneal injection of 50 mg T_1AM/kg increased the blood glucose level and decreased insulin levels. This action was attributed to the stimulation of G_i-protein-coupled α_{2A}-adrenergic receptors since it was inhibited by the α_{2A} antagonist yohimbine, and it was absent in transgenic mice with either α_{2A} receptor knockout or selective β-cell expression of the catalytic subunit of pertussis toxin, a known inhibitor of $G_{i/o}$ signaling. By contrast, in an insulinoma cell line with 200-fold overexpression of the TAAR1 gene, exposure to T_1AM increased rather than decreased insulin secretion. It was concluded that T_1AM stimulates insulin secretion via TAAR1 and inhibits insulin secretion via the α_{2A} receptor. EC_{50}s for these two processes were not provided, and it is uncertain how these effects relate to the shift in fuel metabolism described above.

Another endocrine effect exerted by iodothyronamines was observed as early as 1984, when T_3AM was reported to inhibit prolactin secretion in cultured pituitary cells [12]. At that time the effect was attributed to interference with the adrenergic system, but other iodothyronamines were not tested and the involvement of TAARs, which are now known to be expressed in pituitary, cannot be excluded.

6.7 Neurological Effects

In a mouse model of stroke induced by middle cerebral artery occlusion, intraperitoneal injection of either T_1AM or T_0AM (50 mg/kg) 1 h after the occlusion produced a significant decrease in infarct size [31]. With T_1AM, but not with T_0AM, protection could also be induced by preconditioning, i.e., by administration 2 days before occlusion. In all cases, protection required hypothermia to develop, since it was abolished if body temperature was kept constant by a thermostat-controlled heating pad. The neuroprotective effect of mild hypothermia is well known, although its mechanisms are poorly understood and probably involve both reduced metabolic demand and changes in gene expression. Notably, no protection was achieved in neuronal cultures subjected to simulated normothermic ischemia in vitro, even using very high concentrations (up to 500 μM) of either

T_1AM or T_0AM. Both compounds were actually cytotoxic at concentrations in excess of 50 μM.

Besides their neuroprotective action, a nontranscriptional role as neuromodulators has been proposed for iodothyronamines. A neuromodulator is not a neurotransmitter, but it can modify the response to established neurotransmitters. In synaptosomal preparations T_1AM inhibited dopamine and norepinephrine transporters, thus preventing neuronal reuptake of these neurotransmitters. T_1AM also inhibited the action of vesicular monoamine transporter 2 ($VMAT_2$), the intracellular transporter responsible for loading secretory vesicles with intracellular monoamines for exocytotic release [32]. A neuromodulatory role has also been proposed for trace amines [33] and for thyroid hormone [34, 35], but it is unknown whether these different substances share a common mechanism of action.

6.8 Cardiac Effects

T_1AM shows significant cardiac effects [4, 21]. In the isolated working rat heart model, the addition of T_1AM or T_0AM to the perfusion buffer produced within 30 s a dose-dependent decrease in aortic flow, cardiac output, developed pressure, and heart rate, while coronary flow was unchanged. The effect was persistent for at least 50 min, and it was reversible upon a switch to control perfusion buffer. It was concluded that T_1AM and T_0AM produce both a negative inotropic and a negative chronotropic action. The former is independent of the latter, since it was also observed in paced hearts and in isolated cardiomyocytes. IC_{50} values lay in the microsomal range: with regard to the effect on cardiac output they averaged 27 μM and 94 μM with T_1AM and T_0AM, respectively [21]. Negative inotropic and chronotropic responses can also be elicited in vivo. In mice surgically implanted with radiotelemetric devices, administration of T_1AM (50 mg/kg) produced an immediate bradycardia which persisted for 6–8 h [4]. In the anesthetized rat, intravenous injection of T_1AM (0.5 mg/kg) caused within 1 min a transient decrease in heart rate and aortic pressure (present authors' unpublished observations).

The involvement of TAARs in these cardiac effects was suggested by the observation that similar actions were produced by some trace amines, with the following potency ranking: T_1AM > T_0AM = octopamine = β-phenylethy-lamine > tryptamine, while *p*-tyramine was virtually inactive [36]. This is not the same potency ranking as observed in heterologous cells expressing TAAR1, in which *p*-tyramine and β-phenylethylamine were much more effective than other trace amines [13, 14]. In addition, radioligand binding experiments showed specific and saturable binding sites for [^{3}H]-*p*-tyramine and [^{125}I]-T_1AM, but [^{125}I]-T_1AM was not displaced by *p*-tyramine, while [^{3}H]-*p*-tyramine was displaced by T_1AM [36]. Since at least five TAAR subtypes are expressed in rat heart [21], it seems likely that the cardiac effects are not mediated by TAAR1, but rather by a different subtype. TAAR8a shows the highest expression levels, i.e., about 100-fold higher than TAAR1, and is the most likely candidate.

In the presence of T_1AM, cardiac cAMP levels were unchanged and the functional response to T_1AM was not affected by pertussis toxin, ruling out the involvement of G_s or G_i proteins. Inhibitors of protein kinase C, calcium-calmodulin-dependent protein kinase II, MAP kinases, and phosphatidylinositol-3-phosphate kinase were also ineffective, while the hemodynamic changes were dramatically potentiated by genistein, a tyrosine kinase inhibitor, and blunted by vanadate, a protein phosphatase inhibitor. It was therefore hypothesized that T_1AM modulates the phosphorylation state of critical tyrosine residues (Fig. 6.4), and Western blot experiments with anti-phosphotyrosine antibodies confirmed dephosphorylation of several proteins in the microsomal and cytosolic fractions [21]. The identity of these proteins is still unknown.

While T_1AM has been discovered only recently, T_0AM has been known for a long time and a few reports about its cardiovascular effects have appeared in the literature [6–9]. In the anesthetized dog, T_0AM administration (8–16 mg/kg) produced an increase in heart rate and cardiac inotropic state. The response was remarkably reduced or abolished by adrenergic blockade, and it was suggested that T_0AM induced catecholamine release. Interestingly, after catecholamine depletion and/or adrenergic blockade, T_0AM infusion produced an immediate negative inotropic effect [9], which is consistent with the results obtained in the isolated heart.

Preliminary experiments recently investigated the influence of T_1AM on cardiac ischemic injury. In isolated rat hearts subjected to 30 min of global normothermic ischemia followed by 120 min of reperfusion, pretreatment with T_1AM produced a

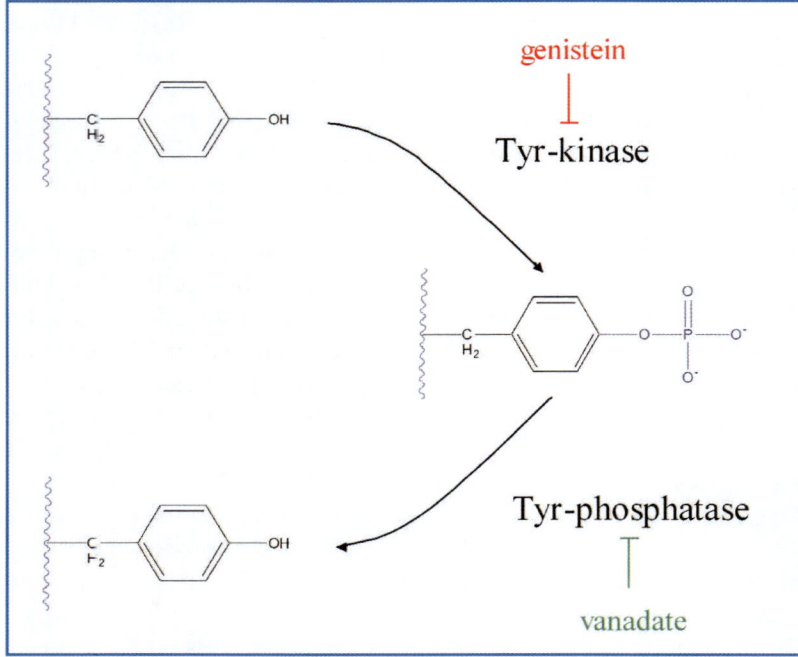

Fig. 6.4 Effects of genistein and vanadate on tyrosine phosphorylation. Since the effect of T_1AM was potentiated by genistein and inhibited by vanadate, the most straightforward hypothesis is that T_1AM promotes the dephosphorylation of tyrosine residues

significant reduction in infarct size [37]. Interestingly, cardioprotection was observed even at submicromolar doses, which did not produce any negative inotropic effect. Therefore, contrary to the neuroprotective action, cardioprotection is independent of hypothermia and can be elicited in the absence of changes in overall cardiac performance. There is also preliminary evidence that in cardiac cells T_1AM can modulate sarcoplasmic reticulum calcium handling [38]. Since calcium is the physiological trigger of muscle contraction and cytosolic calcium overload is a major determinant of ischemic injury, it is possible that calcium homeostasis is the general target of T_1AM, at least in this tissue.

6.9 Open Questions

Taken together, the investigations reviewed above suggest that T_1AM should be regarded as a novel chemical messenger, since it is an endogenous compound, interacts with specific receptors, and produces functional effects. Notably, the effects of T_1AM on cardiac function and body temperature are the opposite of those produced on a longer time scale by thyroid hormone, suggesting that T_3 and its iodothyronamine metabolites act to maintain a balance in homeostasis, with T_1AM and possibly other iodothyronamines acting as a quick brake to the more prolonged effects of T_3. In this view, thyroid hormone signaling may be hypothesized to include three different components:
1. Classical genomic effects, which are mediated by nuclear receptors.
2. Nongenomic effects, which generally have the same functional consequences as the genomic effects and whose underlying transduction pathways remain obscure.
3. Iodothyronamine effects, which are mediated by G-protein-coupled receptors (mostly by TAARs) and generally have opposite functional consequences.

While this picture is attractive, there are still many questions that need to be answered before the hormonal role of T_1AM can be definitely established. The most critical of these relate to T_1AM metabolism, the signaling pathway(s) triggered by T_1AM, and the functional relevance of endogenous T_1AM levels.

As detailed above, it is generally assumed that T_1AM is produced from thyroid hormone by the sequential action of aromatic amino acid decarboxylase and D1 or D2 deiodinases. However, this conclusion has not been directly established, nor is it known to what extent T_1AM is produced in the thyroid or in peripheral organs. Experiments with isolated organs or radiolabeled T_1AM would be necessary to answer these questions.

While it is quite clear that T_1AM can activate TAAR1 in heterologous cells transfected with the TAAR1 gene, there is no definite evidence that any of the functional effects produced by T_1AM is mediated by TAAR1, or by other TAAR subtypes. This will require significant technical advances, particularly the development of specific receptor antagonists or knockout models for specific TAAR subtypes. At present, even specific antibodies for each TAAR subtype are not available; thus, it is virtually impossible to provide conclusive evidence that TAAR proteins are involved in any of the observed biological actions. At this stage, a conservative conclusion is that some effects of T_1AM (particularly, inhibition of insulin secretion) may be attributed to low-affinity interaction with adrenergic receptors, while in other cases (i.e., the hypothermic effect and the cardiac effects) it is hard to envisage a role for adrenergic signaling, and TAAR stimulation appears as the most logical alternative.

In addition, functional effects usually required micromolar concentrations of T_1AM, while the EC_{50} for TAAR1 activation was about 100-fold lower. Differences of one or two orders of magnitude are not uncommonly observed in comparisons of molecular and functional studies, or in vitro and in vivo models, but the reason for this discrepancy should be addressed by further investigations.

It is also unknown what transduction pathways may be coupled to the putative TAAR(s) activated by T_1AM. In heterologous cells expressing TAAR1, T_1AM induced cAMP production. However, most of the observed functional effects of T_1AM are not consistent with cAMP-mediated effects, the possible exception being the stimulation of insulin secretion in pancreatic β cells. Therefore, either TAAR1 is not coupled to G_s proteins, or other TAARs are involved. So far, an attempt to characterize the transduction pathway has been made only in cardiac tissue, where G_s or pertussis-toxin-sensitive $G_{i/o}$ proteins do not play a significant role, while tyrosine dephosphorylation appears to be a critical step.

Finally, there is still no evidence that endogenous T_1AM produces functional effects at physiological concentrations. The average tissue or plasma concentration of T_1AM, as reported in the few available studies published so far, lies in the nanomolar range, while functional effects have been reported at micromolar concentrations. However, the extent of T_1AM binding to proteins, the existence of active transport mechanisms, and the location of enzymes able to produce or catabolize T_1AM are largely unknown. Therefore, the concentration at the receptor level might be substantially different from the average tissue concentration. Here again, a substantial technical advance is needed, namely, the development of a quantitative assay for total and free T_1AM.

6.10 Conclusions

T_1AM is an endogenous derivative of thyroid hormone. There is consistent, although not conclusive, evidence that it is a chemical messenger on its own, producing functional effects through G-protein-coupled receptors, such as the novel receptor class known as TAARs. The heart is a target of T_1AM: micromolar doses of exogenous T_1AM have a negative inotropic and chronotropic action, and there is preliminary evidence of a cardioprotective effect. While the physiological or pathophysiological role of endogenous T_1AM remains to be ascertained, this novel signaling pathway might be an important target for pharmaceutical exploitation.

Key Points

- 3-Iodothyronamine (T_1AM) is an endogenous compound derived from thyroid hormone through decarboxylation and deiodination. It can interact with a novel G-protein-coupled receptor, known as trace-amine-associated receptor 1 (TAAR1).

- TAAR1 and other receptors of this family are expressed in several tissues, including the heart.

- In the heart, exogenous T_1AM produces a negative inotropic and chronotropic action. A cardioprotective effect has been described as well.

- Modulation of calcium homeostasis might be the mechanism underlying the cardiac effects of T_1AM.

- The extracardiac effects of T_1AM described so far include reduction of body temperature, increased lipid versus carbohydrate metabolism, and modulation of insulin secretion.

- While the physiological and pathophysiological role of T_1AM must still be ascertained, this signaling system might allow the development of new therapeutic agents.

References

1. Yen PM (2001) Physiological and molecular basis of thyroid hormone action. Physiol Rev 81:1097–1142
2. Mortoglou A, Candiloros H (2004) The serum triiodothyronamine to thyroxine (T3/T4) ratio in various thyroid disorders and after levothyroxine replacement therapy. Hormones 3:120–126
3. Davis PJ, Leonard JL, Davis FB (2008) Mechanisms of nongenomic actions of thyroid hormone. Front Neuroendocrinol 29:211–218
4. Scanlan TS, Suchland KL, Hart ME et al (2004) 3-Iodothyronamine is an endogenous and rapid-acting derivative of thyroid hormone. Nat Med 10:638–642
5. Tomita K, Lardy HA (1956) Synthesis and biological activity of some triiodinated analogues of thyroxine. J Biol Chem 219:595–604
6. Buu-Hoi NP, Pham-Huu-Chanh, Petit L (1966) Some biological effects of thyronamine. Med Pharmacol Exp 15:17–23
7. Buu-Hoi NP, Pham-Huu-Chanh, Petit L (1969) Thyronamine, a new substance with long-acting positive inotropic effect. Pharmacology 2:281–287
8. Boissier JR, Giudicelli JF, Larno S, Advenier C (1973) Differential inotropic-chronotropic action of thyronamine. Eur J Pharmacol 22:141–149

9. Cotè P, Polumbo RA, Harrison DC (1974) Thyronamine, a new inotropic agent: its cardiovascular effects and mechanism of action. Cardiovasc Res 8:721–730

10. Felt V, Ploc I (1982) Effect of theophylline on binding of triiodothyronine, thyroxine, thyroxamine, tetraiodothyroacetic acid and cortisol in the cytosol of human leukocytes. Endokrinologie 79:315–317

11. Meyer T, Hesch R-D (1983) Triiodothyronamine: a b-adrenergic metabolite of triiodothyronine? Horm Metab Res 15:602–606

12. Cody V, Meyer T, Dohler KD et al (1984) Molecular structure and biochemical activity of 3,5,3'-triiodothyronamine. Endocrine Res 10:91–99

13. Borowsky B, Adham N, Jones KA et al (2001) Trace amines: identification of a family of mammalian G protein-coupled receptors. Proc Natl Acad Sci USA 98:8966–8971

14. Bunzow JR, Sonders MS, Arttamangkul S et al (2001) Amphetamine, 3,4-methylenedioxymethamphetamine, lysergic acid diethylamide, and metabolites of the catecholamine neurotransmitters are agonists of a rat trace amine receptor. Mol Pharmacol 60:1181–1188

15. Lindemann L, Ebeling M, Kratochwil NA et al (2005) Trace amine-associated receptors form structurally and functionally distinct subfamilies of novel G protein-coupled receptors. Genomics 85:372–385

16. Zhu MY, Jurio AV (1995) Aromatic L-amino acid decarboxylase: biological characterization and functional role. Gen Pharmacol 26:681–696

17. Wu SY, Green WL, Huang WS et al (2005) Alternate pathways of thyroid hormone metabolism. Thyroid 15:943–958

18. Bianco AC, Kim BW (2006) Deiodinases: implications of the local control of thyroid hormone action. J Clin Invest 116:2571–2579

19. Piehl S, Heberer T, Balizs G et al (2008) Thyronamines are isozyme-specific substrates of deiodinases. Endocrinology 149:3037–3045

20. Pietsch, CA, Scanlan, TS, Anderson RJ (2007) Thyronamines are substrates for human liver sulfotransferases. Endocrinology 148:1921–1927

21. Chiellini G, Frascarelli S, Ghelardoni S et al (2007) Cardiac effects of 3-iodothyronamine: a new aminergic system modulating cardiac function. FASEB J 21:1597–1608

22. Braulke LJ, Klingenspor M, DeBarber A et al (2008) 3-Iodothyronamine: a novel hormone controlling the balance between glucose and lipid utilisation. J Comp Physiol 178:167–177

23. Regard JB, Kataoka H, Cano DA et al (2007) Probing cell type-specific functions of Gi in vivo identifies GPCR regulators of insulin secretion. J Clin Invest 117:4034–4043

24. Grandy DK (2007) Trace amine-associated receptor 1 – family archetype or iconoclast? Pharmacol Ther 116:355–390

25. Gloriam DEI, Bjarnadóttir TK, Schiöth HB, Fredriksson R (2005) High species variation within the repertoire of trace amine receptors. Ann N Y Acad Sci 1040:323–327

26. Zucchi R, Chiellini G, Scanlan TS, Grandy DK (2006) Trace amine-associated receptors and their ligands. Br J Pharmacol 149:967–978

27. Liberles SD, Buck LB (2006) A second class of chemosensory receptors in the olfactory epithelium. Nature 442:645–650

28. Hart ME, Suchland KL, Miyakawa M et al (2006) Trace amine-associated receptor agonists: synthesis and evaluation of thyronamines and related analogues. J Med Chem 49:1101–1112

29. Tan ES, Miyakawa M, Bunzow JR et al (2007) Exploring the structure–activity relationship of the ethylamine portion of 3-iodothyronamine for rat and mouse trace amine-associated receptor 1. J Med Chem 50:2787–2798

30. Tan ES, Groban ES, Jacobson MP, Scanlan TS (2008) Toward deciphering the code to aminergic G protein-coupled receptor drug design. Chem Biol 15:343–353

31. Doyle KP, Suchland KL, Ciesielski TM et al (2007) Novel thyroxine derivatives, thyronamine and 3-iodothyronamine, induce transient hypothermia and marked neuroprotection against stroke injury. Stroke 38:2569–2576

32. Snead AN, Santos MS, Seal RP et al (2007) Thyronamines inhibit plasma membrane and vesicular monoamine transport. ACS Chem Biol 2:390–398

33. Berry MD (2004) Mammalian central nervous system trace amines. Pharmacologic amphetamines, physiologic neuromodulators. J Neurochem 90:257–271

34. Dratman MB, Gordon JT (1996) Thyroid hormones as neurotransmitters. Thyroid 6:639–647

35. Mason GA, Walker CH, Prange AJ (1993) L-Triiodothyronine: is this peripheral hormone a central neurotransmitter? Neuropsychopharmacology 8:253–258

36. Frascarelli S, Ghelardoni S, Chiellini G et al (2008) Cardiac effects of trace amines: pharmacological characterization of trace amine-associated receptors. Eur J Pharmacol 587:231–236

37. Frascarelli S, Chiellini S, Ghelardoni S et al (2008) Cardioprotection by 3-iodothyronamine, a new endogenous chemical messenger [abstract]. J Mol Cell Cardiol 44:773

38. Borgioni S, Chiellini G, Suffredini S et al (2007) 3-Iodothyronamine affects calcium handling in isolated rat cardiomyocytes [abstract]. J Mol Cell Cardiol 42:S21

Cardiac Thyroid-Hormone Deiodinative Pathways in Ventricular Hypertrophy and Heart Failure

7

Warner S. Simonides

Abstract Many of the cardiac genes that are involved in contractile dysfunction following pathological ventricular remodeling are transcriptionally regulated by thyroid hormone (TH). The phenotype of the pathologically hypertrophied cardiomyocyte suggests that reduced TH signaling contributes to its development. Increased expression of the TH-degrading enzyme deiodinase type 3 (D3) in cardiomyocytes of hypertrophic left or right ventricles has recently been described for different rodent models of heart failure. At least in right ventricular failure, this was associated with a severe, cardiomyocyte-specific hypothyroid condition. D3 expression is transcriptionally stimulated by factors that are implicated in cardiomyocyte hypertrophy, e.g., mitogen-activated protein kinases (MAPK) ERK, and p38 and Smad proteins activated by transforming growth factor-β (TGFβ). Hypoxia-inducible factor 1 (HIF-1) also stimulates D3 transcription. Reduced oxygen tension and subsequent HIF-1 signaling may occur in the hypertrophic cardiomyocyte, and this appears to account for the increased D3 expression in the model of right ventricular failure. It remains to be established whether stimulation of D3 activity and the ensuing local hypothyroid condition with reduction of energy turnover are an adaptive response or contribute to the further deterioration of contractile function and heart failure.

Keywords Thyroid hormone • Triiodothyronine (T$_3$) • Heart failure • Ventricular hypertrophy • Hypothyroid • Deiodinase type 1 (D1) • Deiodinase type 2 (D2) • Deiodinase type 3 (D3) • Pulmonary arterial hypertension • Transforming growth factor-β (TGFβ) • Hypoxia • Hypoxia-inducible factor 1 α subunit (HIF-1α)

7.1 Introduction

The marked differences in cardiac contractility, electrophysiology, and energy metabolism between hypothyroidism and hyperthyroidism illustrate the particular responsiveness of the heart to thyroid hormone (TH) and the wide range of cellular processes affected by it [1]. This is also evident in the perinatal transition from the fetal to the adult cardiac phenotype, which in large part is dependent on the rise of plasma TH levels. Recapitulation of many aspects of the fetal phenotype is a hallmark of pathological remodeling of the heart and is considered to contribute to the contractile dysfunction seen in heart failure [2]. Persistent hemodynamic overload of the heart is the principal cause of chronic heart failure, and the underlying problems include hypertension, aortic stenosis, valvular dysfunction, and loss of ventricular tissue due to myocardial infarction. Left ventricular (LV) failure

W.S. Simonides (✉)
VU University Medical Center Amsterdam,
Institute for Cardiovascular Research Department of Physiology,
Amsterdam, The Netherlands

G. Iervasi, A. Pingitore (eds.), *Thyroid and Heart Failure.*
© Springer-Verlag Italia 2009

is most prevalent, but right ventricular (RV) failure accounts for a considerable percentage of cases of heart failure. RV failure independent of left heart disease is principally caused by pulmonary arterial hypertension, which may result from various conditions. For both ventricles, the increase in ventricular wall stress and accompanying rise in energy turnover trigger a hypertrophic response that is aimed at normalizing wall stress. Hypertrophy may be successfully compensatory, but sustained overload often leads to compromised Ca^{2+} homeostasis, mitochondrial dysfunction, myocyte apoptosis, and interstitial fibrosis, which results in progressive contractile dysfunction and heart failure. The regulation of ventricular remodeling has proved to be exceedingly complex, and numerous interacting signal-transduction pathways have been identified that may drive the characteristic changes in gene expression [3–5]. TH signaling is of interest because of the number of key genes that are regulated by TH and the interaction of nuclear TH receptors (TRs) with trans-acting factors of several signaling cascades that are implicated in ventricular hypertrophy [6]. The similar pattern of cardiac gene expression seen in hypothyroidism and in heart failure suggests that TH signaling is impaired in the failing heart. Possible causes include changes in expression of TRs or their co-factors and the reduction of plasma TH levels. The latter is seen in heart failure, as in other types of severe illness. These issues are discussed elsewhere in this volume; here, the focus is on recent data from rodent models of heart failure showing changes in cardiac TH metabolism that appear to strip the chronically overloaded heart of TH, creating a local hypothyroid condition.

7.2 Thyroid-Hormone Deiodination: Activation and Inactivation

The term "thyroid hormone" is used to refer to both of the iodinated thyronines secreted by the thyroid, 3,5,3',5'-tetraiodothyronine (T_4, or thyroxine) and 3,5,3'-triiodothyronine (T_3). T_4 is the principal secreted product of the thyroid, but it is regarded as a prohormone because of its low biological activity compared to that of T_3, which is the high-affinity ligand of the TRs. Removal of one iodine from an outer-ring position of T_4 to generate T_3 is primarily catalyzed by deiodinase type 2 (D2). Figure 7.1 depicts the principal deiodinative pathways that activate and inactivate TH. The deiodinases form a family of enzymes characterized by the presence of a selenocysteine in the active center of the protein (reviewed in [7]). D2 is present in a number of tissues, including brown adipose tissue (BAT), brain, and pituitary, where it is involved in active regulation of intracellular T_3 levels. The best-studied example of this is the strong induction of D2 in BAT during cold exposure, resulting in a local increase in T_3 that enables the thermogenic response of this tissue. Significant D2 expression is also present in human heart and skeletal muscle, and D2 is considered to be the main source of extrathyroidal T_3 [8]. Deiodinase type 1 (D1) is also capable of outer-ring deiodination, but its affinity for T_4 is three orders of magnitude lower than that of D2. It is primarily expressed in liver and kidney, and although of significance in rodents, the role of D1 in T_3 production in humans is minor under normal circumstances. However, transcription of the DIO1 gene is stimulated by T_3, and in hyperthyroid patients D1 activi-

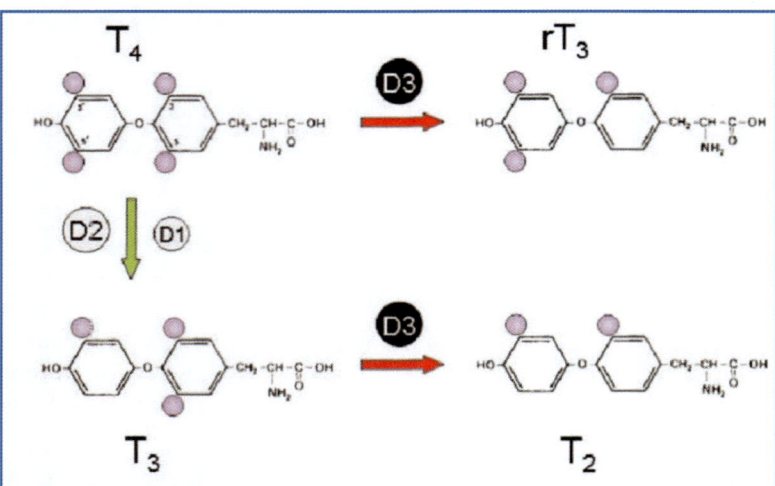

Fig. 7.1 Structure of T_4 (3,5,3', 5'-tetraiodothyronine) and T_3 (3,5,3'-triiodothyronine) and the action of deiodinases type 1, 2, and 3. Removal of iodine (purple spheres) from the outer ring of T_4 by D1 and D2 converts T_4 to the active hormone T_3. Inner-ring deiodination of T_4 and T_3 by D3 generates the biologically inactive metabolites reverse T_3 and T_2, respectively

ty contributes significantly to T_3 production. The physiological role of D1 is mainly in deiodination and subsequent clearance of sulfated T_3 and in deiodination of reverse T_3 (3,3',5'-triiodothyronine, rT_3). Reverse T_3 is the product of removal of the first iodine from the inner ring of T_4, which is also catalyzed by D1, albeit with low efficiency.

The third type of deiodinase (D3) has high affinity for both T_4 and T_3 but is only capable of inner-ring deiodination, generating rT_3 and 3,3'-T_2, respectively. In contrast to D2, the D3 protein is primarily located in the plasma membrane. Extracellular catalytic activity of D3 has been proposed [9], but more recent data show that intracellular T_4 and T_3 are the principal substrate for D3, in line with the reducing environment required for activity [10]. The TH-inactivating activity of D3 is high in placenta and in several embryonic tissues including the heart, but virtually absent in adult tissues, with the exception of various areas and cell types in the brain. The expression of D3 in fetal tissues is thought to be related to the differentiation potential of T_3. Periods of cell proliferation during fetal development require low cellular T_3 levels to prevent differentiation, and tight regulation of tissue T_3 levels appears to be critical for normal early development [11]. Tissue-specific reduction of T_3 is accomplished by induction of D3 or, as has been shown for bone development, by repression of D2 activity [12]. The proliferation-promoting morphogen sonic hedgehog (Shh) is one of the factors that drives the induction of D3 as well as the inactivation of D2 [12, 13]. Shh is a secreted signaling protein that acts through the Gli family of transcription factors, with numerous effects in vertebrate development, including development of the heart [14], and in the adult (patho)physiology. Cell culture studies have shown that several growth factors, serum, and phorbol esters are also potent stimulators of D3 expression [15, 16]. D3 may be reinduced in adult tissues under certain conditions, and, perhaps not surprisingly in the context of cell proliferation, several types of human tumors have been found to express D3. In vascular tumors in infants and adults, as well as in a case of a solitary fibrous tumor, D3 activity reached levels that even resulted in a systemic hypothyroid condition [17–19]. D3 activity was also found to be increased in skeletal muscle and liver of critically ill patients analyzed shortly after death [20]. Combined with reduced muscle D2 activity, this may provide a mechanism for the reduction of plasma T_3 levels that is typically seen in critical illness, i.e., the low-T_3 or nonthyroidal illness syndrome.

7.3 Cardiac Thyroid-Hormone Metabolism

Animal studies have shown that deiodination of T_4 accounts for no more than 7% of cardiac T_3 [21]. In line with this, the activity levels of D1 and D2 are low or undetectable in the rodent heart, as is the activity of D3 [22]. Sabatino et al. [23] reported similarly low levels of D1 and D2 activity in human cardiac tissue, although D2 mRNA expression is considerably higher in human than in rat heart [24]. Cardiac D2 activity may increase during hypothyroidism in the rat [25], but this does not appear to prevent the drop in tissue levels of T_3 in proportion to the very low plasma levels [22]. However, a lesser reduction of plasma T_3 due to iodine deficiency in the rat did not affect cardiac T_3 levels, suggesting an effective compensatory mechanism [26]. This may include D2 activity, but could also include changes in the active uptake of T_3 by the recently identified TH transporters [27].

When considering data on hormone levels and deiodinase activities in ventricular tissue, it should be kept in mind that, although cardiomyocytes make up the bulk of the cell mass, approximately 70% of the cells present in the heart are not cardiomyocytes but fibroblasts, endothelial cells, and vascular smooth muscle cells, among others. A low enzyme activity per gram of cardiac tissue may therefore reflect a high activity in a nonmyocyte cell population, unless cardiomyocyte-specific expression is shown.

7.4 Cardiac Deiodinase Expression in Pathological Ventricular Remodeling

Cardiac deiodinase activities in chronically overloaded ventricles were determined for the first time in a rat model of RV hypertrophy induced by pulmonary arterial hypertension (PAH) [22]. PAH was induced by a single dose of the pyrrolizidine alkaloid monocrotaline. The bioactive metabolite of monocrotaline selectively injures the vascular endothelium of the lung vessels, with progressive pulmonary vasculitis leading to increasing vascular resistance and a gradual rise in arterial pressure. The increase in RV afterload induces ventricular hypertrophy. Depending on the level of PAH, this hypertrophy progresses to a stable compensated state (HYP), or to congestive heart failure (CHF) and death within 4–5 weeks [22, 28]. RV hypertrophy at 4 weeks following induction of PAH was significantly greater in the CHF group compared to the HYP group and this correlated with the extent of changes in gene expression, such as the reduction of mRNA levels of SERCA2a and the shift from the myosin heavy chain (MHC) α to the β isoform, which is a characteristic aspect of pathological remodeling [22, 28]. Plasma T_3 levels were normal in the HYP group but reduced by approximately 60% in the CHF group, indicative of the critical condition of these animals. This reduction in circulating T_3 probably contributed to the almost complete MHCα to MHCβ shift in the right ventricle of these animals, because a partial shift was seen in the left ventricle of CHF animals.

D2 activity was not detectable in ventricular tissue in any group, but a low level of D1 activity was found in the left and right ventricles of control animals. Interestingly, D1 activity was almost absent in the right ventricle of HYP and CHF animals, whereas a small number of experiments suggested reduction of D1 activity in the left ventricle also. The latter could not be confirmed in subsequent studies

(unpublished data), and reduction of the low D1 activity in the right ventricle appears to be an aspect of hypertrophy. However, D1 activity is not considered relevant for cardiac TH metabolism, since the maximum observed level amounted to less than 0.1% of that found in the livers of these animals [22].

Unexpectedly, significant D3 activity was found in control hearts. Moreover, this activity increased threefold in the right ventricle of the HYP group and more than fivefold in that of the CHF group, with no change in activity in the left ventricles of the same hearts (Fig. 7.2). High D3 activity was therefore associated with overt heart failure and impending death in these animals, whereas moderate induction levels were associated with the development of stable compensatory RV hypertrophy. Subsequent analysis of this model has shown an average tenfold stimulation of RV D3 activity in the CHF group, which corresponds to approximately 20% of the level of D3 activity found in brains of these rats [29] (see also Fig. 7.4). Trivieri et al. [30] reported increased D3 activity in the hypertrophic left ventricle due to pressure overload (aortic constriction, mouse), but activity levels were not presented in that study.

Using a rat model of myocardial infarction (MI), Olivares et al. [31] conducted a 12-week analysis of LV remodeling. Chronic heart failure was observed, with reduced ejection fraction and increased LV end-diastolic diameters. D3 activity was observed in the

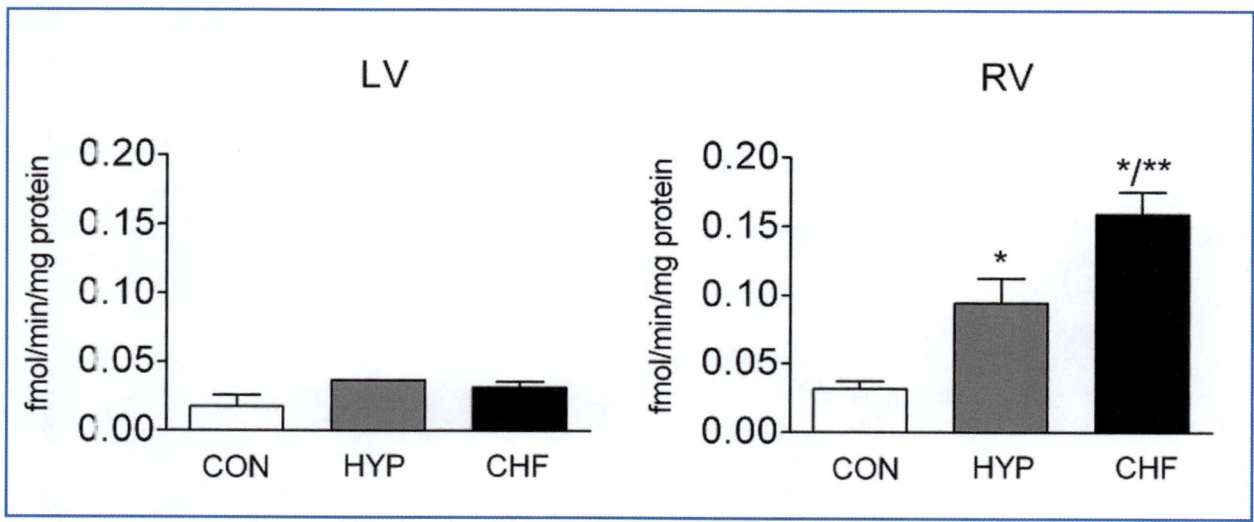

Fig. 7.2 Stimulation of D3 enzyme activity in the right ventricle of rats suffering from pulmonary arterial hypertension. The increase in hemodynamic load induces right ventricular (*RV*) hypertrophy which was either successfully compensated (*HYP* group) or progressed to overt congestive heart failure (*CHF* group). Note that the D3 activity remains low in the left ventricles (*LV*) of the same hearts. * $p < 0.05$ vs. CON; ** $p < 0.05$ vs. HYP. (Reprinted from [22] with permission. Copyright 2002, The Endocrine Society)

infarcted left ventricle at 1 week following myocardial infarction (MI) and the level of activity was identical to that shown previously for the right ventricle (RV) in the study by Wassen et al. [22]. The authors suggested that, as in the D3-expressing tumors mentioned above, this activity is responsible for the transient decrease in plasma T_3 levels seen during the first 3 weeks following MI. However, D3 activity was not determined at later time points, which could have supported this suggestion. Furthermore, it needs to be established whether the reported specific D3 activity in cardiac tissue, which is at least two orders of magnitude lower than that reported for the large tumors [18, 19], is sufficient to reduce systemic TH levels. The suggestion of transient post-MI expression of D3 is in fact not supported by a recent study by Pol et al. [32], who analyzed post-MI LV remodeling and D3 expression in the mouse. Also in this model, induction of D3 was found in the hypertrophic, noninfarcted area of the left ventricle (LV) at 1 week, and LV function was severely reduced from the 1st week after MI onward, with increased LV end-diastolic and end-systolic diameters and reduced fractional shortening. However, D3 activity remained high at 4 and 8 weeks after MI, as depicted in Fig. 7.3. The activity levels were again similar to those reported in the rat RV and LV studies, and although LV function was compromised in these mice, they did not succumb to heart failure. Importantly, using immunohistochemistry and validated D3 antibodies, this study also showed for the first time that D3 protein in the hypertrophic left ventricle is localized to cardiomyocytes (Fig. 7.3).

7.5 Consequences of Cardiac D3 Expression in Pathological Ventricular Remodeling

Cardiac TH levels in hypertrophy have so far only been determined in the PAH model of RV failure [29]. Total tissue levels in the left and right ventricles are largely proportional to the plasma levels and were consequently reduced in CHF animals in that study, with plasma T_4 and T_3 reduced by 60%. However, T_3 levels of the hypertrophic right ventricle were 35% lower than in the left ventricle of the same heart, in line with the high D3 activity in the right ventricle. The lesser or absent role of T_4 uptake in the rat cardiomyocyte, mentioned earlier, was indicated by a low ratio of tissue T_4 to plasma T_4, i.e., 0.12 vs 2.00 for T_3, and no effect on the T_4 level in the hypertrophic right ventricle.

The question of whether the right-ventricle-specific reduction of total tissue T_3 actually affects T_3-dependent transcription in the cardiomyocyte was assessed using an in vivo T_3-transcription probe. The probe consisted of a reporter plasmid in which the firefly luciferase gene is placed under the control of a T_3-responsive minimal promoter that has no cardiac-specific regulatory sequences. Direct injection of the plasmid, together with a normalization plasmid expressing *Renilla* luciferase, into the free wall of the right and left ventricles leads to transfection of cardiomyocytes. Analysis of tissue luciferase activities after 5 days gives a measure of T_3-dependent transcriptional activity. It is not known which membrane property of the contracting

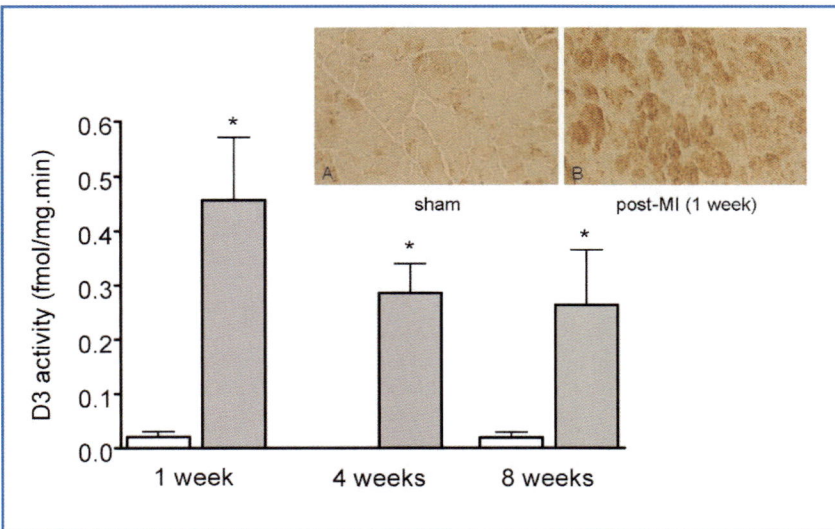

Fig. 7.3 Stimulation of D3 enzyme activity in the left ventricle of mice following myocardial infarction (*MI*). MI was induced by permanent ligation of the left coronary artery. D3 activity was determined in the left ventricle of sham-operated animals and in the noninfarcted, remodeling part of the left ventricle of animals with MI. The degree of LV dilation and reduction of contractile function following MI was the same at 1, 4, and 8 weeks. The *insert* shows cross-sections of the left ventricle of a sham-operated mouse and a mouse with MI at 1 week, stained for D3 using the polyclonal anti-D3 antibody 718 [18]. *White column* sham, *gray column:* MI; * $p < 0.05$ vs. sham. (Reprinted from [32] with permission)

myocyte is responsible for the uptake of plasmid DNA, but important for the interpretation of these data is that other cell types present in the myocardium are not transfected. Validation of the probe showed a 50% reduction of firefly luciferase activity in hearts of animals that were hypothyroid (plasma T_3: 0.03 nM) compared to euthyroid controls (plasma T_3: 0.94 nM). Analysis of CHF animals showed that normalized firefly luciferase activity was reduced by 45% in the hypertrophic right ventricle compared to the activity in the left ventricle of the same heart, which remained at euthyroid levels (Fig. 7.4). This right-ventricle-specific reduction of T_3-dependent luciferase activity, together with the results described above, suggests that D3 expression in the hypertrophic RV cardiomyocyte reduces cellular T_3 content to a level equal to that seen in severe systemic hypothyroidism. However, at this point it cannot be ruled out that other changes in the hypertrophic cardiomyocyte contribute to a reduction of T_3-dependent transcription. For example, changes in TR expression levels, including differential effects on the $\alpha 1$, $\alpha 2$, and $\beta 1$ isoforms, have been reported in models of LV remodeling following MI [33] and due to pressure overload [34, 35]. Although contractile function in a model of LV pressure overload was improved by increasing car-

diac TR expression through viral transfection [36], the relevance of TR changes is not clear, and both increased and decreased expression of TR have been suggested to suppress T_3 signaling.

A reduction of cellular T_3 levels as a principal cause of the local hypothyroid condition of hypertrophic cardiomyocytes is supported by the study of Trivieri et al. [30]. A mouse model of inducible, cardiac-specific overexpression of D2 was used to test the effect of increased cardiac T_3 signaling on the development of LV hypertrophy and dysfunction due to aortic constriction. In control mice, overexpression of D2 increased total cardiac T_3 levels by approximately 25%, which coincidentally indicates that cardiomyocyte uptake of T_4 is not negligible. The increase in T_3 levels had the expected effect on protein levels of T_3-responsive genes, resulting in enhancement of contractile function. When these animals were then subjected to aortic constriction, LV hypertrophy developed, but without the characteristic decrease in SERCA2a and increase in $MHC\beta$ expression seen in wild-type mice. Measurements of Ca^{2+} transients and contractility of cardiomyocytes also indicated preservation of function in the D2-overexpressing hearts. D3 expression was reported to be increased fivefold in the hypertrophic left ventricle, and although cardiac

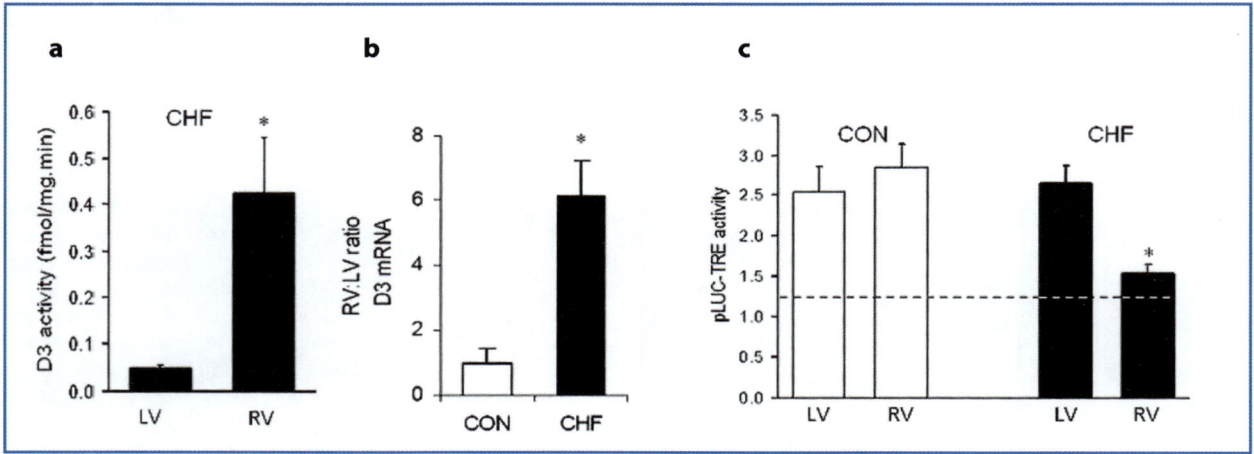

Fig. 7.4 In vivo T_3-dependent transcriptional activity in left and right ventricles of control rats and animals suffering from CHF induced by pulmonary arterial hypertension (see Fig. 7.1). **a** Stimulation of D3 mRNA expression in the right ventricle of CHF rats determined by quantitative RT-PCR and expressed as the average ratio between RV and LV D3 mRNA levels of individual hearts. **b** Ventricular D3 enzyme activity in these animals; the right-ventricle-specific reduction of T_3-dependent transcriptional activity is shown in **c**. This activity was assessed by *in vivo* transfection of a T_3-responsive firefly luciferase expression vector (pLucTRE) together with a control vector expressing *Renilla* luciferase for normalization. The horizontal line indicates the level of activity seen in left ventricle and right ventricle of rats that were rendered hypothyroid, i.e., plasma T_3 and T_4 levels were more than 96% and 99% lower, respectively, compared to control levels. * $p < 0.05$ vs LV CHF (*A, C*) or vs CON (*B*). (Reprinted from [29] with permission)

T_3 levels were not determined, the fact that D2 activity could prevent the changes in T_3-responsive gene expression suggests reduced tissue T_3 levels in the hypertrophic left ventricle of wild-type mice.

7.6 Regulation of Cardiac D3 Expression in Pathological Ventricular Remodeling

Cell culture studies have identified a number of factors that stimulate D3 activity through transcriptional activation of the *DIO3* gene either directly or in combination with other factors [7, 8]. These include serum, phorbol esters and several growth factors, i.e., fibroblast, epidermal, and transforming growth factor (FGF, EGF, TGFβ). The effect of TGFβ was analyzed in detail in various nontransformed human cell types by Huang et al. [15]. Transcriptional stimulation of the *DIO3* gene by TGFβ signaling was mediated by the Smad family of *trans*-activating factors. These proteins are phosphorylated by TGFβ-activated cell surface receptor kinases and migrate to the nucleus to activate target genes. Combinations of different Smad isoforms synergistically activated the promoter of the *DIO3* gene, but only in those cell types that expressed D3 endogenously, such as hepatocarcinoma cells and skeletal muscle myocytes, indicating that other, cell-specific factors are required. Furthermore, the stress-activated branch of the mitogen-activated protein kinase (MAPK) system, i.e., p38 MAPK, as well as the extracellular responsive kinase (ERK) MAPK, synergized with the TGFβ route to stimulate D3 expression. These observations may be particularly relevant for understanding the stimulation of D3 activity in the heart, since TGFβ has long been known to play a role in the development of ventricular hypertrophy and adverse remodeling [37]. Moreover, p38 and ERK MAPKs, together with the c-Jun N-terminal kinases (JNKs), are important signaling cascades modulating transcription in pathological hypertrophy of the cardiomyocyte [3]. Stimulation of D3 expression in the PAH model of RV failure indeed appears to be transcriptional, with reports of a sixfold increase in D3 mRNA levels [22, 29] (see Fig. 7.4). In addition, activation of p38 MAPK was found in the pressure-overloaded right ventricle [28]. Similarly, p38 MAPK activity is increased following MI, and blocking it attenuates pathological LV remodeling [38]. Consequently,

these pathways are potential candidates for the stimulation of D3 activity, suggesting that re-expression of D3 is part of the phenotypic changes in hypertrophy that also include other fetal characteristics.

The recent finding that the *DIO3* gene is a direct target of hypoxia-inducible factor 1 (HIF-1) adds another level of complexity to the regulation of cardiac D3 expression, suggesting it is part of an adaptive response [29]. HIF-1 signaling constitutes a general cellular response to reduced oxygen availability, entailing changes in energy metabolism and stimulation of vascularization [39]. These HIF-1 effects are aimed at reducing cellular oxygen consumption while stimulating oxygen delivery. HIF-1 is a transcriptional activator consisting of a constitutively expressed HIF-1β subunit and a HIF-1α subunit. The stability of HIF-1α is oxygen-dependent; under normoxic conditions it is ubiquinated and degraded, resulting in low levels of HIF-1. As cellular oxygen tension drops, HIF-1α accumulates, and hence HIF-1, which then activates a large number of genes that are mostly involved in glucose metabolism and angiogenesis. Neovascularization is mediated by up-regulation of vascular endothelial growth factor (VEGF) expression. Cardiac ischemia due to impaired coronary circulation is a potent stimulator of the HIF-1 response, but cellular hypoxia can also occur in hypertrophy when capillary density and oxygen diffusion distances become limiting factors for the enlarged cardiomyocytes [40]. For instance, Sano et al. [41] showed that HIF-1 activity is required for adaptive LV hypertrophy and angiogenesis in a mouse model of transverse aortic constriction. Similarly, in the PAH model of RV hypertrophy increased nuclear HIF-1α was found in cardiomyocytes [40], as well as increased VEGF expression [28]. In this model, stimulation of HIF-1α levels was shown to be restricted to the hypertrophic right ventricle and to be associated with the right-ventricle-specific stimulation of D3 mRNA expression and enzyme activity [29]. Analysis in that study of the effect of hypoxia on D3 expression in various cell types indicated direct transcriptional regulation of the *DIO3* gene by HIF-1. Hypoxic culture conditions increased D3 activity in rat neonatal cardiomyocytes, but also in human neurons (SK-N-AS cells), rhesus monkey hepatocytes (NCLP6E cells), and human choriocarcinoma cells (JEG-3). Induction of D3 activity was dynamic, with transient exposure to hypoxia resulting in a transient increase in D3 mRNA and activity. Finally, ChiP analysis using SK-N-AS cells cultured under conditions of increased expression of HIF-1α and D3 indicated that HIF-1α interacts directly with the *DIO3* promoter. The 5'-flanking region of the *DIO3* gene indeed contains a conserved HIF-1-binding site, or hypoxia response element, which characterizes genes that are regulated by HIF-1. This suggests that D3 induction is part of the cellular response to hypoxia, which is supported by the observation that D3 activity reduces T_3-dependent metabolic rate in cultured cells [29].

In contrast to extracellularly activated signaling cascades in cardiac hypertrophy, HIF-1 signaling would restrict the induction of D3 to only those cells that would benefit from a reduction in energy turnover. The mixed pattern of D3-positive and D3-negative cardiomyocytes seen in the study of Pol et al. [32] seems to support this. However, the picture is complicated by the observation of rapid HIF-1α accumulation under normoxic conditions following an increase in ventricular wall tension, a common trigger of cardiac hypertrophy [42]. Stretch-activated channels signaling through the phosphatidylinositol 3-kinase pathway appear to be responsible for the HIF-1 response, and HIF-1

may therefore be a factor in early hypertrophic signaling as well as in the adaptive response to hypoxia at later stages of remodeling. To further complicate matters, TGFβ signaling is likely to potentiate HIF-1 signaling, since Smad proteins synergize with HIF-1α on responsive promoters [43]. The factors and pathways that are implicated in the regulation of cardiac D3 expression are depicted schematically in Figure 7.5.

7.7 Implications and Future Directions

Increasing the energy efficiency of the stressed heart through reduction of T_3-dependent metabolism can be considered adaptive. However, when the changes in gene expression include those that are implicated in the development of the pathological phenotype, as is the case for a number of T_3-dependent genes such as SERCA2a, the adaptive response may become part of the problem. The latter is still the current view concerning the possible involvement of reduced T_3 signaling in heart failure, but the stable induction of D3 in the post-MI left ventricle [32] and results from the original study by

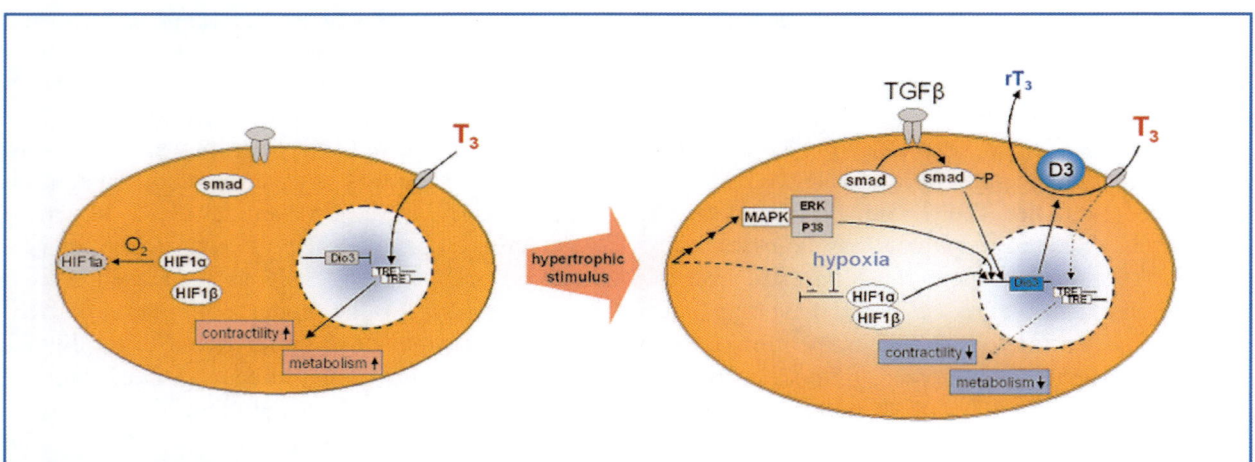

Fig. 7.5 Some of the pathways that may contribute to the expression of D3 in the overloaded, hypertrophic heart. A normal cardiomyocyte is depicted on the *left*. T_3 is taken up by specific transporters, and genes that are transcriptionally regulated by T_3 are characterized by the presence in their promoters of thyroid hormone response elements (TRE), to which the T_3 receptor binds. Examples are MHCα and SERCA2a, whose enzyme activities determine rates of contraction and relaxation. HIF-1α is degraded under normoxic conditions, whereas HIF-1β is stable. Transition to the hypertrophic cardiomyocyte, depicted on the *right,* may be triggered by various stimuli (see text for details). Several of the signaling pathways converge on the mitogen-activated protein kinases (MAPK) ERK and p38. The enlarged cell may develop a hypoxic core, resulting in stabilization of HIF-1α and dimerization with HIF-1β to form the HIF-1 complex. HIF-1α is possibly also directly stabilized as a result of hypertrophic signaling. Activation of cell surface receptor kinases by TGFβ leads to phosphorylation of Smad proteins. Nuclear translocation of the phosphorylated factors, together with HIF-1 and phosphorylated ERK and p38, results in the synergistic stimulation of transcription of the *DIO3* gene. D3 activity converts T_3 to the inactive metabolite reverse T_3, resulting in reduced T_3 signaling and a concomitant reduction of contractile activity and energy turnover

Wassen et al. [22] suggest that the timing and extent of D3 induction are critical factors in turning an adaptive into a maladaptive response. In the latter study, ventricles that developed stable compensatory hypertrophy showed significantly less induction of D3 activity than did ventricles in which hypertrophy progressed to failure (Fig. 7.2). TGFβ signaling may play a role in further increasing the D3 induction in this model, since this signaling is suggested to increase in the transition from compensatory hypertrophy to failure [44, 45]. Given the stimulation of *DIO3* gene transcription by HIF-1 signaling as well as by various signaling cascades implicated in hypertrophy, additional studies are needed to delineate which factors drive D3 expression during the course of pathological ventricular remodeling.

Taken together, the data from several different models of cardiac overload suggest that induction of D3 activity and reduction of cellular T_3 signaling are aspects of pathological hypertrophy. Although it is tempting to infer a causal relationship between these aspects, there are no data as yet to confirm this. One problem is that there are no selective inhibitors of D3 activity. A transgenic approach using cardiac-specific conditional knockout of D3 expression would be the optimal way to test the relevance of D3 activity for the development of adaptive or maladaptive ventricular hypertrophy. Finally, D3 immunohistochemistry of human ventricular biopsies needs to be done as a first step in assessing whether induction of D3 plays a role in pathological hypertrophy and heart failure in humans.

Key Points

- T_3 regulates multiple genes that are involved in contractile dysfunction and heart failure following pathological ventricular hypertrophy.

- Reduced cardiac T_3 signaling may contribute to the development of the phenotype of pathological hypertrophy.

- Expression of the T_3-degrading enzyme deiodinase type 3 (D3) is stimulated in cardiomyocytes of hypertrophic left or right ventricles in different rodent models of heart failure.

- Induction of D3 activity is associated with a severe, cardiomyocyte-specific hypothyroid condition in at least one model of heart failure.

- Cardiac D3 expression is transcriptionally stimulated by hypoxia-inducible factor 1 (HIF-1) and by signaling cascades that are implicated in cardiomyocyte hypertrophy.

- It needs to be established which factors drive D3 expression during the course of pathological ventricular remodeling and whether this is an adaptive or ultimately a maladaptive response.

References

1. Klein I, Ojamaa K (2001) Thyroid hormone and the cardiovascular system. N Engl J Med 344:501–509
2. Rajabi M, Kassiotis C, Razeghi P, Taegtmeyer H (2007) Return to the fetal gene program protects the stressed heart: a strong hypothesis. Heart Fail Rev 12:331–343
3. Frey N, Olson EN (2003) Cardiac hypertrophy: the good, the bad and the ugly. Annu Rev Physiol 65:45–79
4. Molkentin JD (2004) Calcineurin-NFAT signalling regulates the cardiac hypertrophic response in coordination with the MAPKs. Cardiovasc Res 63:467–475
5. Selvetella G, Hirsch E, Notte A et al (2004) Adaptive and maladaptive hypertrophic pathways: points of convergence and divergence. Cardiovasc Res 63:373–380
6. Muller A, Simonides WS (2005) Regulation of myocardial SERCA2a expression in ventricular hypertrophy and heart failure. Future Cardiol 1:543–553
7. Gereben B, Zavacki AM, Ribich S et al (2008) Cellular and molecular basis of deiodinase-regulated thyroid hormone signaling. Endocr Rev 29:898–938
8. Maia AL, Kim BW, Huang SA et al (2005) Type 2 iodothyronine deiodinase is the major source of plasma T3 in euthyroid humans. J Clin Invest 115:2524–2533
9. Baqui M, Botero D, Gereben B et al (2003) Human type 3 iodothyronine selenodeiodinase is located in the plasma membrane and undergoes rapid internalization to endosomes. J Biol Chem 278:1206–1211
10. Friesema EC, Kuiper GG, Jansen J et al (2006) Thyroid hormone transport by the human monocarboxylate transporter 8 and its rate-limiting role in intracellular metabolism. Mol Endocrinol 20:2761–2772

11. Bianco AC, Kim BW (2006) Deiodinases: implications of the local control of thyroid hormone action. J Clin Invest 116:2571–9

12. Dentice M, Bandyopadhyay A, Gereben B et al (2005) The Hedgehog-inducible ubiquitin ligase subunit WSB-1 modulates thyroid hormone activation and PTHrP secretion in the developing growth plate. Nat Cell Biol 7:698–705

13. Dentice M, Luongo C, Huang S et al (2007) Sonic hedgehog-induced type 3 deiodinase blocks thyroid hormone action enhancing proliferation of normal and malignant keratinocytes. Proc Natl Acad Sci USA 104:14466–14471

14. Gianakopoulos PJ, Skerjanc IS (2005) Hedgehog signaling induces cardiomyogenesis in P19 cells. J Biol Chem 280:21022–21028

15. Huang SA, Mulcahey MA, Crescenzi A et al (2005) TGF-b promotes inactivation of extracellular thyroid hormones via transcriptional stimulation of type 3 iodothyronine deiodinase. Mol Endocrinol 19:3126–3136

16. Gereben B, Zeold A, Dentice M et al (2008) Activation and inactivation of thyroid hormone by deiodinases: local action with general consequences. Cell Mol Life Sci 65:570–590

17. Huang SA, Tu HM, Harney JW et al (2000) Severe hypothyroidism caused by type 3 iodothyronine deiodinase in infantile hemangiomas. N Engl J Med 343:185–189

18. Huang SA, Fish SA, Dorfman DM et al (2002) A 21-year-old woman with consumptive hypothyroidism due to a vascular tumor expressing type 3 iodothyronine deiodinase. J Clin Endocrinol Metab 87:4457–4461

19. Ruppe MD, Huang SA, Jan de Beur SM (2005) Consumptive hypothyroidism caused by paraneoplastic production of type 3 iodothyronine deiodinase. Thyroid 15:1369–1372

20. Peeters RP, Wouters PJ, Kaptein, van Toor H, Visser TJ, Van der Berghe G (2003) Reduced activation and increased inactivation of thyroid hormone in tissues of critically ill patients. J Clin Endocrinol Metab 88:3202–3211

21. Escobar-Morreale HF, Obregon MJ, Escobar del Rey F et al (1999) Tissue-specific patterns of changes in 3,5,3?-tri-iodo-L-thyronine concentrations in thyroidectomized rats infused with increasing doses of the hormone. Which are the regulatory mechanisms? Biochimie 81:453–462

22. Wassen FW, Schiel AE, Kuiper GG et al (2002) Induction of thyroid hormone-degrading deiodinase in cardiac hypertrophy and failure. Endocrinology 143:2812–2815

23. Sabatino L, Iervasi G, Ferrazzi P et al (2000) A study of iodothyronine 5'-monodeiodinase activities in normal and pathological tissues in man and their comparison with activities in rat tissues. Life Sci 68:191–202

24. Dentice M, Morisco C, Vitale M et al (2003) The different cardiac expression of the type 2 iodothyronine deiodinase gene between human and rat is related to the differential response of the Dio2 genes to Nkx-2.5 and GATA-4 transcription factors. Mol Endocrinol 17:1508–21

25. Wagner MS, Morimoto RJ, Dora JM et al (2003) Hypothyroidism induces type 2 iodothyronine deiodinase expression in mouse heart and testis. J Mol Endocrinol 31:541–550

26. Pedraza PE, Obregon MJ, Escobar-Morreale HF et al (2006) Mechanisms of adaptation to iodine deficiency in rats: thyroid status is tissue specific. Its relevance for man. Endocrinology 147:2098–2108

27. Friesema EC, Jansen J, Milici C, Visser TJ (2005) Thyroid hormone transporters. Vitam Horm 70:137–167

28. Buermans HPJ, Redout EM, Schiel AE et al (2005) Microarray analysis reveals pivotal divergent mRNA expression profiles early in the development of either compensated ventricular hypertrophy or heart failure. Physiol Genomics 21:314–323

29. Simonides WS, Mulcahey MA, Redout EM et al (2008) Hypoxia-inducible factor induces local thyroid hormone inactivation during hypoxic-ischemic disease in rats. J Clin Invest 118:975–983

30. Trivieri MG, Oudit GY, Sah R et al (2006) Cardiac-specific elevations in thyroid hormone enhance contractility and prevent pressure overload-induced cardiac dysfunction. Proc Natl Acad Sci USA 103:6043–6048

31. Olivares EL, Marassi MP, Fortunato RS et al (2007) Thyroid function disturbance and type 3 iodothyronine deiodinase induction after myocardial infarction in rats a time course study. Endocrinology 148:4786–4792

32. Pol C, Zuidwijk M, Deel E et al (2008) Left ventricular myocardial infarction in mice induces sustained cardiac deiodinase type III activity. XXVIII European Section Meeting of the International Society for Heart Research, Medimond International Proceedings, Bologna, Italy, pp 57–60

33. Pantos C, Mourouzis I, Xinaris C et al (2007) Time-dependent changes in the expression of thyroid hormone receptor alpha 1 in the myocardium after acute myocardial infarction: possible implications in cardiac remodelling. Eur J Endocrinol 156:415–24

34. Kinugawa K, Yonekura K, Ribeiro RC et al (2001) Regulation of thyroid hormone receptor isoforms in physiological and pathological cardiac hypertrophy. Circ Res 89:591–598

35. Kinugawa K, Minobe WA, Wood WM et al (2001) Signaling pathways responsible for fetal gene induction in the failing human heart: evidence for altered thyroid hormone receptor gene expression. Circulation 103:1089–1094

36. Belke DD, Gloss B, Swanson EA, Dillmann WH (2007) Adeno-associated virus-mediated expression of thyroid hormone receptor isoforms-alpha1 and -beta1 improves contractile function in pressure overload-induced cardiac hypertrophy. Endocrinology 148:2870–2877

37. Rosenkranz S (2004) TGF-b1 and angiotensin networking in cardiac remodeling. Cardiovasc Res 63:423–432

38. See F, Thomas W, Way K et al (2004) p38 mitogen-activated protein kinase inhibition improves cardiac function and attenuates left ventricular remodeling following myocardial infarction in the rat. J Am Coll Cardiol 44:1679–1689

39. Semenza GL (2004) O2-regulated gene expresson: transcriptional control of cardiorespiratory physiology by HIF-1. J Appl Physiol 96:1173–1177

40. Des Tombes AL, van Beek-Harmsen BJ, Lee-de Groot MBE, van der Laarse WJ (2002) Calibrated histochemistry applied to oxygen supply and demand in hypertrophied myocardium. Microsc Res Tech 58:412–420

41. Sano M, Minamino T, Toko H et al (2007) p53-induced inhibition of Hif-1 causes cardiac dysfunction during pressure overload. Nature 446:444–448

42. Kim CH, Cho YS, Chun YS et al (2002) Early expression of myocardial HIF-1alpha in response to mechanical stresses: regulation by stretch-activated channels and the phosphatidylinositol 3-kinase signaling pathway. Circ Res 90:E25–33

43. Euler-Taimor G, Heger J (2006) The complex pattern of

SMAD signaling in the cardiovascular system. Cardiovasc Res 69:15–25

44. Boluyt MO, O'Neill L, Meredith AL et al (1994) Alterations in cardiac gene expression during the transition from stable hypertrophy to heart failure: marked upregulation of genes encoding extracellular matrix components. Circ Res 75:23–32

45. Lim H, Zhu YZ (2006) Role of transforming growth factor-b in the progression of heart failure. Cell Mol Life Sci 63:2584–2596

Koichiro Kinugawa, Mark Y. Jeong, Michael R. Bristow
and Carlin S. Long

Abstract Although it is well-accepted that alterations in thyroid function occur in patients with heart failure, this was ascribed previously to "euthyroid-sick" syndrome rather than real hypothyroidism. This has been called into question by a series of reports that implicate a primary change in the myocardial response to thyroid hormone as being responsible, at least in part, for the changes in myocardial form and function seen in the failing heart. Based on our findings that myocardial thyroid hormone receptor (TR) isoform expression is altered in patients with heart failure, our group has focused on the possibility that these changes in TR expression are responsible for certain aspects of the failure phenotype. In this regard TR isoforms were found to have differential effects on the cardiac myocyte phenotype. Specifically, TRα is linked to cardiac myocyte growth that is dependent upon the p38MAPK family. In contrast, TRβ has little effect on cardiac myocyte growth, limits p38 activation, and stimulates a number of the known thyroid-responsive cardiac myocyte genes. We conclude from these investigations that changes in the expression of TR isoforms play a direct role in myocardial growth and gene expression in heart failure. Furthermore, manipulation of the TH:TR axis in an isoform-specific manner may represent a new therapeutic approach to congestive heart failure (CHF) and may complement treatment profiles already in use for this syndrome.

Keywords Heart failure • Gene expression • Thyroid hormone • Cardiac hypertrophy • Thyroid receptor • Myosin heavy chain • Sarcoplasmic reticulum Ca^{2+}ATPase

8.1 Introduction

There are a number of changes in the gene profile exhibited by the heart under circumstances of pathological stress that in many ways mimic those seen in patients with overt hypothyroidism. Moreover, there are also changes in the expression of key members of the thyroid hormone:thyroid hormone receptor (TH:TR) signaling pathway in patients with heart failure. Notably, under circumstances of both hypothyroidism and heart failure alterations in contractile and relaxation properties are seen that may be a direct result of these changes in gene expression. It is tempting to speculate that correcting an imbalance in the TH:TR axis could be associated with beneficial changes in gene expression and function in heart failure patients. However, before such an approach can be considered, the mechanism(s) responsible for the effect of thyroid

C.S. Long (✉)
Division of Cardiology, University of Colorado,
Denver, CO, United States

G. Iervasi, A. Pingitore (eds.), *Thyroid and Heart Failure.*
© Springer-Verlag Italia 2009

hormone on cardiac growth, which remains controversial, should be clarified. Specifically, although it was thought that thyroid hormone causes cardiac hypertrophy mainly through its increase in myocardial work load, work from both our group and others indicates that thyroid hormone has a direct effect on cardiac myocyte hypertrophy in an in vitro system in which no increase in work load occurs. In this chapter, we describe the thyroid-receptor-specific mechanism of cardiac hypertrophy induced by thyroid hormone in this cell culture system.

8.2 The Myocardial Gene Program of the Failing Human Heart Resembles That Seen in Hypothyroidism

The gene program that characterizes the hypertrophic and failing heart in a number of experimental models is often referred to as the "fetal" gene program because it recapitulates a genetic profile reminiscent of that seen during early embryonic development. Specifically, while expression of the skeletal-muscle-specific genes β-myosin heavy chain (β-MyHC) and skeletal α-actin increases, that of the adult cardiac-muscle-specific genes α-myosin heavy chain (α-MyHC) and sarcoplasmic reticulum Ca^{2+}ATPase (SERCA2a) decreases. Similarly, expression of both atrial and brain natriuretic peptides (ANP and BNP), sensitive markers of cardiac hypertrophy and dysfunction, also increase [1]. Although these changes have been most frequently studied in animal models of pathological growth, similar changes are also see in the human heart. Even though the β-MyHC isoform predominates in the heart, recent work indicates that α-MyHC expression is, in fact, decreased in the failing human ventricle, an observation that may explain, at least in part, some of the contractile abnormalities seen in the failing heart [2, 3]. Indeed, in rodents, the ratio of ATPase activity between α and β isoforms is approximately 2, but in humans it is about 10 (Bristow et al., unpublished observations), suggesting that even small changes in α-MyHC significantly impact contractile activity in the human heart. We have measured the expression of α-MyHC in end-stage failing human hearts [2–4]. In nonfailing human hearts, α-MyHC accounted for approx. 7% of total MyHC protein [4]. In failing human hearts, α-MyHC protein was not at all detectable, which was consistent with the idea that decreases in α-MyHC are important in the failing property. These changes in MyHC isoform expression in human failing heart have been consistently observed by a number of independent investigators, as has the decrease in SERCA expression and an increase in the natriuretic peptides in patients with dilated cardiomyopathy [3, 5]. Curiously, this pattern of gene expression is also seen in the hypothyroid heart. This led to our original hypothesis, that alterations in myocardial TR expression and/or effect are involved in the development and/or maintenance of the pathological cardiac myocyte gene program.

As suggested above, these changes in gene expression have been extensively investigated in experimental animals and isolated myocardial cells, particularly from the rat. With respect to the changes in MyHC and SERCA expression described above, it is likely that one of the key determinants of the rapid changes in MyHC isoform composition (and possible alterations in calcium handling) in the neonatal heart relates to alterations in thyroid hormone levels in the neonate and the fact that both α-MyHC and SERCA2a genes contain thyroid-responsive elements (TREs) in their 5'-promoter region [6–8]. The TRE is a consensus DNA sequence that binds TRs either as a monomer, homodimer, or, in most cases, as a heterodimer with the retinoid X receptor (RXR) [9, 10]. Although a substantial percentage of cellular TRs are expressed in nuclei, cytoplasmic TRs may have an equally important role [11]. However, since the chromosomal DNA containing these TRE motifs is limited to the nuclear compartment of the cell, in exploration of TR action on TREs, the focus must be primarily on TRs in the nucleus, where these dimers are usually bound to the TRE "waiting" for thyroid hormone. In this un-liganded state, TRs are associated with a number of transcriptional repressors, such as the histone deacetylases (HDACs), which inhibit downstream gene expression [12]. Once thyroid hormone enters the nucleus and binds with TR, this liganded TR recruits and interacts with transcriptional activators such as the histone acetyltransferases (HATs) [12], resulting in transcriptional activation of downstream gene expression. This is the predominant mechanism of transcriptional activation for the α-MyHC and SERCA2a genes, and such TREs are often referred to as "positive" TREs since their association with both TR and ligand results in an up-regulation of gene expression.

In contrast, some thyroid-responsive genes, like the β-MyHC isoform, which is markedly diminished after birth in rodents, undergo repression in response to ligand. The decreased expression of β-MyHC is also dependent upon TR binding to specific DNA motifs in these repressed genes; such sequences are commonly referred to as "negative" TREs in that their action in response to ligand is primarily a negative/repression pattern [13]. In contrast to the positive TRE, less is known about the nature of this kind of negative TRE, in which ligand binding results in gene repression.

What has been discussed thus far are mechanisms that are developmentally regulated by thyroid hormone in myocyte-specific gene expression. The fetal heart expresses higher β-MyHC and lower α-MyHC/SERCA2a and this pattern is reversed in the postnatal heart. As noted previously, however, the fetal gene program is also expressed in the adult heart in response to various pathological stimuli, including hypertension, valvular disease, and ischemia/infarction, and in response to a number of neurohumoral factors (e.g., angiotensin II, catecholamines, endothelin), all of which are known to induce pathologic myocardial hypertrophy [14–16] but notably are not induced under circumstances of physiological growth, which is also characterized by larger myocytes but with enhanced contractile function [16, 17]. Pathological hypertrophy usually results in diminished myocardial function, i.e., heart failure, and the increase in β-MyHC accompanied by the decrease in α-MyHC and SERCA2a may explain, at least in part, the depressed contractile/relaxation function, normally seen in hypertrophied/failing heart (reviewed in [18, 19]). In contrast, physiological hypertrophy is associated with enhanced expression of the adult gene program, i.e., increased α-MyHC and SERCA2a and decreased β-MyHC expression [16].

For a number of years, our research group, like others, has pursued the idea that reversal of the fetal gene program may improve depressed myocardial function in pathological hypertrophy. Although this idea has been proposed for some time [20], the focus on the TH:TR axis in this regard has received much less attention. Notably Chang et al. [15] reported that thyroid hormone reversed systolic and diastolic function in the pathological hypertrophied heart in vivo. Improvement was associated with isoform switching back to the α-MyHC isoform as

well as increases in SERCA2a. This "rescue" of the myocyte gene program has also been confirmed in vitro [16]. Only recently, however, have studies suggested that the alterations in these thyroid-responsive genes extend to alterations in the expression of the thyroid receptors themselves.

8.3 TR Expression in Pathological/Physiological Hypertrophy

The first suggestion that TRs might themselves be involved in the pathological growth and abnormal gene profile came from an appreciation of the similarity between the fetal gene program, the hypothyroid heart, and the myocardial gene program seen in the resistance to thyroid hormone (RTH) syndrome which results from an alteration in TRβ action [7, 21]. Therefore, we hypothesized that in failing heart the fetal gene program may be induced, at least in part, by a deficiency in thyroid hormone signaling in cardiac myocytes. However, circulating levels of thyroid hormone are not consistently altered in heart failure patients. Thus, if thyroid signaling is altered under these circumstances, it must occur somewhere downstream in the pathway, such as the level of the TR/TRE. To test this hypothesis, we measured TR expression in both human and rodent heart under several different circumstances of myocardial growth.

It is generally accepted that TRs have four major isoforms: $TR\alpha_1$, $TR\alpha_2$, $TR\beta_1$, and $TR\beta_2$ [9]. $TR\alpha_1$ and $TR\alpha_2$ are alternatively spliced from the TRα gene locus, and $TR\beta_1$ and $TR\beta_2$ from the TRβ gene locus. Although $TR\beta_2$ is exclusively expressed in pituitary gland, the other three isoforms are ubiquitously expressed throughout the body, including the heart. $TR\alpha_2$ has a distinct feature in that it lacks the thyroid-hormone-binding domain and thus acts as naturally occurring repressor for positive TRE function [22].

As shown in Figure 8.1, we identified expression of $TR\alpha_1$, $TR\alpha_2$, and $TR\beta_1$ in rat heart, but, as expected, failed to find any expression of $TR\beta_2$ [16]. Exercise-induced physiological hypertrophy in rat (voluntary wheel-running) resulted in the expression of an adult gene program in the heart, i.e., α-MyHC and SERCA2a were increased, while β-MyHC was decreased. Investigating of TR isoform expression in this model of physiological hypertrophy showed an increase in TRβ₁ with no changes in either TRα₁ or TRα₂ expression (Fig. 8.1a). Thyroid hormone treatment of cultured myocytes also induced the adult gene program and modest hypertrophy, and we confirmed TRβ₁ up-regulation in this in vitro model of physiological hypertrophy (Fig. 8.1b). In contrast, we observed marked induction of the fetal gene program in the hypertrophied/failing rat heart induced by ascending aortic banding, i.e., up-regulation of β-MyHC and skACT with down-regulation of α-MyHC and SERCA2a. In the same heart, expression of TRα₁ and TRβ₁ was also decreased (Fig. 8.1a). These phenomena were confirmed in cultured rat cardiac myocytes in which the fetal gene program was induced along with marked hypertrophy by phenylephrine treatment (Fig. 8.1c). Moreover, expression of the pathological fetal gene program was reversed by thyroid hormone and was accompanied by up-regulation of TRβ₁ but not

TRα₁ (Fig. 8.1c). These data suggested that the hypothyroid-like features of the fetal gene program are also associated with decreased expression of functional TRs, whereas the hyperthyroid-like gene program is accompanied by increased expression of at least one of the functional TRs. Therefore, it seems rational to hypothesize that the altered signaling at the level of TR expression is one of the mechanisms leading to the distinct gene expression pattern in cardiac myocytes.

With this experimental data in hand, we next measured TR isoform expression in human hearts, where we identified a similar expression pattern to the rat including distinct signals for TRα₁, TRα₂, and TRβ₁, but no TRβ₂ (Fig. 8.2a) [23]. However, in contrast to rodent failing hearts, in which we observed down-regulation of all three TR isoforms, in human failing hearts TRα₁ was decreased but TRα₂ was up-regulated (Fig. 8.2a,b). The TRβ sig-

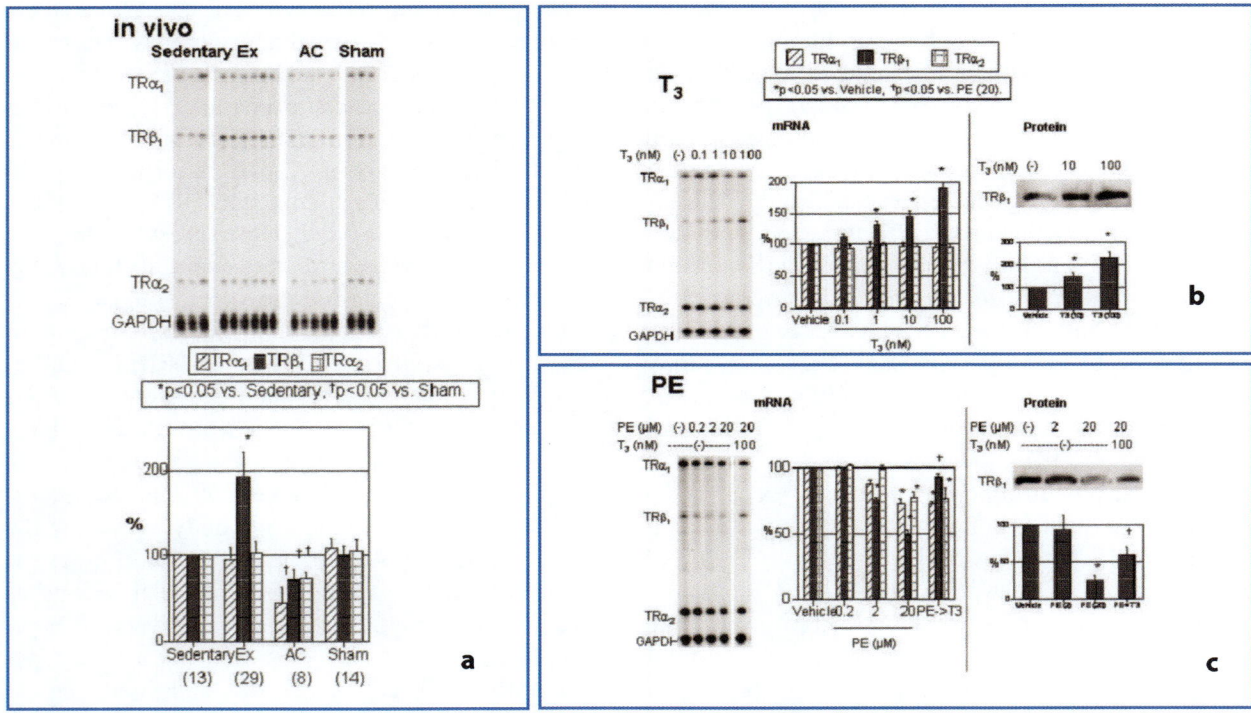

Fig. 8.1 Regulation of thyroid hormone receptor (TR) isoforms in vivo (**a**) and in culture (**b, c**). **a** Hypertrophy was induced in adult male rats by voluntary running exercise (*Ex*) for 10 weeks or ascending aortic constriction (*AC*) for 4 weeks, and left ventricular TR isoform mRNAs were assayed. A representative gel is shown with mean values from the indicated numbers of rats, normalized to the sedentary control group shown below. **b, c** Cultured neonatal rat cardiac myocytes were treated with (**b**) triiodothyronine (*T₃*) or (**c**) phenylephrine (*PE*) for 72 h, and TR isoform mRNAs were assayed in 10 μg total RNA by RNase protection (*left and middle*). Alternatively, cells were treated for 120 h, and TRβ₁ protein in equal numbers of myocyte nuclei was quantified by Western blot (*right*). In the "PE+T₃" groups, cells treated with 20 μmolPE/l were also treated with 100 nmolT₃/l for the final 24 h (mRNA) or 72 h (protein). Representative gels are shown; mean data are from five cultures for mRNA and three cultures for protein. (Adapted from [16])

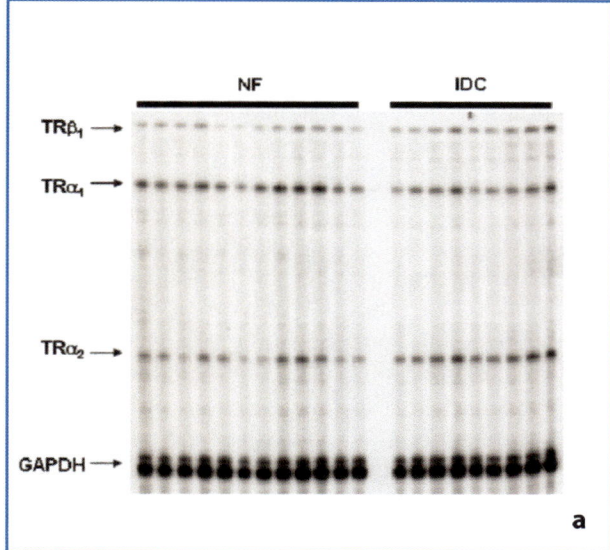
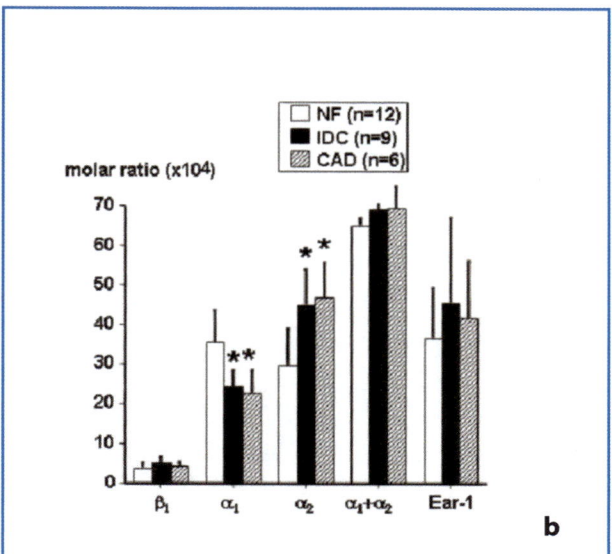

Fig. 8.2 TR expression in human heart. **a** Representative RNase protection assay (2.5 days' exposure) using probes specific for TRα1/α2 and TRβ1. Each lane was loaded with 10 μg total RNA extracted from nonfailing hearts (*NF*) or hearts with idiopathic dilated cardiomyopathy (*IDC*). GAPDH probe was used as an internal loading control. **b** mRNA expression determined by RNase protection assay was quantified by counting the radioactivity of each specific band for each mRNA species. Counts were converted to molar amount with several coefficients, such as specific activity of each probe, and normalized to GAPDH molecules. *$p < 0.01$ vs. NF. *CAD* coronary artery disease. (Adapted from [23])

nal was very low at baseline and not convincingly changed. Since TRα2 is a naturally occurring dominant-negative isoform, the conceptual model remains the same in which the hypothyroid-like gene program may be caused by attenuated thyroid hormone signaling at the level of TR expression.

8.4 Isoform-Specificity of TR in Thyroid-Hormone-Induced Cardiac Hypertrophy

Since we had observed distinct alterations in TR isoform expression under circumstances of both physiological and pathological growth stimuli which appeared to be regulated in concert with the expression of the pathological gene program, we next investigated the possibility that the individual TR isoforms have distinct effects on cardiac myocyte growth and the expressed gene program. As a prelude to these studies, we were interested in exploring the subcellular localization of the individual TR isoforms as well as the possibility that the TRs themselves had unique effects, reflecting both genomic and extranuclear, nongenomic targets as has been recently described for a number of nuclear

hormone receptors. For example, the estrogen hormone receptor (ER) is a well-characterized nuclear hormone receptor that possesses both nuclear and extranuclear nongenomic activities. Estrogen's vasodilatory effect is too rapid to be attributed to ER-induced gene expression. Recent reports describe cell membrane ER that interact with phosphatidylinositol-3 kinase (PI-3 kinase) [24] with subsequent phosphorylation of endothelial nitric oxide synthase (eNOS) [25]. This ER-PI-3 kinase modulation of eNOS likely accounts for the rapid nongenomic effect of estrogen as a vasodilator. A similar mechanism has also been described for the thyroid hormone receptor where, in vascular smooth muscle cells, nongenomic thyroid hormone activity decreases vascular tone by altering the activities of various ion channels [26]. In endothelial cells, extranuclear TRα1 also interacts with PI-3 kinase to increase phosphorylation of eNOS [27]. Given the evidence arguing for significant nonnuclear TR effects, it is plausible to postulate that interactions of cytosolic TR with other signaling molecules are involved in cardiac myocyte growth and gene expression.

As noted previously, in studies of neonatal rat ventricular myocytes in primary culture, T3 treatment leads to a significant increase in protein synthesis and expression of the adult-specific gene profile, i.e., up-regulation of αMHC and SERCA2a and down-regulation of βMHC [16]. The prevailing thought is that gene expression and myocyte hypertrophy are obligate processes, i.e., gene expression begets hypertrophy. Contrary to this view, GC-1 [28], a relatively specific TRβ agonist, is ineffective as a myocyte hypertrophic agent [16] compared to T_3 (EC_{50} for protein synthesis: triiodothyronine [T_3] 0.1 nmol/l, GC-1 2 nmol/l), but its effect on gene expression is similar to that of T_3 (up-regulation of αMHC and SERCA2a, and down-regulation of βMHC). These findings suggested that thyroid hormone isoforms do, in fact, have differential effects in the myocyte; specifically, thyroid-hormone-induced cardiac hypertrophy is due to the activity of $TR\alpha_1$, while $TR\beta_1$ appears to be mainly involved in the transcription of thyroid-hormone-responsive genes.

To address this possibility further, we developed three adenoviral delivery constructs to overexpress $TR\alpha_1$, $TR\alpha_2$, or $TR\beta_1$ proteins (AdTRα1, AdTRα2, AdTRβ1) [11]. In support of the hypothesis that there are TR isoform-specific effects in the heart, infection with AdTRα1 resulted in a dose-dependent increase in protein synthesis [11], while neither AdTRα2 nor AdTRβ1 caused an increase in protein synthesis even when expressed at very high levels. As expected, the expression of thyroid-hormone-responsive genes also showed TR-isoform-specific differences (Fig. 8.3). Overexpression of $TR\beta_1$ induces the adult-specific gene profile similar to T_3, while overexpression of $TR\alpha_1$ induces the pathological gene profile (up-regulation of βMHC, ANP, BNP, skeletal actin, and down-regulation of αMHC and SERCA2a). As shown in Figure 8.4, localization patterns of TR isoforms in the myocyte also show isoform-specific differences. The expression of TRα is noted in both the cytosol and the nucleus even at low levels of AdTRα1 or AdTRα2 infection, while the expression of $TR\beta_1$ is predominantly nuclear (cytosolic expression is only noted at multi-

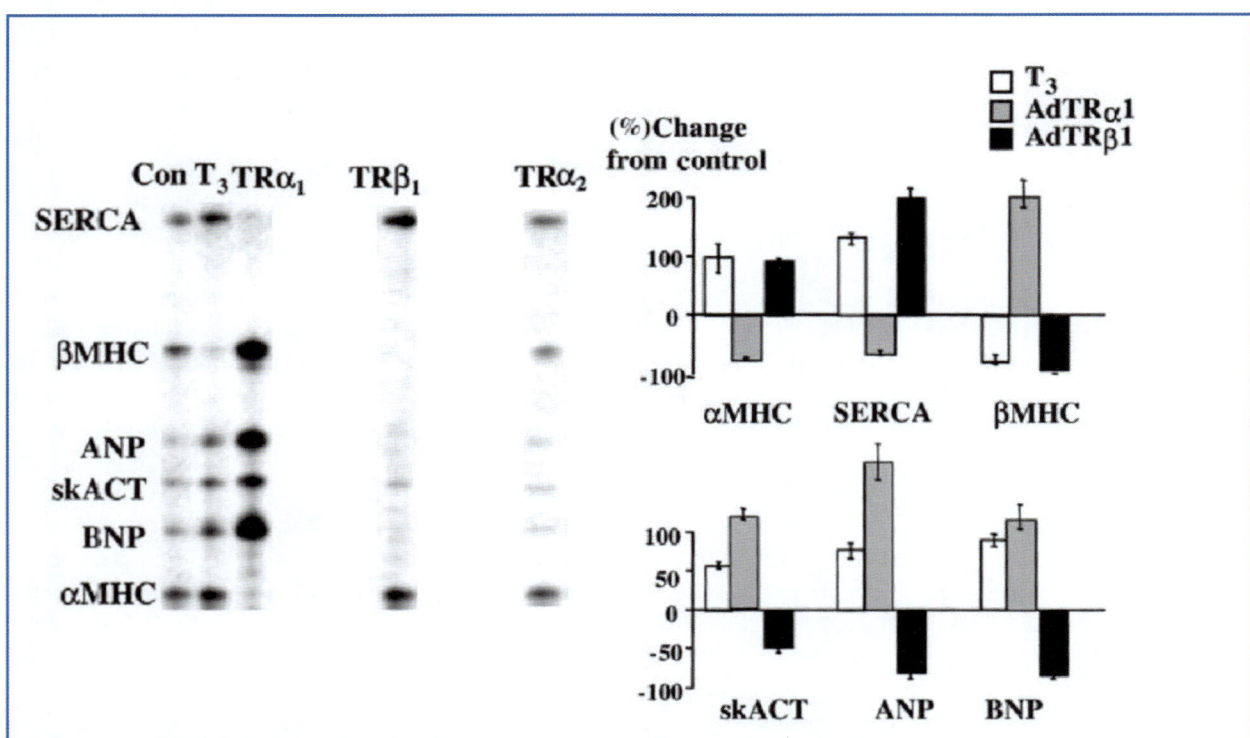

Fig. 8.3 TR-isoform-specific changes in the cardiac myocyte gene program. Cells were treated with AdβGal at 50 multiplicity of infection (MOI), with or without T_3 (100 nM), for 72 h and compared with cells infected with AdTRα1 or AdTRα2, or AdTRβ1 at 50 MOI. Values of the corresponding AdβGal group were set at 100%, and data are presented as percentage change from 100% (n = 3–4); i.e., a value of 0% equals no change from AdβGal-infected cells and 100% represents a doubling of signal. All signals were corrected for RNA loading using an internal GAPDH signal. (Reproduced from [11])

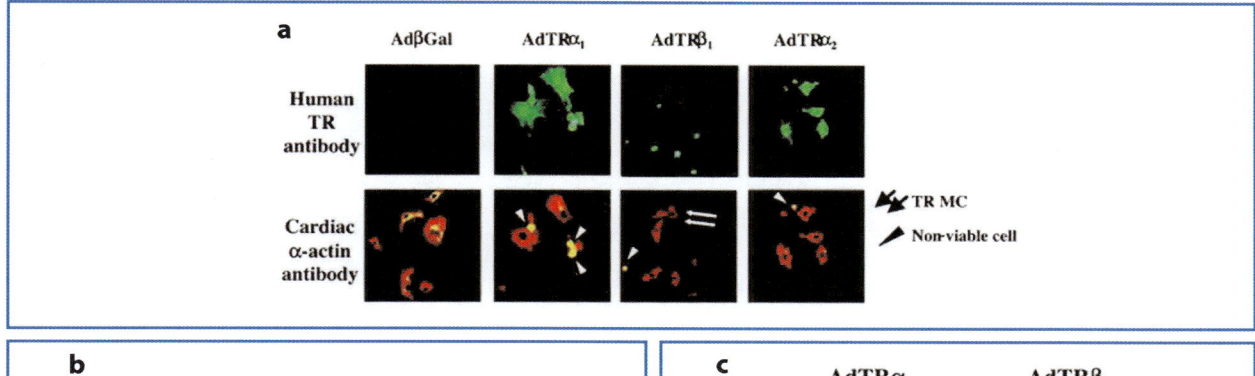

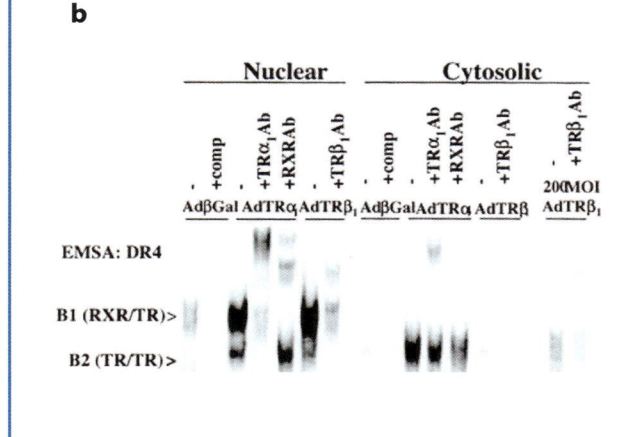

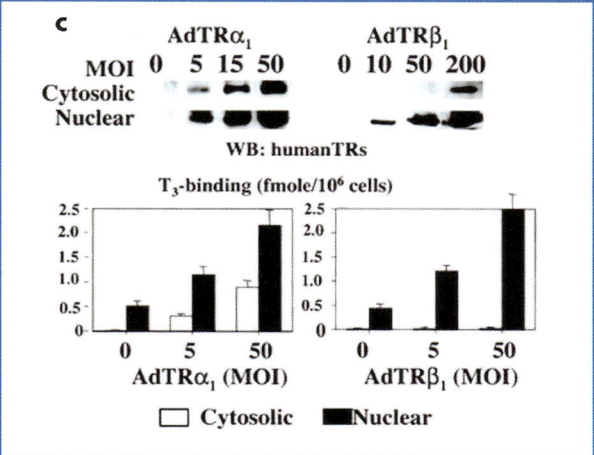

Fig. 8.4 Cardiac myocyte expression of human TRs. **a** Immunostaining. Neonatal rat cardiac myocytes (*MC*) were exposed to adenovirus at 100 MOI for 72 h. Less than 5% of cells were sarcomeric-actin-negative (nonmyocytes). A myocyte without expression of human TRβ1 is identified (*double white arrows*). Note the restriction of TRβ1 expression to the nucleus of these cells while both TRα1 and TRα2 appear to be distributed in nuclear and cytoplasmic compartments. **b** Electrophoretic mobility shift assay for the DR4 (direct repeat-4) thyroid-responsive element (TRE). Cells were exposed to adenovirus at 50 MOI for 48 h. B1 and B2 consist of heterodimers of retinoid X receptor (RXRα, β, or γ) and TR (one molecule of each), and homodimers of TRs (two TR molecules), respectively. No monomer binding was observed. Competitor lanes were with unlabeled oligonucleotide. **c** Quantification and subcellular location of human TR overexpression in neonatal rat cardiac myocytes. Myocytes were infected with the individual AdTRs at the indicated MOIs for 48 h. Fractionated cell extracts were prepared and subjected to Western blotting with human-specific TR antibodies in the *upper panels* (hence no rat TR is detected in uninfected lanes). In the binding experiments, cell extracts from equal numbers of cells were subjected to [^{125}I]T$_3$-binding assay as described previously [33]. Notably, expression of TRα1 was readily found in both nuclear and cytoplasmic fractions, while AdTRβ1 expression was generally limited to the nucleus. (Reproduced from [11])

plicity of infection > 200). Taken together, we conclude that the effects of thyroid hormone involve a complex interaction of different TR isoforms with the genomic effect of T$_3$ being mediated by preferential activity of TRβ1 in the nucleus while the myocyte hypertrophic response is mediated by both cytosolic and nuclear TRα1 effects.

To characterize the mechanism behind thyroid-hormone-mediated myocyte hypertrophy and gene expression in cultured cardiac myocytes, we investigated the interactions of T$_3$ with mitogen-activated protein kinases (MAPK). MAPK comprise three families of protein kinases: extracellular signal-related kinases (ERK), c-Jun N-terminal kinases (JNK), and p38 kinase. All of them have been reported to play a role in myocardial hypertrophy and gene expression. Somewhat unexpectedly, we found that TRα1 interacts with transforming-growth-factor-activating kinase 1 (TAK1), MAPK kinase 3/6 (MKK3/6), and p38MAPK [11], but not with JNK or ERK pathways, and the TRα1 interaction with TAK1 was localized to the cytosol (Fig. 8.5a–c). p38MAPK is a strong inducer of both myocyte hypertrophy and the fetal gene program [29], and in the neonatal cardiac myocyte culture system overexpression of TRα1 leads to expression of the fetal gene program in a p38-dependent pathway [11]. TRα2 also binds TAK1, but the TRα2-TAK1 complex does not activate downstream signaling cascades, consistent with the repressor property of TRα2. On the other hand, we did not observe any TRβ1 interaction with TAK1 in the cytosol (Fig. 8.5a), and its cellular action appears to be exclusively in the nucleus. AdTRβ1 infection results in expression of the adult-specific gene program with attenuation of cardiac hypertrophy (Fig. 8.3

and [11]). Importantly, TRβ1 inhibited p38MAPK activation in the nuclei (Fig. 8.5d,e), indicating that TRβ1 is able to "suppress" the pathological gene expression induced by TRα1/p38MAPK activation. In summary, T3-induced myocyte hypertrophy appears to be mediated by the cytosolic interaction of TRα1 and TAK1/p38MAPK, while the induction of the adult-specific gene profile is due to the nuclear activity of TRβ1, where this TR isoform directly activates the transcription of thyroid-hor-

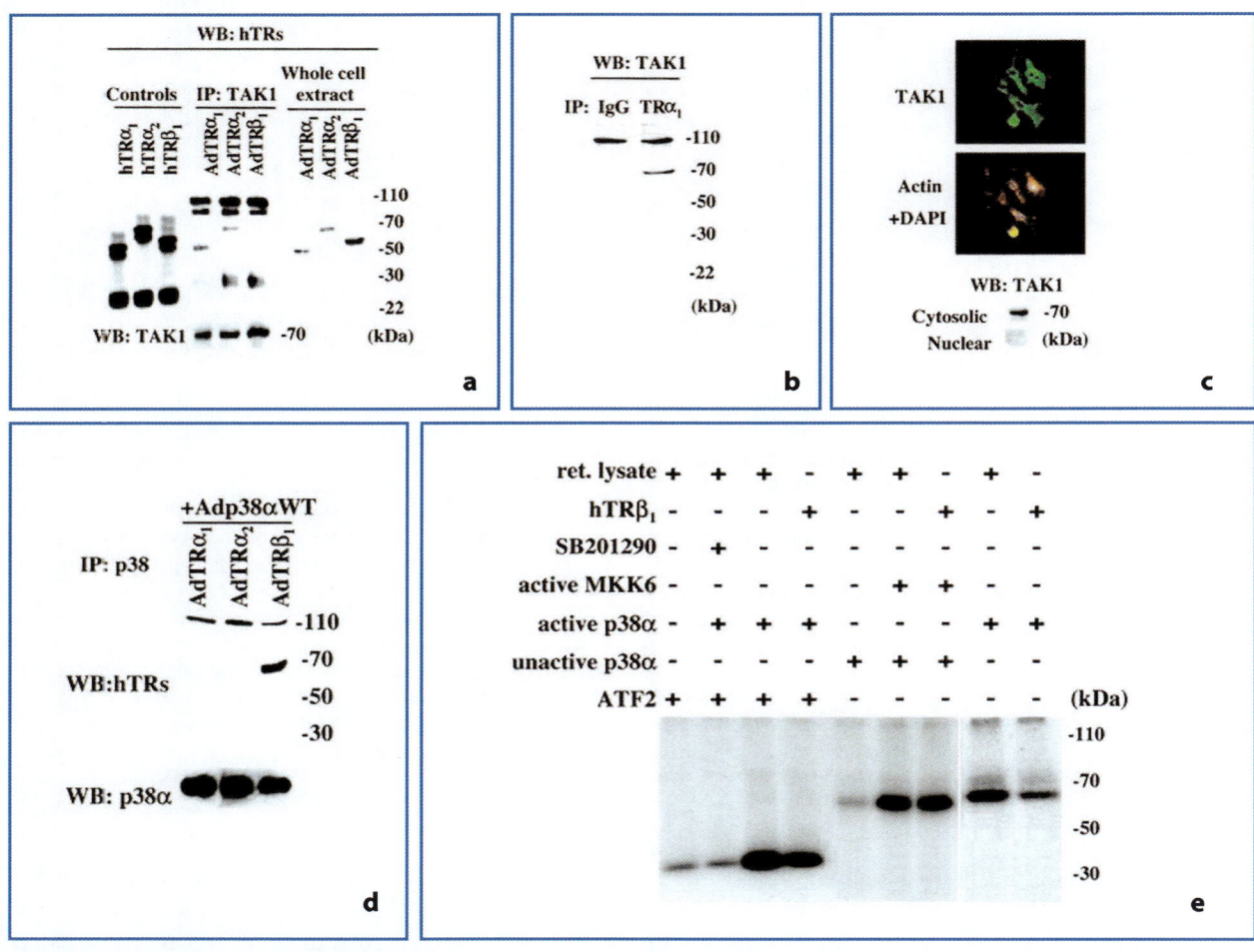

Fig. 8.5 Cytosolic TRα1 interacts with TAK1 (**a–c**) and nuclear TRβ1 inhibits p38 activation (**d, e**). **a** TRα1 and TRα2 , (but not TRβ1) interact with TAK1. *Lanes 1-3* Human-specific TR antibody was validated for Western blotting with control human TRs synthesized in rabbit reticulocyte lysate [TRα1 (~48 kDa), TRα2 (~58 kDa), and TRβ1 (~52 kDa)]. Doublets represent lysate-specific in vitro processing and are not seen in AdTR-infected cells. *Lanes 4-6* Myocytes were infected with AdTRs at 50MOI for 24 h followed by immunoprecipitation of endogenous TAK1. This was subjected to Western blotting for TR. *Lanes 7-9* Expression of human TRs in each sample was confirmed using the same antibody. **b** Whole-cell extract from uninfected cells was immunoprecipitated with rabbit IgG or rat-specific TRα1 antibody, and subjected to Western blotting for TAK1. **c** Western blotting and immunofluorescence microscopy for endogenous cardiac myocyte TAK1 expression. **d, e** TRβ1 (but not TRα1 and TRα2) interacts with p38 and diminishes its kinase activity. Cells were infected with AdTRs and Adp38αWT for 24 h. Total p38 was immunoprecipitated and subjected to Western blotting for human TR (C1). **e** In vitro synthesized human TRβ1 or control rabbit reticulocyte lysate was mixed with active MKK6 or active p38α (~68 kDa and their activities measured on unactive recombinant GST-p38α (~64 kDa) or GST-ATF2 (~40 kDa), respectively. SB202190 was used at 10 Nm

mone-responsive genes and inhibits the pathological effects of p38MAPK.

Although reversing the fetal gene program with thyroid hormone may lead to functional improvement in the failing myocardium, thyroid hormone also possesses deleterious effects on the heart that may limit its therapeutic use for clinical heart failure (tachycardia, increased oxygen consumption, arrhythmogenesis). It is tempting to speculate that targeting the TH:TR axis and/or use of specific TR agonists will thwart the deleterious effects of thyroid hormone treatment in heart failure while maintaining the salutary effects on gene program and myocardial function (reviewed in [30, 31]). In this regard, further studies are needed to clearly identify the extent to which TRα_1 interacts with TAK1 and other kinases. Considering the variety of cellular action of thyroid hormone, it will be important to identify cytosolic TR interactions with other signaling molecules. Better characterization of cytosolic activity and identification of specific nuclear TRβ1-specific agonism may provide novel treatment strategies for heart failure. This latter possibility is particularly germane as TR-specific agonists are currently being explored clinically for their metabolic effects (reviewed in [32]).

8.5 Conclusions

The fetal gene program is an important feature of the failing heart, resembles the gene expression pattern seen in the hypothyroid heart, and is also associated with decreased expression of functional TRs themselves. In contrast, physiological hypertrophy exhibits a more "hyperthyroid-like" gene program and is accompanied by the increased expression of specific functional TRs. Expression of individual TR isoforms in a cell culture model of cardiac myocyte hypertrophy indicates that there are isoform-specific effects on both cardiac myocyte growth and the gene program. This work indicates that nuclear TRs are critically important for specific gene regulation; thyroid-hormone-induced hypertrophy is mediated, at least in part, by cytosolic TR (α_1) as a function of its ability to bind to and activate members of the p38MAPK signaling cascade. As heart failure is a clinical syndrome of ever increasing importance around the world, the development of novel approaches to this problem that target alterations in the cardiac myocyte gene program by directly promoting a more physiological response in terms of myocyte contractility will be a welcome addition.

Key Points

- The gene expression pattern in the hypertrophied and failing heart is frequently called the fetal gene program and is similar to that seen in hypothyroidism.

- Thyroid receptor expression is altered in the failing human heart and in several experimental models of pathological growth.

- Thyroid hormone treatment induces the expression of a physiological gene program in the cardiac myocyte and is associated with enhanced contractility.

- Individual thyroid receptors exhibit isoform-specific effects on cardiac myocyte growth and the gene program in cell culture.

- The TRα_1 isoform has a direct nongenomic effect on cardiac myocyte growth through its binding to an upstream member of the p38MAPK family TAK1.

- The TRβ_1 isoform does not bind TAK1 and has genomic effects that result in a more physiological gene program with little hypertrophic growth.

- Exploiting isoform-specific effects of thyroid hormone receptors on the cardiac myocyte may represent a unique therapeutic approach to the clinical syndrome of heart failure.

References

1. van Bilsen M and Chien KR, (1993) Growth and hypertrophy of the heart: towards an understanding of cardiac specific and inducible gene expression. Cardiovasc Res 27:1140–1149

2. Nakao K, Minobe W, Roden R et al (1997) Myosin heavy chain gene expression in human heart failure. J Clin Invest 100:2362–2370

3. Lowes BD, Minobe W, Abraham WT et al (1997) Changes in gene expression in the intact human heart. Downregulation of alpha-myosin heavy chain in hypertrophied, failing ventricular myocardium. J Clin Invest 100:2315–2324

4. Miyata S, Minobe W, Bristow MR et al (2000) Myosin heavy chain isoform expression in the failing and nonfailing human heart. Circ Res 86:386–390

5. Lowes BD, Gilbert EM, Abraham WT et al (2002) Myocardial gene expression in dilated cardiomyopathy treated with beta-blocking agents. N Engl J Med 346:1357–1365

6. Dillmann WH (1990) Biochemical basis of thyroid hormone action in the heart. Am J Med 88:626–630

7. Klein I, Ojamaa K (2001) Thyroid hormone and the cardiovascular system. N Engl J Med 344:501–509

8. van Tuyl M, Blommaart PE, de Boer PA et al (2004) Prenatal exposure to thyroid hormone is necessary for normal postnatal development of murine heart and lungs. Dev Biol 272:104–117

9. Lazar MA (1993) Thyroid hormone receptors: multiple forms, multiple possibilities. Endocr Rev 14:184–193

10. Ribeiro RC, Apriletti JW, West BL et al (1995) The molecular biology of thyroid hormone action. Ann N Y Acad Sci 758:366–389

11. Kinugawa K, Jeong MY, Bristow MR et al (2005) Thyroid hormone induces cardiac myocyte hypertrophy in a thyroid hormone receptor alpha1-specific manner that requires TAK1 and p38 mitogen-activated protein kinase. Mol Endocrinol 19:1618–1628

12. Xu L, Glass CK and Rosenfeld MG (1999) Coactivator and corepressor complexes in nuclear receptor function. Curr Opin Genet Dev 9:140–147

13. Morkin E (1993) Regulation of myosin heavy chain genes in the heart. Circulation 87:1451–1460

14. Izumo S, Nadal-Ginard B, Mahdavi V (1988) Protooncogene induction and reprogramming of cardiac gene expression produced by pressure overload. Proc Natl Acad Sci U S A 85:339–343

15. Chang KC, Figueredo VM, Schreur JHM et al (1997) Thyroid hormone improves function and Ca2+ handing in pressure overload hypertrophy: association with increased sarcoplasmic reticulum Ca2+-ATPase and a-myosin heavy chain in rat hearts. J Clin Invest 100:1742–1749

16. Kinugawa K, Yonekura K, Ribeiro RC et al (2001) Regulation of thyroid hormone receptor isoforms in physiological and pathological cardiac hypertrophy. Circ Res 89:591–598

17. Crawford MH and O'Rourke RA (1979) The athlete's heart. Adv Intern Med 24:311–329

18. Bristow MR (1998) Why does the myocardium fail? Insights from basic science. Lancet 352(Suppl 1):SI8–14

19. Inesi G, Prasad AM, Pilankatta R (2008) The Ca2+ ATPase of cardiac sarcoplasmic reticulum: physiological role and relevance to diseases. Biochem Biophys Res Commun 369:182–187

20. Izumo S, Lompre AM, Matsuoka R et al (1987) Myosin heavy chain messenger RNA and protein isoform transitions during cardiac hypertrophy: interaction between hemodynamic and thyroid hormone-induced signals. J Clin Invest 79:970–977

21. Weiss RE, Refetoff S (2000) Resistance to thyroid hormone. Rev Endocr Metab Disord 1:97–108

22. Izumo S, Mahdavi V (1988) Thyroid hormone receptor alpha isoforms generated by alternative splicing differentially activate myosin HC gene transcription [published erratum appears in Nature (1988) 335:744]. Nature 334:539–542

23. Kinugawa K, Minobe WA, Wood WM et al (2001) Signaling pathways responsible for fetal gene induction in the failing human heart:evidence for altered thyroid hormone receptor gene expression. Circulation 103:1089–1094

24. Simoncini T, Hafezi-Moghadam A, Brazil DP et al (2000) Interaction of oestrogen receptor with the regulatory subunit of phosphatidylinositol-3-OH kinase. Nature 407:538–541

25. Chen Z, Yuhanna IS, Galcheva-Gargova Z et al (1999) Estrogen receptor alpha mediates the nongenomic activation of endothelial nitric oxide synthase by estrogen. J Clin Invest 103:401–406

26. Davis PJ, Davis FB (1996) Nongenomic actions of thyroid hormone. Thyroid 6:497–504

27. Hiroi Y, Kim HH, Ying H et al (2006) Rapid nongenomic actions of thyroid hormone. Proc Natl Acad Sci U S A 103:14104–14109

28. Chiellini G, Apriletti JW, Yoshihara H et al (1998) A high-affinity subtype-selective agonist ligand for the thyroid hormone receptor. Chem Biol 5:299–306

29. Sugden PH (2001) Signalling pathways in cardiac myocyte hypertrophy. Ann Med 33:611–622

30. Pantos C, Mourouzis I, Xinaris C et al (2008) Thyroid hormone and "cardiac metamorphosis": potential therapeutic implications. Pharmacol Ther 118:277–294

31. Pingitore A, Iervasi G (2008) Triiodothyronine (T3) effects on cardiovascular system in patients with heart failure. Recent Patents Cardiovasc Drug Discov 3:19–27

32. Brenta G, Danzi S, Klein I (2007) Potential therapeutic applications of thyroid hormone analogs. Nat Clin Pract Endocrinol Metab 3:632–640

33. Ribeiro RC, Apriletti JW, Yen PM et al (1994) Heterodimerization and deoxyribonucleic acid-binding properties of a retinoid X receptor-related factor. Endocrinology 135:2076–2085

Pharmacological Effects of Amiodarone and Dronedarone on Cardiac Thyroid Hormone Receptors

9

Wilmar M. Wiersinga

Abstract Amiodarone, via its main metabolite desethylamiodarone, exerts competitive inhibition of T_3 binding to thyroid hormone receptor protein α_1 ($TR\alpha_1$) and noncompetitive inhibition of T_3 binding to thyroid hormone receptor protein β_1 ($TR\beta_1$) in vitro. Dronedarone, via its main metabolite debutyldronedarone, exerts competitive inhibition of T_3 binding to $TR\alpha_1$ in vitro, but not of T_3 binding to $TR\beta_1$. Mechanisms of inhibition of T_3-dependent gene expression by desethylamiodarone include inhibition of T_3 binding to TR, inhibition of coactivator binding to TR, and inhibition of TR binding to the thyroid hormone response element (TRE). Tissue concentrations of desethylamiodarone and debutyldronedarone obtained in vivo are of the same order of magnitude as their IC_{50} values for inhibition of T_3 binding to TR obtained in vitro. Experimental animal studies demonstrated that amiodarone acts as an antagonist to both $TR\alpha_1$ and $TR\beta_1$ in vivo, whereas dronedarone acts as a selective $TR\alpha_1$ antagonist. Amiodarone induces a local hypothyroid condition in the heart, evident from a lower heart rate, lengthening of the QTc interval, and decreased SERCA2a and αMHC and increased βMHC gene expression (all closely resembling the changes in systemic hypothyroidism). Dronedarone may also act by inducing a local hypothyroid-like condition in the heart, evident from a lower heart rate, lengthening of the QTc interval, and decreased αMHC gene expression (all $TR\alpha_1$-mediated), although it does not change SERCA2a and βMHC gene expression (which are $TR\beta_1$-mediated).

Keywords Amiodarone • Dronedarone • Thyroid hormone receptor • Receptor antagonist • Heart • Electrocardiogram • Myosin heavy chain • Sarcoplasmic reticulum Ca^{2+} ATPase • Liver • LDL receptor • Iodothyronine-5^1-deiodinase

9.1 Introduction

Amiodarone was introduced in the early 1970s as an anti-anginal drug [1] but is nowadays mostly used as a highly effective antiarrhythmic drug for the treatment of atrial and ventricular cardiac rhythm disturbances [2]. Amiodarone contains 37% organic iodine by weight. During biotransformation of the drug, pharmacological quantities of iodine are released, giving rise to iodine excess. In susceptible patients, iodine excess may cause iodide-induced hypothyroidism or iodide-induced thyrotoxicosis. A destructive type of thyrotoxicosis is frequently seen, caused by the cytotoxic effects of amiodarone and its main metabolite desethylamiodarone (DEA) on thyrocytes [3]. Dronedarone, a new antiarrhythmic drug that is structurally related to amiodarone (Fig. 9.1), lacks an iodine moiety and thus amiodarone's iodine-related organ toxicity. Electrophysiological

W.M. Wiersinga (✉)
Department of Endocrinology and Metabolism, Academic Medical Center, University of Amsterdam, Amsterdam, The Netherlands

G. Iervasi, A. Pingitore (eds.), *Thyroid and Heart Failure*.

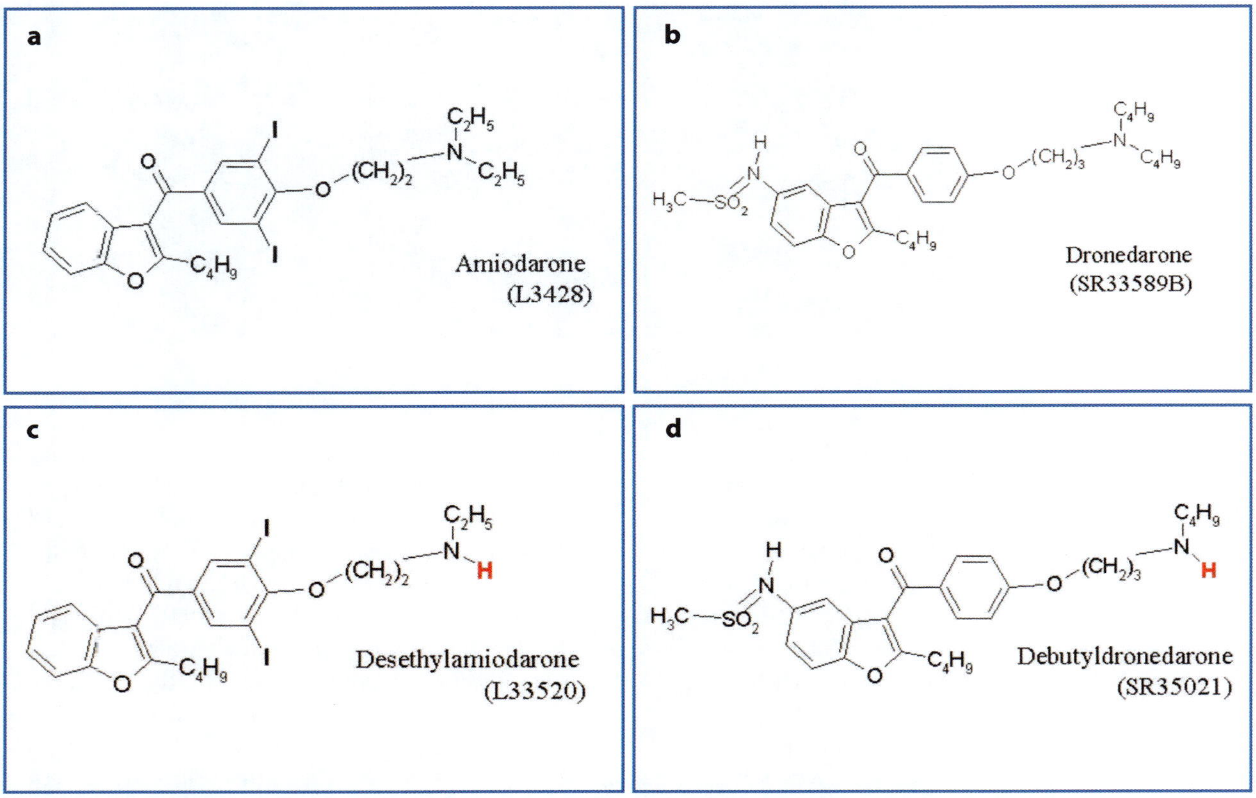

Fig. 9.1 Chemical structures of amiodarone, dronedarone, and their main metabolites desethylamiodarone and debutyldronedarone

studies showed that drone-darone shares amiodarone's multichannel blocking effects, inhibiting transmembrane Na^+, K^+, and Ca^{2+} channels, and slow L-type calcium channels, as well as its antiadrenergic effects [4]. Drone-darone possesses both rate-control and rhythm-control properties and has proved safe and effective in preventing recurrence of atrial fibrillation. So far, no association has been reported between drone-darone treatment and the occurrence of hypo- or hyperthyroidism.

Early on, similarities were observed between the effects of amiodarone treatment and hypothyroidism. Both conditions induce bradycardia, lengthening of the cardiac action potential, and depression of myocardial oxygen consumption. It has therefore been hypothesized that the cardiac effects of amiodarone can be explained–at least partly–by the induction of a local hypothyroid-like condition in the heart [1]. The cardiac effects of amiodarone are observed in all patients treated with the drug irrespective of ambient thyroid-stimulating hormone (TSH) levels, and thus have nothing to do with the occasionally observed direct effects of amiodarone on the thyroid gland resulting in sys-

temic hypothyroidism. Possible mechanisms by which amiodarone may induce cardiac hypothyroidism are inhibition of conversion of T_4 into the active hormone T_3 by 5^1-deiodinase, inhibition of transport of T_4 and T_3 through the plasma membrane, inhibition of T_3 binding to its nuclear receptors, and down-regulation of specific isoforms of the nuclear thyroid hormone receptors [5]. In this chapter, we review the effects of amiodarone and dronedarone with regard to thyroid hormone receptors (TR), specifically in the heart.

9.2 In Vitro Inhibition of T_3 Binding to TR

DEA, but not amiodarone, inhibits the binding of T_3 to the thyroid hormone receptor protein β_1 (TRβ_1) in vitro [6]. Lineweaver–Burk analysis indicates noncompetitive inhibition. Plots of the intercepts of Lineweaver–Burk plots versus DEA concentration are linear, giving a K_i of 30 μM for the binding of DEA to the occupied receptor. Plots of the slopes versus inhibitor concentration are parabolic, indicating a progressively stronger effect of DEA on the unoccupied receptor as concentrations rise. This preference for the unoccupied receptor is reflected in experiments that show a progressive loss of T_3 binding when the receptor is incubated for increasing periods with DEA before T_3 is added. DEA, but not amiodarone, likewise decreases the binding of T_3 to the thyroid hormone receptor α_1 (TRα_1) in vitro in a dose-dependent manner. However, Lineweaver–Burk plots clearly indicate competitive inhibition by DEA with regard to TRα_1 [7].

In vitro experiments with dronedarone revealed that dronedarone has no effect on the binding of T_3 to TRβ_1; at a high concentration of 100 μM, it decreases T_3 binding to TRα_1 by 14%. The major metabolite of dronedarone, debutyldronedarone, is much more potent than the parent drug: at 100 μM it decreases T_3 binding to TRα_1 by 77% and to TRβ_1 by 25% [8]. The decrease in binding is dose-dependent, and Langmuir analysis indicated that inhibition of T_3 binding to TRα_1 by debutyldronedarone is competitive in nature. IC_{50} values are given in Table 9.1.

Taken together, the results of in vitro experiments can be summarized as follows:

1. The major metabolites DEA and debutyldronedarone, rather than their respective parent drugs amiodarone and dronedarone, are capable of inhibiting the binding of T_3 to TR.
2. DEA is a more potent inhibitor than debutyldronedarone, and inhibition of T_3 binding to TRα_1 is more pronounced than inhibition of its binding to TRβ_1.
3. DEA and debutyldronedarone are competitive inhibitors of T_3 binding to TRα_1 but DEA is a noncompetitive inhibitor of T_3 binding to TRβ_1.
4. DEA is an effective antagonist of T_3 binding to TRα_1 and TRβ_1, but debutyldronedarone appears to be a selective TRα_1 antagonist.

Table 9.1 IC_{50} values for inhibitory effects of desethylamiodarone and debutyldronedarone on the binding of T_3 to thyroid hormone receptors α_1 (TRα_1) and β_1 (TRβ_1)[a]

	Desethyl-amiodarone	Debutyl-dronedarone	
TRα1	30 ± 3.9	59 ± 4.1	$p < 0.01$
TRβ1	71 ± 3.4	280 ± 29	$p < 0.01$
	$p < 0.01$	$p < 0.01$	

[a] IC_{50} values (μM) are given as mean ± standard error of the mean [6–8]

9.3 In Vitro Studies on the Mechanism of Inhibition

To gain further insight into the inhibition by DEA of T_3 binding to TRα_1 and TRβ_1, we studied the effects of various amiodarone analogs and of various mutations in TRβ_1. The results of experiments with amiodarone analogs on the structure–function relationship of inhibition of T_3 binding to TR implied that (1) the size of the diethyl-substituted nitrogen group and of the two bulky iodine atoms in the amiodarone molecule hamper the binding of amiodarone at the T_3 binding site of TR, and (2) differences in the hormone-binding domain of TRα_1 and TRβ_1 likely to account for the competitive or noncompetitive nature of inhibition of T_3 binding by amiodarone analogs [9]. To gain insight into the position of the binding site of DEA on TRβ_1, we investigated naturally occurring and artificial mutants in the ligand-binding domain of TRβ_1. Mutant E457A causes a change from a negatively charged amino acid to a hydrophobic amino acid, enhancing the affinity for DEA. Mutant R429Q, located in helix 11, causes an electrostatic potential change from positive to uncharged, also resulting in greater affinity for DEA. Inhibition of T_3 binding to mutated TRβ_1 by DEA was noncompetitive in nature, with IC_{50} values (17 ± 3 μM for E457A, and 32 ± 7 μM for R429Q) significantly lower than those of the wild-type (56 ± 15 μM) [10]. It is postulated that aminoacids R429 and E457 are at or close to the binding site for DEA, and that DEA does not bind in the T_3 binding pocket itself, in line with the noncompetitive nature of the inhibition of T_3 binding to TRβ_1 by DEA.

The binding site of DEA may thus be on the outside surface of the TRβ_1 protein, overlapping the regions where coactivators and corepressors bind. Here, DEA could influence the interaction of TRβ_1 with coactivator GRIP1 (glucocorticoid receptor interacting protein-1). The T_3-dependent binding of GRIP1 to TRβ_1 is indeed disrupted by DEA [11]. A DEA dose experiment showed that DEA acts like an antagonist under "normal" conditions (at 0.1 μM T_3 and 5 DEA μmol/l) but as an agonist under extreme conditions (at 0 and 1 nM T_3 and > 0.1 mM DEA). Comparable results are obtained in NIH3T3 cells transiently transfected with TRβ and the reporter construct ME-TRE-TK-CAT (containing the nucleotide sequence of the thyroid hormone response element TRE of malic enzyme ME, thymidine kinase, and chloramphenicol acyltransferase) [12]. ME-TRE-TK-CAT activity is increased 12.5-fold by the addition of 1 T_3 µmol/l to the culture medium, 3.4-fold by the addition of 1 DEA µmol/l, and 18.9-fold by the addition of both T_3 and DEA. The data suggest a synergistic effect of DEA with T_3 on ME-TRE rather than the postulated inhibitory action, most likely caused by overexpression of transfected TR into the cells. In experiments with a limited amount of $TR\beta_1$, addition of 1 DEA µmol/l decreased T_3-dependent expression of the reporter gene by 50%. The inhibiting effect of DEA was partially due to a reduced binding of TR to ME-TRE, as assessed by gel mobility shift assay.

It appears that DEA can act as an agonist or as an antagonist with regard to TR depending on the ambient concentrations of the drug itself, T_3, and TR. The conditions encountered in the living organism favor an antagonistic effect of DEA. First, DEA concentrations in rat tissues after treatment with amiodarone 100 mg/kg per day orally for 2 weeks are in the micromolar range (liver 18 µmol/kg, heart 14 µmol/kg), close to the IC_{50} values of DEA [13]. Human tissue samples obtained at autopsy from patients treated with amiodarone also display high DEA concentrations (liver 3815 µmol/kg, heart 274 µmol/kg) [3]. Second, T_3 concentrations in rat tissues after treatment with amiodarone 30 mg/kg per day orally for 3 weeks are four to five times lower than in control animals (liver 2 vs. 10 nmol/kg, heart 1 vs. 4 nmol/kg) [14]. The occupancy of nuclear T_3 receptors by hormone will be rather low in all likelihood, favoring the inhibitory effect of DEA [6, 7]. Third, $TR\alpha_1$ and $TR\beta_1$ gene expression is decreased in the atria and ventricles of rats treated with amiodarone or dronedarone [15]. It should be added that inhibition of 5^1-deiodinase alone cannot explain all the effects of amiodarone treatment: administration of iopanoic acid, a drug exerting similar inhibitory effects on 5^1-deiodinase, reproduces the effects of amiodarone only in part [16].

In summary then, the results of in vitro studies suggest several mechanisms by which DEA could induce a local hypothyroid-like condition in the heart:
1. Dose-dependent inhibition of T_3 binding to TR, enhanced by low ambient tissue T_3 concentrations
2. Dose-dependent inhibition of coactivator binding to TR
3. Dose-dependent inhibition of TR binding to TRE
It has not been studied whether the same mech-

anisms operate with respect to debutyldronedarone, except for its demonstrated inhibitory effect on T_3 binding to $TR\alpha_1$. Treatment with dronedarone does not appear to influence 5^1-deiodinase [8].

9.4 In Vivo Studies Comparing Amiodarone and Dronedarone

Experimental animal studies have tested two hypotheses. Based upon the in vitro inhibitory effects on nuclear T_3 binding, the first hypothesis was that amiodarone, via its metabolite DEA, acts as a $TR\alpha_1$ and $TR\beta_1$ antagonist in vivo and that dronedarone, via its metabolite debutyldronedarone, acts as a selective $TR\alpha_1$ antagonist. Based on similarities in the cardiac effects of amiodarone and hypothyroidism, the second hypothesis was that both amiodarone and dronedarone induce a local hypothyroid-like condition in the heart.

The first hypothesis was tested by treating rats with either amiodarone or dronedarone (100 mg/kg per day orally for both drugs) for 2 weeks and comparing T_3-dependent TR-isoform-specific gene expression in liver and heart [8]. In the liver, $TR\beta_1$ is much more abundant than $TR\alpha_1$. Expression of the LDL receptor gene [17, 18] and 5^1-deiodinase activity [19] are T_3-dependent and mediated mainly by $TR\beta_1$. Amiodarone but not dronedarone would be expected to reduce the concentration and activity of these liver proteins. In the heart, $TR\alpha_1$ represents 70% and $TR\beta_1$ the remaining 30% of TR in ventricular myocytes [20]. The heart–in contrast to the liver–is thus viewed as a $TR\alpha_1$-predominant organ. Heart rate and the QTc interval on the electrocardiogram are both influenced by T_3, an effect mediated via $TR\alpha_1$ [21, 22]. The expectation is that amiodarone and dronedarone would lower heart rate and lengthen the QTc interval to a similar extent. In the liver, the results were as expected. Amiodarone but not dronedarone treatment decreased LDL receptor protein concentration and thereby increased serum total and LDL cholesterol. Also, amiodarone but not dronedarone treatment reduced liver 5^1-deiodinase activity associated with a decrease in serum T_3. On the ECG, QTc interval was indeed similarly lengthened in amiodarone-treated and dronedarone-treated animals (0.141 vs. 0.142 ms, respectively) as compared to controls (0.114 ms). Heart rate in the amiodarone group was also lower than in controls (351 vs. 382 beats per minute, respectively). Heart rate in the dronedarone group was not lower than in controls (390 vs. 382 bpm) in this study [8], but in another study it was (296 vs. 381 bpm) [23]. Tissue concentrations of dronedarone and debutyldronedarone are known from animal studies in rabbits treated with dronedarone 20 mg/kg per day orally for 3 weeks [24]. The myocardial dronedarone content is 23 μmol/kg, and of debutyldronedarone 6 μmol/kg of the same order of magnitude as amiodarone and DEA concentrations in rat hearts. In view of the higher doses of dronedarone, 90–100 mg/kg per day given orally for 2 weeks [8, 23], it is likely that debutyldronedarone tissue concentrations were sufficiently high to exert an antagonistic effect on $TR\alpha_1$. The collective data support the hypothesis that amiodarone (via DEA) acts as a $TR\alpha_1$ and $TR\beta_1$ antagonist in vivo and that dronedarone (via debutyldronedarone) acts as a selective $TR\alpha_1$ antagonist.

The second hypothesis was explored by evaluating the effect of amiodarone and dronedarone on T_3-dependent expression of a number of cardiac genes involved in cardiac contractility. T_3-responsive genes in cardiac myocytes include sarcoplasmic reticulum Ca^{2+}-ATPase (SERCA2a) and its inhibitor phospholamban (which regulate the uptake of calcium into the sarcoplasmic reticulum during diastole), α-myosin heavy chain (αMHC), the fast myosin with higher ATPase activity, and β-myosin heavy chain (βMHC), the slow myosin [2]. Administration of T_3 results in up-regulation of SERCA2 and αMHC and down-regulation of βMHC [25]. The opposite is observed in hypothyroidism: down-regulation of SERCA2 and αMHC and up-regulation of βMHC [23, 26]. The decreased cardiac contractility associated with hypothyroidism results in part from changes in the expression of these cardiac genes [2]. Previous studies suggested that $TR\alpha_1$ is linked to αMHC transcription and $TR\beta_1$ to βMHC and SERCA2 [27]. One would thus expect amiodarone treatment to be associated with down-regulation of SERCA2 and αMHC and up-regulation of βMHC, whereas dronedarone treatment would result in down-regulation of αMHC only.

Amiodarone treatment in rats (100 mg/kg per day orally for 2 weeks) decreased SERCA2 and αMHC and increased βMHC gene expression in the heart relative to controls [8], which is in agreement with other reports in the literature [26, 28]. Dronedarone treatment in rats (90–100 mg/kg per day orally for 2 weeks) had no effect on SERCA2

and βMHC, but decreased αMHC in one study [8, 23]. The results once again underline the inhibitory effects of amiodarone mediated by $TR\alpha_1$ and $TR\beta_1$, whereas antagonism of dronedarone is restricted to $TR\alpha_1$. The studies further support the hypothesis that a local hypothyroid-like condition in the heart is induced by amiodarone. Hypothyroidism has been associated with increased tolerance of the myocardium to ischemia. Propylthiouracil-induced hypothyroidism results in increased postischemic functional recovery of isolated rat hearts, which may–at least partly–be attributed to tissue hypothyroidism [29]. This in turn may be explained by less energy consumption in the hypothyroid myocardium due to predominant expression of slow βMHC, while myocardial glycogen content is increased. Decreased energy demands and increased energy availability are the main mechanisms of protection by hypothyroidism.

Whether dronedarone also induces a local hypothyroid-like condition in the heart is less clear. Although the lower heart rate, the lengthening of the QTc interval, and the fall in αMHC resemble hypothyroidism, βMHC and SERCA2 levels do not change (Table 9.2). However, Pantos et al. observed a higher myocardial glycogen content in dronedarone-treated rats (just as in hypothyroid rats) relative to controls [23]. In addition, they noted reduced contractility, suppression of ischemic contracture, and a decrease of postischemic left ventricular end-diastolic pressure and lactate dehydrogenase release after ischemia–reperfusion in dronedarone-treated animals. These authors thus concluded that dronedarone treatment results in cardioprotection by selectively mimicking hypothyroidism.

Table 9.2 Influence of hypothyroidism, amiodarone, and dronedarone on T3-dependent cardiac effects

	Hypothyroidism	Amiodarone	Dronedarone
$TR\alpha_1$-mediated effects			
Heart rate	Lower	Lower	Lower
QTc interval	Longer	Longer	Longer
αMHC	Lower	Lower	Lower
$TR\beta_1$-mediated effects			
βMHC	Higher	Higher	No change
SERCA2	Lower	Lower	No change

Key Points

- Amiodarone, via its main metabolite desethylamiodarone, exerts competitive inhibition of T_3 binding to $TR\alpha_1$ and noncompetitive inhibition of T_3 binding to $TR\beta_1$ in vitro.

- Dronedarone, via its main metabolite debutyldronedarone, exerts competitive inhibition of T_3 binding to $TR\alpha_1$ in vitro, but not of T_3 binding to $TR\beta_1$.

- Mechanisms of inhibition of T_3-dependent gene expression by desethylamiodarone include inhibition of T_3 binding to TR, inhibition of coactivator binding to TR, and inhibition of TR binding to TRE.

- Tissue concentrations of desethylamiodarone and debutyldronedarone obtained in vivo are of the same order of magnitude as their IC_{50} values for inhibition of T_3 binding to TR obtained in vitro.

- Experimental animal studies demonstrated that amiodarone acts as an antagonist to both $TR\alpha_1$ and $TR\beta_1$ in vivo, whereas dronedarone acts a selective $TR\alpha_1$ antagonist.

- Amiodarone induces a local hypothyroid condition in the heart, evident from a lower heart rate, lengthening of the QTc interval, and decreased SERCA2a and αMHC and increased βMHC gene expression (all closely resembling changes in systemic hypothyroidism).

- Dronedarone may also act by inducing a local hypothyroid-like condition in the heart, evident from a lower heart rate, lengthening of the QTc interval, and decreased αMHC expression (all $TR\alpha_1$-mediated), although it does not change SERCA2a and βMHC gene expression (which are $TR\beta_1$-mediated).

References

1. Singh BN, Vaughan Williams EM (1970) The effect of amiodarone, a new anti-anginal drug, on cardiac muscle. Br J Pharmacol 39:657–667
2. Klein I, Danzi S (2007) Thyroid disease and the heart. Circulation 116:1725–1735
3. Wiersinga WM (1997) Amiodarone and the thyroid. In: Weetman AP, Grossman A (ed) Pharmacotherapeutics of the thyroid gland. Handbook of experimental pharmacology, vol 128. Springer, Berlin, pp 225–287
4. Wegener FT, Ehrlich JR, Hohnloser SH (2006) Dronedarone: an emerging agent with rhythm- and rate- controlling effects. J Cardiovasc Electrophysiol 17(Suppl 2):S17-S20
5. Kahaly GJ, Dillman W (2005) Thyroid hormone action in the heart. Endocr Rev 26:704–728
6. Bakker O, van Beeren HC, Wiersinga WM (1994) Desethylamiodarone is a noncompetitive inhibitor of the binding of thyroid hormone to the thyroid hormone β_1-receptor protein. Endocrinology 134:1665–1670
7. Van Beeren HC, Bakker O, Wiersinga WM (1995) Desethylamiodarone is a competitive inhibitor of the binding of thyroid hormone to the thyroid hormone α_1-receptor protein. Mol Cell Endocrinol 112:15–19
8. Van Beeren HC, Jong WM, Kaptein E et al (2003) Dronedarone acts as a selective inhibitor of $3,5,3^1$-triiodothyronine binding to thyroid hormone receptor-alpha 1: in vitro and in vivo evidence. Endocrinology 144:552–558
9. Van Beeren HC, Bakker O, Wiersinga WM (1996) Structure–function relationship of the inhibition of the $3,5,3^1\alpha$-triiodothyronine binding to the alpha 1- and beta 1-thyroid hormone receptor by amiodarone analogs. Endocrinology 137:2807–2814
10. Van Beeren HC, Bakker O, Chatterjee VK, Wiersinga WM (1999) Effect of mutations in the beta 1-thyroid hormone receptor on the inhibition of T3 binding by desethylamiodarone. FEBS Lett 450:35–38
11. Van Beeren HC, Bakker O, Wiersinga WM (2000) Desethylamiodarone interferes with the binding of co-activator GRIP to the beta 1 thyroid hormone receptor. FEBS Lett 481:213–216
12. Bogazzi F, Bartalena L, Brogioni S et al (2001) Desethylamiodarone antagonizes the effect of thyroid hormone at the molecular level. Eur J Endocrinol 145:59–64
13. Plomp TA, Wiersinga WM, Maes RA (1985) Tissue distribution of amiodarone and desethylamiodarone in rats after repeated oral administration of various amiodarone dosages. Arzneimittelforschung 35:1805–1810
14. Schröder-van der Elst JP, van der Heide D (1990) Thyroxine, T3, and reverse T3 concentrations in several tissues of the rat: effects of amiodarone and desethylamiodarone on thyroid hormone metabolism. Endocrinology 127:1656–1664
15. Stoykov I, Van Beeren HC, Moorman AF et al (2007) Effect of amiodarone and dronedarone administration in rats on thyroid hormone-dependent gene expression in different cardiac components. Eur J Endocrinol 156:695–702

16. Meese R, Smitherman TC, Croft CH et al (1985) Effect of peripheral thyroid hormone metabolism on cardiac arrhythmias. Am J Cardiol 55:849–851

17. Hudig F, Bakker O, Wiersinga WM (1998) Amiodarone decreases gene expression of low-density lipoprotein receptor at both the mRNA and the protein level. Metabolism 47:1052–1057

18. Bakker O, Hudig F, Meyssen S, Wiersinga WM (1998) Effects of triiodothyronine and amiodarone on the promotor of the human LDL receptor gene. Biochem Biophys Res Commun 249:517–521

19. Yu J, Koenig RJ (2000) Regulation of hepatocyte thyroxine 5^1-deiodinase by T3 and nuclear receptor coactivators as a model of the sick euthyroid syndrome. J Biol Chem 275:38296–38301

20. Swanson EA, Gloss B, Belke D et al (2003) Cardiac expression and function of thyroid hormone receptor β and its PV mutant. Endocrinology 144:4820–4825

21. Johansson C, Vennström B, Thoren P (1998) Evidence that decreased heart rate in thyroid hormone receptor-α_1 deficient mice is an intrinsic defect. Am J Physiol 275:R640–R646

22. Gloss B, Trost S, Bluhm W et al (2001) Cardiac ion channel expression and contractile function in mice with deletion of thyroid hormone receptor alpha or beta. Endocrinology 142:544–550

23. Pantos C, Mourouzis I, Malliopoulou V et al (2005) Dronedarone administration prevents body weight gain and increases tolerance of the heart to ischemic stress: a possible involvement of thyroid hormone receptor α1. Thyroid 15:16–23

24. Sun W. Sarma JS, Singh BN (1999) Electrophysiological effects of dronedarone (SR33589), a noniodinated benzofuran derivative, in the rabbit heart: comparison with amiodarone. Circulation 100:2276–2281

25. Danzi S, Ojamaa K, Klein I (2003) Triiodothyronine-mediated myosin heavy chain gene transcription in the heart. Am J Physiol Heart Circ Physiol 284:H2255–H2262

26. Franklyn JA, Green NK, Gammage MD et al (1989) Regulation of α- and β-myosin heavy chain messenger RNAs in the myocardium by amiodarone and by thyroid status. Clin Sci 76:463–467

27. Kinugawa K, Yonekura K, Ribeiro RCJ et al (2001) Regulation of thyroid hormone receptor isoforms in physiological and pathological cardiac hypertrophy. Circ Res 89:591–598

28. Bagchi N, Brown TR, Schneider DS, Benerjee SK (1987) Effect of amiodarone on the rat heart myosin isoenzymes. Circ Res 60:621–625

29. Pantos C, Mourouzis I, Xinaris C et al (2008) Thyroid hormone and "cardiac metamorphosis": potential therapeutic implications. Pharmacol Ther 118:277–294

Changes in Thyroid Hormone Metabolism and Gene Expression in the Failing Heart: Therapeutic Implications

10

Sara Danzi and Irwin Klein

Abstract Thyroid hormone has profound effects on the heart and cardiovascular system. The cellular and systemic changes that occur with hypothyroidism include blood pressure changes, alterations in lipid metabolism, decreased cardiac contractility, and increased systemic vascular resistance. The resulting increased hypercholesterolemia and diastolic hypertension predispose these patients to atherosclerotic cardiovascular and coronary artery disease. Heart failure is associated with low-T_3 syndrome, resulting from alterations in thyroid hormone metabolism. This nonthyroidal illness may cause cardiovascular alterations similar to the changes described for hypothyroidism. New research suggests that T_3 treatment of patients with heart failure and low-T_3 syndrome improves some of the clinical manifestations of heart failure.

Keywords Elderly • Atrial fibrillation • Skeletal muscle • Subclinical thyroid disease • Myocardial infarction • Cardiac myocyte • Low-T_3 syndrome • Nonthyroidal illness • Heart failure • Deiodinase • Hyperlipidemia • LDL cholesterol • Amiodarone • Pulmonary hypertension • Autoimmune • Analogues • Hypertrophy • QT

10.1 Introduction

The most prevalent and clinically relevant signs and symptoms of both hyperthyroidism and hypothyroidism are the cardiovascular manifestations [1–3]. These include palpitations as well as changes in blood pressure, cardiac output, contractility, and systemic vascular resistance (SVR) (Fig. 10.1) [1,4]. It is not surprising, therefore, that alterations in thyroid hormone metabolism that often accompany heart failure (HF) may in turn contribute to the pathophysiology of that disease. While hypothyroidism is associated with an increased incidence of diastolic dysfunction and diastolic hypertension, hyperthyroidism is associated with systolic hypertension and an overall decline in mean arterial pressure. Contrary to the decreased SVR evident in hyperthyroidism, pulmonary pressures may rise, leading to pulmonary hypertension. This chapter discusses the role of thyroid hormone in maintaining normal cardiac function and the effects of thyroid disease on the heart, in order to better understand the contribution of impaired thyroid hormone metabolism in the pathophysiology and clinical outcomes associated with HF. Lastly, we review the preclinical and clinical evidence to support the therapeutic utility of triiodothyronine (T_3) in treating HF.

S. Danzi (✉)
North Shore University Hospital, Department of Medicine and the Feinstein Institute for Medical Research, Manhasset, NY, United States

G. Iervasi, A. Pingitore (eds.), *Thyroid and Heart Failure*.
© Springer-Verlag Italia 2009

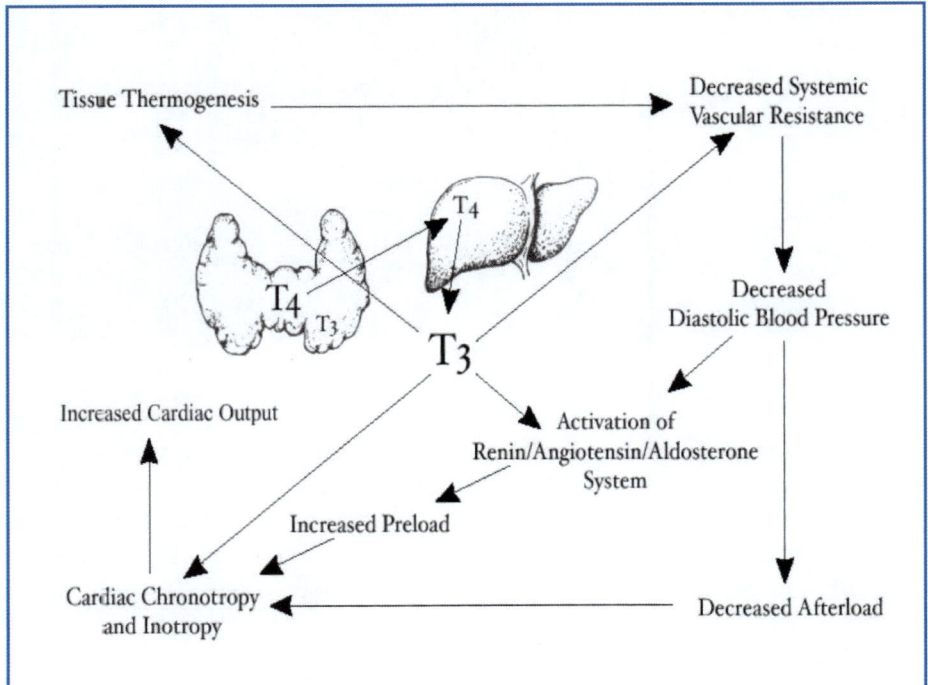

Fig. 10.1 Effects of thyroid hormone on cardiovascular hemodynamics. T_3 affects tissue thermogenesis, systemic vascular resistance, blood volume, cardiac contractility, heart rate, and cardiac output. (Reproduced from [7] with permission from Elsevier)

10.2 Hypothyroidism

The clinical signs and symptoms of hypothyroidism include weight gain, cold intolerance, dry skin, fatigue, bradycardia, narrowed pulse pressure, and diastolic hypertension [5,6]. Overt hypothyroidism affects approximately 5% of the adult female population and is associated with increased SVR, decreased cardiac contractility, decreased cardiac output, and accelerated atherosclerosis [7]. In elderly patients, symptoms may include hypothermia, altered mental status, depression, pericardial and pleural effusions, and myopathy [8]. In addition, the risk of developing HF increases in this age group.

The cardiovascular findings of hypothyroidism, however, are more subtle than those of hyperthyroidism. The blood pressure changes, alterations in lipid metabolism, decreased cardiac contractility, and increased SVR that accompany hypothyroidism are caused by decreased thyroid hormone action on multiple organs, including the heart, liver, and peripheral vasculature, and are potentially reversible with thyroid hormone replacement. There is also an increase in serum creatine kinase to levels as high as 10 times normal in anywhere from 15% to 50% of patients [1]. Hypothyroidism is associated with other atherosclerotic cardiovascular disease risk factors and with coronary artery disease, most likely because of the increased hypercholesterolemia and diastolic hypertension seen in these patients [9, 10].

10.3 Hyperthyroidism

An excess of endogenous thyroid hormone causes hyperthyroidism and results in an array of signs and symptoms that are diametrically opposite to those of hypothyroidism. Most patients with hyperthyroidism present with cardiac manifestations that include palpitations, tachycardia, exercise intolerance, dyspnea on exertion, widened pulse pressure, and atrial fibrillation, especially in older patients [11]. With atrial fibrillation, cardiovascular manifestations become more severe and rate-related HF may occur [12]. In longstanding hyperthyroidism, exercise intolerance may also result from skeletal muscle weakness [13]. While atrial fibrillation may be the most significant supraventricular arrhythmia, sinus tachycardia is the most common rhythm disturbance and is recorded in almost all patients with hyperthyroidism. Other rhythm disturbances, such as ventricular tachycardia, are relatively uncommon and may be the result of underlying heart disease.

Cardiac contractility is enhanced and resting heart rate is increased in hyperthyroidism. Cardiac output is increased due to the combined effect of increased resting heart rate, contractility, and blood volume, with a decrease in SVR. Many of the signs of HF, including neck vein distension and peripheral edema, may be due to right heart strain as a result of pulmonary hypertension. Although thyrotoxicosis is often associated with decreased SVR and decreased mean arterial pressure, a subset of patients, especially the elderly, will experience hypertension, in part because they have decreased arterial compliance with increased cardiac output [14–16].

Cardiovascular hemodynamics are altered in all thyroid disease states. T_3 regulates the basal metabolic rate (BMR) by increasing oxygen consumption in peripheral tissues and tissue thermogenesis. Metabolic demands, as well as direct effects of T_3, can affect SVR and lead to increased blood flow to peripheral tissues with increased cardiac output. Older patients with hyperthyroidism may have an even greater increase in systolic blood pressure because of the loss of elastic components of the larger (capacitance) arteries [17]. The effect of thyroid hormone on blood pressure homeostasis extends into the euthyroid range. Diastolic function, as measured by isovolumic relaxation time, varies across the entire spectrum of thyroid function (Fig. 10.2).

While hyperthyroidism and hypothyroidism are both associated with altered blood pressure, a low-sodium diet in patients with untreated hypothyroidism, but not hyperthyroidism, was shown to beassociated with a fall in diastolic blood pressure. Renin levels also vary with alterations in thyroid status, demonstrating that different mechanisms are responsible for the increased blood pressure that can occur in patients with hypothyroidism and hyperthyroidism [18].

Several of the cardiovascular manifestations of hyperthyroidism mimic those of a hyperadrenergic state. However, catecholamine metabolism is normal in hyperthyroidism [19]. Many of these changes are the result of T_3-mediated effects on vascular endothelial and smooth muscle cells, including endothelial nitric oxide production. T_3 may act to increase atrial natriuretic peptide expression and renin synthesis and secretion, all of which may contribute to the hemodynamic changes described above [20].

10.4 Subclinical Thyroid Disease

Subclinical hypothyroidism is defined by a thyroid-stimulating hormone (TSH) concentration above the normal range, with serum total and free T_3 and T_4 levels within the normal range. Similarly, subclinical hyperthyroidism is defined by a TSH concentration below the normal range with normal serum T_3 and T_4 levels.

Lipid profile changes are evident in subclinical hypothyroidism. Even with mildly elevated TSH levels (< 10 mIU/l), subclinical hypothyroidism has been shown to be associated with changes in the lipid profile significant enough to raise cardiovascular risk [21]. In addition, the abnormal presence of C-reactive protein, a risk factor for heart disease, is increased in subclinical hypothyroidism, as are atherosclerosis, coronary heart disease, and myocardial infarction risks [22]. While the suitability of treatment of subclinical hypothyroidism with appropriate doses of L-thyroxine (T_4) has been controversial, the benefits of restoring TSH levels to normal can be considered sufficient to outweigh the risks [2]. Rendering such patients euthyroid results in an improvement of many modifiable cardiovascular risk factors [23].

Patients with subclinical hyperthyroidism may have no clinical signs or symptoms; however, studies show that they are at risk of many of the cardiovascular manifestations associated with overt hyper-

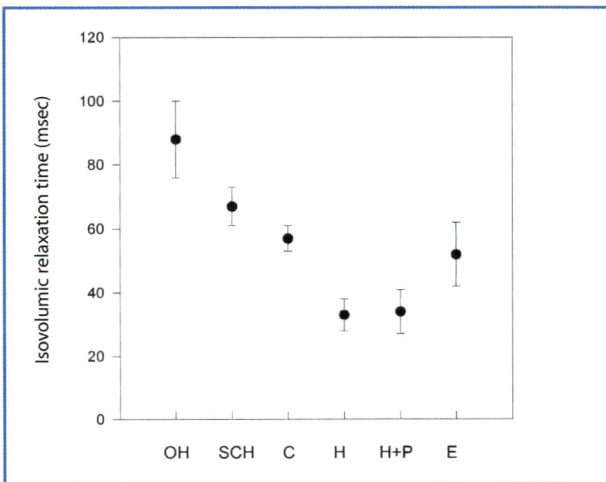

Fig. 10.2 Thyroid status and isovolumic relaxation time. Isovolumic relaxation time as a measure of diastolic function is altered across the spectrum of thyroid status. *OH* hypothyroidism, *SCH* subclinical hypothyroidism, *C* control, *H* hyperthyroidism, *H+P* hyperthyroidism plus β-adrenergic blockade (propranolol), *E* hyperthyroidism after treatment to restore euthyroidism. (Reproduced from [7] with permission from Elsevier)

thyroidism. Subclinical hyperthyroidism carries the same or greater relative risk of atrial fibrillation as does overt disease [24]. In a 10-year cohort study of older patients, low TSH was associated with a marked increased risk of cardiovascular mortality and atrial fibrillation [25], as subsequently confirmed by similar studies [9].

10.5 Cellular Mechanisms of Thyroid Hormone Action

The classic cellular thyroid hormone effects, the regulation of cell-specific gene transcription, are mediated by thyroid hormone receptors (TRs) encoded by two genes, TRα and TRβ (Fig. 10.3) [4]. Multiple splice variants mediate the genomic actions of T_3. TRs bind to thyroid hormone response elements (TREs) in the promoter regions of positively regulated genes [26, 27]. In the presence of T_3, transcription is induced, and in the absence of T_3, transcription is repressed. Negatively regulated genes are expressed in the opposite manner, but may not require upstream

TREs [28]. There is no single mechanism by which all T_3-mediated negatively regulated genes are expressed. The myosin heavy chain (MHC) genes α and β are well-studied thyroid-hormone-responsive genes that are positively and negatively regulated, respectively, by T_3. β-MHC is induced in the absence of T_3 and repressed in its presence due to an antisense RNA that is expressed from the downstream β/α intergenic promoter region in the opposite direction of the β-MHC gene [29, 30].

The model for α-MHC activation and repression, like that of other positively regulated genes, involves two sequential steps requiring assembly of protein complexes at the promoter [31]. Retinoid X receptor (RXR) is a common heterodimer partner for the TRs. In the first step, TR/RXR heterodimers bind to TRE sequences and recruit histone acetyltransferases (HATs), which facilitate chromatin remodeling. In the second step, the HATs are exchanged for coactivator complexes that function to activate transcription by recruiting the RNA polymerase II transcription machinery. In the absence of T_3, TRs recruit histone deacetylases (HDACs) to the TREs and actively repress transcription. Chromatin remodeling caused by histone hypoacetylation is associated with repression.

Genes positively regulated by thyroid hormone encode important cardiac proteins, including the fast myosin heavy chain of the contractile apparatus, α-MHC; the calcium transporter, sarcoplasmic-reticulum calcium-activated ATPase (SERCA2); the sodium–potassium ATPase (Na^+/K^+ ATPase); and the β1-adrenergic receptor. Many are negatively regulated, including the counterparts to the α-MHC and SERCA2 genes, β-MHC and phospholamban (PLB), respectively. These genes are regulated in an opposite manner in response to T_3 and other hemodynamic stimuli [1].

T_3 mediates extranuclear, nongenomic effects on the cardiac myocyte and on the systemic vasculature, including changes in membrane ion channels for sodium, potassium, and calcium, effects on actin polymerization, and a variety of intracellular signaling pathways in the heart and vascular smooth muscle cells [32, 33].

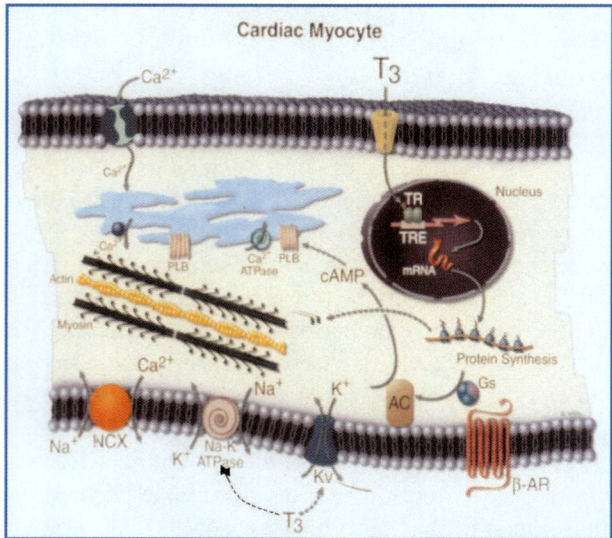

Fig. 10.3 T_3 effects on the cardiac myocyte. T_3 has both genomic and nongenomic effects on the cardiac myocyte. Genomic mechanisms involve T_3 binding to TRs, which regulate transcription of specific cardiac genes. Nongenomic mechanisms include direct modulation of membrane ion channels as indicated by the dashed arrows. *AC* adenylyl cyclase, *β-AR* β adrenergic receptor, *Gs* guanine nucleotide binding protein, *Kv* voltage-gated potassium channels, *NCX* sodium calcium exchanger, *PLB* phospholamban. (Reproduced from [1] with permission)

10.6 Thyroid Hormone Metabolism

In overt hypothyroidism, TSH is elevated and serum T_4 and T_3 are low. Treatment is accomplished with replacement doses of l-T_4 which is then metabolized to T_3 in peripheral organs such as the liver, kidney, and skeletal muscle. This peripheral conversion, especially in human skeletal muscle, is accomplished by 5'-monodeiodinase enzymes and is responsible for the majority of serum T_3.

Two of the three deiodinases are responsible for the conversion of T_4 to the physiologically active form of the hormone, T_3 [34]. The type 1 5'-monodeiodinase (D1) in the liver and kidney together with the type 2 enzyme (D2) in skeletal muscle are responsible for generating the circulating plasma levels of T_3 [35, 36].

In a variety of chronic illnesses, the rate of thyroid hormone metabolism may be impaired, leading to reduced levels of serum T_3 but with normal T_4 and TSH. This low-T_3 syndrome is referred to as nonthyroidal illness. When serum T_3 levels are reduced as a result of chronic illness, caloric restriction, or trauma, there are resulting changes in cardiac gene expression and function similar to those observed with classic primary hypothyroidism [37]. Some organs, such as the brain, readily transport and metabolize T_4 while other organs, such as the heart, do not and are more vulnerable to reduced serum T_3 levels. In turn, reversal of these changes in the cardiac phenotype can be accomplished with T_3 but not T_4 treatment.

10.7 Heart Failure and Thyroid Hormone

The parallels between hypothyroidism and HF are numerous (Table 10.1). Hypothyroidism results in impaired left ventricular contractile function, increased SVR, low cardiac output, and changes in cardiac gene expression, similar to those seen with HF.

Table 10.1 Similarities between hypothyroidism and heart failure

Characteristics	Hypothyroidism	HF
Cardiac output	↓	↓
Cardiac contractility	↓	↓
Serum T_3 levels	↓	↓
Ischemic heart disease	±	+++
Systemic vascular resistance	↑	Variable
Response to thyroid hormone	+++	?

The conversion of T_4 to T_3 is impaired after cardiac surgery, acute myocardial infarction (MI), and in HF in proportion to the severity of the heart disease, as assessed by the New York Heart Association functional classification [38]. Recently published studies reported that approximately 30% of patients with HF have low-T_3 syndrome. Low serum T_3 is a strong predictor of death in patients with heart disease and in fact is a stronger predictor of mortality than is ejection fraction [39].

Decreased expression of both D1 and D2 has been implicated in the development of the low-T_3 syndrome in HF [35, 40]. A recent study reported that in cardiac tissue, activity of type 3 deiodinase (D3), which converts T_4 and T_3 to the inactive compounds reverse T_3 (rT_3) and diiodothyronine (T_2), respectively, was increased in the infarcted myocardium after induced MI, resulting in low serum T_3 levels in the experimental animals [36, 41].

In animal models, the low-T_3 syndrome can be produced by caloric restriction, resulting in impaired cardiac contractility. Restoration of normal serum T_3 levels by administration of exogenous T_3 re-establishes normal cardiac function. Hypertension or MI can lead to HF with systolic or diastolic dysfunction along with the low-T_3 syndrome. Low serum T_3 levels can further impair cardiac function. Data suggest that replacement with T_3 restores normal function. Saline-treated animals do not show a similar pattern of improvement.

The cardiac myocyte has limited, if any, ability to convert T_4 to T_3 intracellularly and relies on serum T_3. Thus, with low-T_3 syndrome, the myocardium becomes relatively hypothyroid. Therefore, the changes observed in the low-T_3 syndrome can be reversed with T_3 but not T_4 replacement.

The relationship between hypothyroidism and hyperlipidemia became evident with the observation, over 40 years ago, that hypothyroid patients had elevated serum lipid levels. While thyroid hormone can alter cholesterol metabolism through multiple mechanisms, including a decrease in biliary excretion, the proposed primary mechanism for hyperlipidemia is an accumulation of LDL cholesterol due to a reduction in the number and/or activity of LDL cell surface receptors, resulting in decreased catabolism of LDL [42]. If untreated, the dyslipidemia together with the diastolic hypertension associated with hypothyroidism may further predispose the patient to atherosclerosis [43].

Amiodarone, a commonly used iodine-containing antiarrhythmic drug for the treatment of both atrial and ventricular cardiac rhythm disturbances, can cause changes in thyroid function resulting in either hypothyroidism or hyperthyroidism [44]. The latter is a much more difficult clinical dilemma to manage. Patients with pre-existing thyroid disease are at greater risk of developing amiodarone-induced thyroid dysfunction of either type.

Pulmonary hypertension, defined by a pulmonary arterial pressure greater than 25 mmHg at rest and 30 mmHg during exercise, can be associated with both hypothyroidism and hyperthyroidism. It has been suggested that the autoimmune component is the link because pulmonary hypertension can occur with Hashimoto's and Graves' diseases. Pulmonary hypertension and atrioventricular valve regurgitation have been documented in hyperthyroidism with a surprisingly high prevalence [45]. Several case reports have documented that hyperthyroidism can present as right HF [46]. The reasons for this are unclear. It is possible that the decreased SVR that occurs in hyperthyroidism does not occur in the pulmonary vasculature. The pulmonary hypertension usually resolves after treatment.

10.8 Thyroid Hormone Treatment of Heart Failure

Based upon the cardiovascular actions of thyroid hormone and the alterations in thyroid hormone metabolism that accompany HF, it was hypothesized that thyroid hormone treatment, specifically with T_3, improve or reverses the altered cardiovascular physiology arising from a variety of cardiac disease states (Fig. 10.4) (Table 10.2). Early studies by Morkin and colleagues first hinted at the potential for thyroid hormone to improve cardiac contractility and cardiac output in the post-MI vertebrate animal model [47]. While some benefits were observed, these did not lead to the same degree of improvement as was recently reported from our laboratory and others [48, 49]. Since it is T_3 and not T_4 which is active at the level of the cardiac myocyte and on vascular smooth muscle and endothelial cells to enhance cardiac output, studies which do not provide T_3 in a physiological replacement method or which use nonquantitative replacement with either T_4 or a combination of T_4 and T_3 are inherently limited in their effectiveness [50, 51].

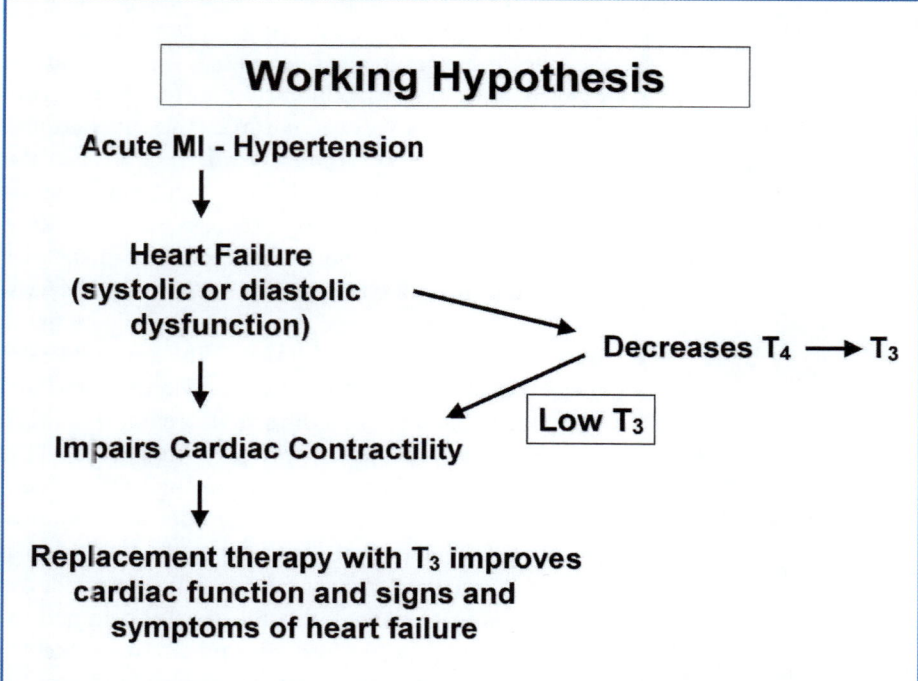

Fig. 10.4 Preclinical and clinical rationale for the role of T_3 treatment in the management of the signs and symptoms of heart failure. *MI* myocardial infarction

Table 10.2 Potential benefits of T_3 treatment in heart failure

Restore serum T_3 to normal	Improve skeletal muscle function
Positive inotropic agent	Synergism with other HF treatments
Positive lusitropic agent	Antiarrhythmic effect on QT interval
Decrease SVR	Promote reverse remodeling
Improve diastolic function	Maintain systolic function
Oxygen cost of T_3-mediated increases in cardiac work less than standard inotropic agents	

Several authors have studied the effects of thyroid hormone to improve cardiac contractility and reverse remodeling in pathological states, including post-MI, hypertensive cardiomyopathy, and a variety of genetic myopathic states. In addition, thyroid hormone has been utilized in the immediate post-MI model to study its effects on necrotic and apoptotic cell death. In essentially every model, when T_3 is provided in a physiological replacement dose there is an improvement in cardiac function and a restoration of the preinfarct genotype. As noted above, when compared to the normal mammalian heart, the failing heart has an alteration in gene expression which is indistinguishable from that seen with experimental hypothyroidism [52]. Thus, the rationale for thyroid hormone treatment to provide for reverse remodeling of this pathologically altered myocardium is validated. The changes in left ventricular (LV) function in the post-MI heart are similar to those of hypothyroidism. Studies designed to assess T_3 treatment have included measures of diastolic as well as systolic function to best reflect the functional activity of SERCA2.

Thyroid hormone analogues including 3,5-diiodothyropropionic acid (DITPA) have been studied in both the rat and rabbit HF models. Despite the inability to demonstrate classic nuclear effects of DITPA on myocyte gene expression, the changes in SVR and cardiac performance suggested a potential therapeutic benefit. However recent studies of DITPA in human trials have failed to confirm these experimental findings [53].

In a rat post-MI model of HF, we have observed a rapid fall in serum T_3 accompanying the decrease in LV systolic function and pathological hypertrophy (Fig. 10.5) [49]. Analysis of LV gene expression demonstrated a fall in α-MHC with a rise in β-MHC and a decrease in SERCA2a. T_3 treatment,

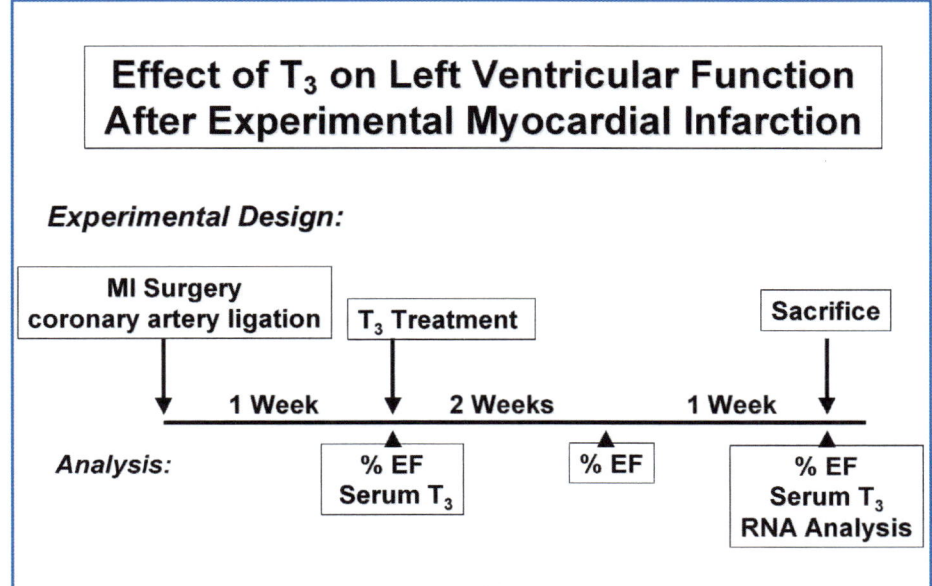

Fig. 10.5 Experimental time course of the preclinical studies to determine the effects of T_3 treatment on serum T_3 levels, cardiac function, and cardiac phenotype after coronary artery ligation to produce myocardial infarction

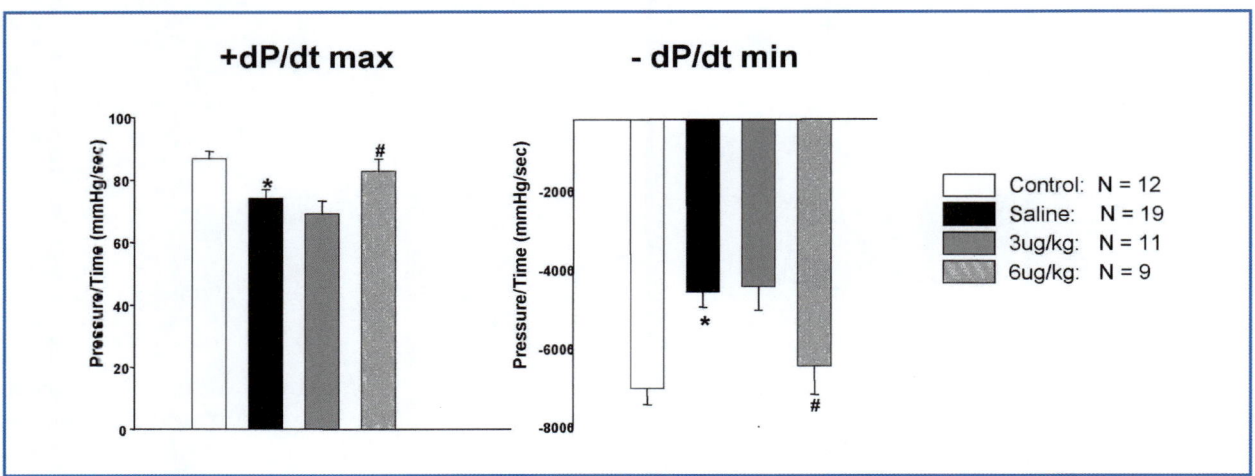

Fig. 10.6 Effects of T_3 replacement on systolic (+dP/dt) and diastolic (−dP/dt) function in the rodent model of acute myocardial infarction produced by coronary artery ligation. T_3 was administered by constant infusion at 3 or 6 µg/kg per day. * versus control ($p < 0.05$), # versus saline ($p < 0.05$). (Data from [48])

provided as a constant infusion to restore serum T_3 levels to normal, led to an improvement in LV systolic function and a decrease in LV mass, with restoration of the normal LV phenotype. This occurred with no increase in heart rate or ventricular irritability. Recently, Henderson et al. extended these studies to include in vivo monitoring of heart rate, atrial and ventricular irritability, and more extensive measures of LV function [48]. They observed that T_3 treatment improved both diastolic and systolic performance in association with partial reversal of the pathological genotype (Fig. 10.6).

10.9 Human Heart Failure Studies

In the first evaluation of changes in thyroid hormone metabolism accompanying human HF, Hamilton et al. showed that acute T_3 treatment produced improvement in cardiovascular hemodynamics [54]. The changes they observed were similar to those reported by Klemperer et al., who used bolus T_3 treatment followed by a 6-h infusion to study the effects of thyroid hormone treatment after coronary artery bypass graft surgery [55]. In both studies, T_3 could be administered safely without untoward effects on cardiac ischemia or rate. There have been multiple anecdotal reports of the ability of T_3 to enhance cardiovascular hemodynamics in brain-dead organ donors, heart transplant recipients, and patients presenting with viral myocarditis.

However, in each report, the benefits of T_3 were observed in the absence of case controls. Chowdhury et al. prospectively studied the effects of T_3 infusion to restore serum T_3 levels to normal in children undergoing surgery for congenital heart disease [56]. In these prospectively randomized studies the benefits of T_3 used to decrease the need for inotropic support and to improve the postoperative recovery were demonstrated.

Most recently the cardiovascular research group in Pisa has prospectively studied the effects of 72 h of T_3 infusion to improve cardiac function in HF patients with low serum T_3 [57]. They demonstrated for the first time the benefit in both cardiovascular performance and in neuroendocrine measures of HF, including B-type (or brain) natriuretic peptide (BNP), norepinephrine and aldosterone for this novel form of treatment. As in all preceding studies there were no untoward effects of intravenous T_3 infusion on measures of cardiac ischemia or atrial or ventricular irritability. In fact, T_3 treatment of these HF patients produced a significant decrease in heart rate commensurate with the improvement in cardiac function.

Based upon the cellular mechanisms of T_3 action, thyroid hormone treatment of HF would be expected to improve diastolic function through a lusitropic mechanism while also lowering SVR. This combination of effects would be especially attractive in long-term treatment and would be expected to act synergistically with both β-adrenergic blockade and angiotensin-converting-enzyme inhibitors. T_3 is also capable of restoring QT intervals to normal and may act in this manner to decrease ventricular irritability and ventricular tachycardia. Restoration of low T_3 levels to normal may also result in improved skeletal muscle function and psychiatric and neuropsychological measures similar to those obtained in the treatment of hypothyroidism. Last, and most important, is the fact that these gains in cardiac performance and cardiovascular hemodynamics are accomplished with no untoward increase in myocardial oxygen consumption.

In the studies by Pingitore et al. T_3 replacement was accomplished by intravenous infusion to restore serum T_3 levels to normal [57]. Due to the short half life of T_3 and the known pharmacokinetics of oral T_3 absorption it is not possible to reproduce similar physiological replacement with the existing formulations of T_3. Novel delivery techniques, including a modified-release, orally absorbed T_3 preparation, may be able to overcome this treatment limitation.

Key Points

- Hypothyroidism is associated with hyperlipidemia, increased systemic vascular resistance, decreased cardiac contractility, and reduced ejection fraction as well as skeletal muscle weakness.

- Thyroid hormone uniquely acts as a lusitropic agent, promoting cardiac relaxation, and therefore hypothyroidism may lead to diastolic dysfunction.

- Thyroid hormone metabolism is altered in heart failure, leading to the low-T_3 syndrome.

- Parallels between heart failure and hypothyroidism are numerous.

- A low serum T_3 concentration is a strong predictor of death in patients with heart disease.

- T_3 replacement in animal models of post-myocardial infarction and heart failure improved cardiac function.

- Studies of T_3 replacement in adults after coronary artery bypass surgery and in children after surgery to repair congenital heart defects demonstrated improved postoperative recovery.

- Infusion of T_3 over 72 h to heart failure patients with low-T_3 syndrome provided benefits in cardiovascular performance and neuroendocrine measures.

- In essentially all preclinical and clinical studies of T_3 replacement in heart failure, no untoward effects were documented.

References

1. Klein I, Danzi S (2007) Thyroid disease and the heart. Circulation 116:1725–1735
2. Klein I, Ojamaa K (2001) Thyroid hormone and the cardiovascular system. N Engl J Med 344:501–509
3. Dillmann WH (2002) Cellular action of thyroid hormone on the heart. Thyroid 12:447–452
4. Kahaly GJ, Dillmann WH (2005) Thyroid hormone action in the heart. Endocrine Rev 26:704–728
5. Levey GS, Klein I (1994) Disorders of the thyroid. In: Stein's Textbook of medicine, 2nd edn. Little Brown, Boston, pp 1383–1396
6. Crowley WF Jr, Ridgway EC, Bough EW et al (1977) Noninvasive evaluation of cardiac function in hypothyroidism. Response to gradual thyroxine replacement. N Engl J Med 296:1–6
7. Klein I (2008) Endocrine disorders and cardiovascular disease. In: Libby P, Bonow R, Mann D, Zipes D (eds) Braunwald's Heart disease, 8th edn. Saunders, Philadelphia, pp 2033–2047
8. Danzi S, Klein I (2006) Treatment of hypertension and thyroid disease. In: Mohler ER, Townsend RR (eds) Advanced therapy in hypertension and vascular disease. BC Decker, Hamilton, Ontario, Canada, pp 354–360
9. Cappola AR, Ladenson PW (2003) Hypothyroidism and atherosclerosis. J Clin Endocrinol Metab 88:2438–2444
10. Danzi S, Klein I (2003) Thyroid hormone and blood pressure regulation. Curr Hypertens Rep 5:513–520
11. Biondi B, Palmieri EA, Lombardi G, Fazio S (2002) Effects of thyroid hormone on cardiac function: the relative importance of heart rate, loading conditions, and myocardial

contractility in the regulation of cardiac performance in human hyperthyroidism. J Clin Endocrinol Metab 87:968–974

12. Nakazawa H, Lythall DA, Noh J et al (2000) Is there a place for the late cardioversion of atrial fibrillation? A long-term follow-up study of patients with post-thyrotoxic atrial fibrillation. Eur Heart J 21:327–333

13. Olsen B, Klein I, Benner R et al (1991) Hyperthyroid myopathy and the response to treatment. Thyroid 1:137–141

14. Napoli R, Biondi B, Guardasole V et al (2001) Impact of hyperthyroidism and its correction on vascular reactivity in humans. Circulation 104:3076–3080

15. Prisant LM, Gujral JS, Mulloy AL (2006) Hyperthyroidism: a secondary cause of isolated systolic hypertension. J Clin Hypertens 8:596–599

16. Palmieri EA, Fazio S, Palmieri V et al (2004) Myocardial contractility and total arterial stiffness in patients with overt hyperthyroidism: acute effects of beta1-adrenergic blockade. Eur J Endocrinol 150:757–62

17. Asvold BO, Bjoro T, Nilsen T, Vatten LJ (2007) Association between blood pressure and serum TSH concentration within the reference range: a population-based study. J Clin Endocrinol Metab 92:841–5

18. Marcisz C, Jonderko G, Kucharz EJ (2001) Influence of short-time application of a low sodium diet on blood pressure in patients with hyperthyroidism or hypothyroidism during therapy. Am J Hypertens 14:995–1002

19. Hoit BD, Khoury SF, Shao Y et al (1997) Effects of thyroid hormone on cardiac b-adrenergic responsiveness in conscious baboons. Circulation 96:592–598

20. Laragh JH, Sealey JE (2003) Relevance of the plasma renin hormonal control system that regulates blood pressure and sodium balance for correctly treating hypertension and for evaluating ALLHAT. Am J Hypertens 16:407–415

21. Hak AE, Pols HA, Visser TJ et al (2000) Subclinical hypothyroidism is an independent risk factor for atherosclerosis and myocardial infarction in elderly women: the Rotterdam Study. Ann Intern Med 132:270–278

22. Razvi S, Ingoe L, Keeka G et al (2007) The beneficial effect of l-thyroxine on cardiovascular risk factors, endothelial function and quality of life in subclinical hypothyroidism: randomised, crossover trial. J Clin Endocrinol Metab 92:1715–1723

23. Biondi B, Klein I (2004) Hypothyroidism as a risk factor for cardiovascular disease. Endocrine 24:1–14

24. Auer J, Scheibner P, Mische T et al (2001) Subclinical hyperthyroidism as a risk factor for atrial fibrillation. Am Heart J 142:838–842

25. Sawin CT, Geller A, Wolf PA et al (1994) Low serum thyrotropin concentrations as a risk factor for atrial fibrillation in older persons. N Engl J Med 331:1249–1252

26. Brent G (1994) The molecular basis of thyroid hormone action. N Engl J Med 331:847–853

27. Lazar MA, Chin WW (1990) Nuclear thyroid hormone receptors. J Clin Invest 86:1777–1782

28. Hu X, Lazar MA (2000) Transcriptional repression by nuclear hormone receptors. Trends Endocrinol Metab 11:6–10

29. Haddad F, Bodell PW, Qin AX et al (2003) Role of antisense RNA in coordinating cardiac myosin heavy chain gene switching. J Biol Chem 278:37132–37138

30. Danzi S, Klein S, Klein I (2008) Differential regulation of myosin heavy chain genes a and b in the rat atria and ventricles: role of antisense RNA. Thyroid 18:761–768

31. Wu Y, Koenig RJ (2000) Gene regulation by thyroid hormone. Trends Endocrinol Metab 11:207–211

32. Davis PJ, Davis FB (2002) Nongenomic actions of thyroid hormone on the heart. Thyroid 12:459–466

33. Hiroi Y, Kim H-H, Ying H et al (2006) Rapid nongenomic actions of thyroid hormone. Proc Natl Acad Sci USA 103:14104–14109

34. Bianco AC, Salvatore D, Gereben B et al (2002) Biochemistry, cellular and molecular biology, and physiological roles of the iodothyronine selenodeiodinases. Endocrine Rev 23:38–89

35. Maia AL, Kim BW, Huang SA et al (2005) Type 2 iodothyronine deiodinase is the major source of plasma T3 in euthyroid humans. J Clin Invest 115:2524–2533

36. Bianco AC, Larsen PR (2005) Cellular and structural biology of the deiodinases. Thyroid 15:777–786

37. Katzeff HL, Powell SR, Ojamaa K (1997) Alterations in cardiac contractility and gene expression during low-T3 syndrome: prevention with T3. Am J Physiol 273:E951–956

38. Schmidt-Ott UM, Ascheim DD (2006) Thyroid hormone and heart failure. Curr Heart Fail Rep 3:114–119

39. Pingitore A, Landi P, Taddei MC et al (2005) Triiodothyronine levels for risk stratification of patients with chronic heart failure. Am J Med 118:132–136

40. Yu J, Koenig RJ (2006) Induction of type 1 iodothyronine deiodinase to prevent the nonthyroidal illness syndrome in mice. Endocrinology 147:3580–3585

41. Olivares EL, Marassi MP, Fortunato RS et al (2007) Thyroid function disturbance and type 3 iodothyronine deiodinase induction after myocardial infarction in rats: a time course study. Endocrinology 148:4786–4792

42. Duntas LH (2002) Thyroid disease and lipids. Thyroid 12:287–293

43. Thompson GR, Soutar AK, Spengel FA et al (1981) Defects of receptor-mediated low density lipoprotein catabolism in homozygous familial hypercholesterolemia and hypothyroidism in vivo. Proc Natl Acad Sci U S A 78:2591

44. Harjai KJ, Licata AA (2006) Effects of amiodarone on thyroid function. Ann Intern Med 126:63–73

45. Marvisi M, Zambrelli P, Brianti M et al (2006) Pulmonary hypertension is frequent in hyperthyroidism and normalizes after therapy. Eur J Intern Med 17:267–271

46. Paran Y, Nimrod A, Goldin Y, Justo D (2006) Pulmonary hypertension and predominant right heart failure in thyrotoxicosis. Resuscitation 69:339–341

47. Morkin E, Pennock G, Spooner PH et al (2002) Pilot studies on the use of 3,5-diiodothyropropionic acid, a thyroid hormone analog, in the treatment of congestive heart failure. Cardiology 97:218–225

48. Henderson KK, Danzi S, Klein I, Samarel A (2009) Physiological replacement of T3 improves left ventricular function in an animal model of myocardial infarction-induced congestive heart failure. Circ Heart Fail (in press)

49. Ojamaa K, Kenessey A, Shenoy R, Klein I (2000) Thyroid hormone metabolism and cardiac gene expression after acute myocardial infarction in the rat. Am J Physiol 279:E1319–1324

50. Thomas TA, Kuzman JA, Anderson BE et al (2005) Thyroid hormones induce unique and potentially beneficial changes in cardiac myocyte shape in hypertensive rats near heart failure. Am J Physiol Heart Circ Physiol 288:H2118–2122

51. Khalife WI, Tang YD, Kuzman JA et al (2005) Treatment of subclinical hypothyroidism reverses ischemia and prevents myocyte loss and progressive LV dysfunction in hamsters with dilated cardiomyopathy. Am J Physiol Heart Circ Physiol 289:H2409–2415

52. Danzi S, Klein I (2004) Thyroid hormone and the cardiovascular system. Minerva Endocrinol 29:139–150

53. Morkin E, Pennock GD, Spooner PH et al (2002) Clinical and experimental studies on the use of 3,5-diiodothyropropionic acid, a thyroid hormone analogue, in heart failure. Thyroid 12:527–533

54. Hamilton MA, Stevenson LW, Luu M, Walden JA (1990) Altered thyroid hormone metabolism in advanced heart failure. J Am Coll Cardiol 16:91–95

55. Klemperer J, Klein I, Gomez M et al (1995) Thyroid hormone treatment after coronary-artery bypass surgery. New Engl J Med 333:1522–1527

56. Chowdhury D, Parnell VA, Ojamaa K et al (1999) Usefulness of triiodothyronine (T3) treatment after surgery for complex congenital heart disease in infants and children. Am J Cardiol 84:34–36

57. Pingitore A, Galli E, Barison A et al (2008) Acute effects of triiodothyronine (T3) replacement therapy in patients with chronic heart failure and low-T3 syndrome: a randomized, placebo-controlled study. J Clin Endocrinol Metab 93:1351–1358

Thyroid-Hormone-Regulated Cardiac Metabolism in Normal and Failing Heart

11

Michael A. Portman

Abstract Thyroid hormones regulate multiple metabolic processes in cardiomyocytes that can impact the failing heart. Recent data suggest that thyroid hormone receptors play an important role in nongenomic regulation as well as in transcription. Myocardial energy metabolism shows a balance between ATP production and utilization. Thyroid hormone regulates this balance through multiple processes. Accordingly, thyroid hormone can control the cellular environment by modifying the cellular energy state, which in turn influences processes such as transport and protein synthesis. Here we review thyroid hormone's direct action on metabolism and ligand-dependent control through the nuclear receptors.

Keywords Cardiac metabolism • Glucose • Fatty acid • Substrate oxidation • ATP synthase

11.1 Introduction

Metabolism in the heart is an exquisite balance between the primary substrate oxidation pathways in order to provide energy in the form of adenosine triphosphate (ATP) to the contractile machinery. The concept is rapidly emerging that abnormalities in cardiac metabolism can exacerbate or even cause various forms of heart failure. These abnormalities extend from disruptions in enzyme systems controlling oxidative phosphorylation to shifts in enzymes regulating intermediary substrate metabolism.

Disturbances in thyroid hormone (TH) homeostasis during heart failure are discussed in other chapters. TH controls cardiac metabolism through transcriptional and post-transcriptional processes. While TH controls metabolism primarily within the mitochondria. However, T_3 also modifies substrate transport across the sarcolemma and the mitochondrial membrane. A general outline of mitochondrial metabolism is shown in Figure 11.1. Decreases in circulating TH levels or in the expression of cardiac thyroid hormone receptors impact metabolic pathways during heart failure [1, 2]. Here review thyroid hormone modulation of cardiac metabolism through transcriptional and post-transcriptional (nongenomic) pathways.

11.2 Efficiency of ATP Hydrolysis

Myocardial oxidative phosphorylation and mitochondrial membrane transport systems efficiently supply ATP for use by energy-consuming processes in the cardiomyocyte. Disruption of these systems can lead to thermodynamic instability and relative cardiac energy starvation during heart failure. The ATP production rate generally matches the overall rate of ATP hydrolysis in the mature heart in vivo if carbon substrate and oxygen supplies are ample. However, in the mature heart, the phosphorylation potential $[ATP/(ADP \cdot P_i)]$

M.A. Portman (✉)
University of Washington and Seattle Children's Hospital, Seattle, WA, United States

G. Iervasi, A. Pingitore (eds.), *Thyroid and Heart Failure*.
© Springer-Verlag Italia 2009

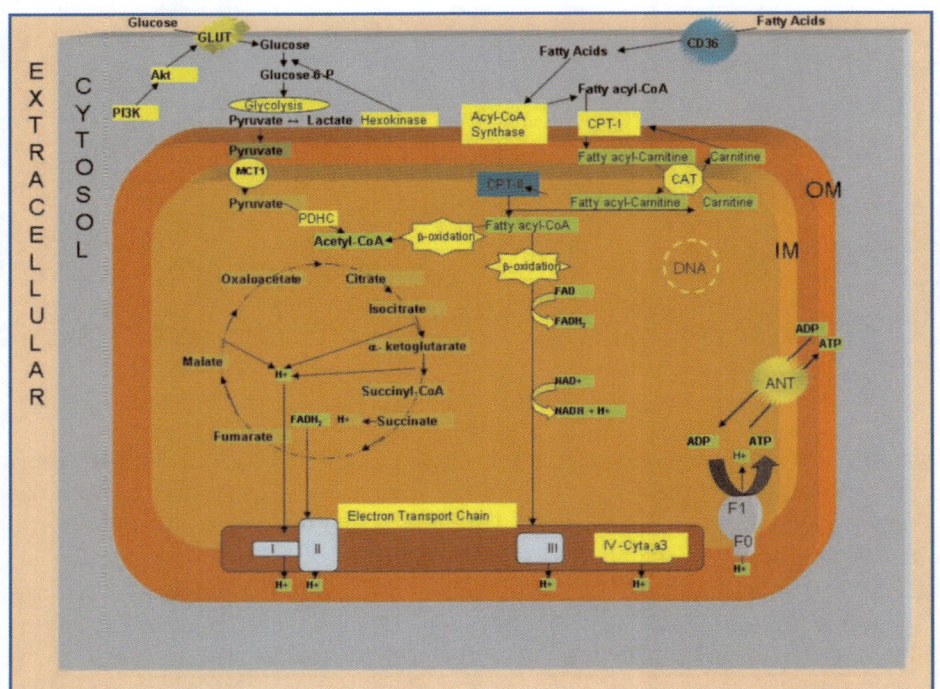

Fig. 11.1 The major metabolic pathways and oxidative phosphorylation. Enzymes and pathways highlighted in yellow are candidates for thyroid hormone regulation. *OM* outer mitochondrial membrane, *IM* inner mitochondrial membrane, *GLUT* glucose transporter, *ANT* adenine nucleotide translocator, *CD36* fatty acid transporter CD36, *CPT-I* carnitine palmitoyl transferase I, *CAT* carnitine acylcarnitine translocase, *PDHC* pyruvate dehydrogenase complex, *MCT* monocarboxylate transporter. F1 and F0 are components of the ATP synthase

diminishes at near-maximal workloads, indicating that a transition in respiratory control occurs. The reduction in phosphorylation potential presumably represents a shift to ADP-dependent respiratory regulation through the adenine nucleotide translocator, the site of ATP/ADP exchange [3]. Proton nuclear magnetic resonance measurements of myoglobin saturation in the mature pig heart indicated that reduced phosphorylation potential at a very high work state is not caused by limited oxygen supply [4–6].

ATP hydrolysis releases the free energy stored in the high-energy phosphate bonds of ATP. Although this is a negative value, the change in free energy state due to release of inorganic phosphate (P_i) by ATP hydrolysis is a positive value. The free energy of ATP hydrolysis (ΔG_{ATP}) is related to the phosphorylation potential [ATP]/[ADP][P_i]] and can be calculated by [7]:

$$\Delta G_{ATP} \text{ (kJ/mol)} = \Delta G° + RT \ln ([ADP][Pi]/[ATP]) \quad \text{(Eq. 11.1)}$$

where $\Delta G°$ (−30.5 kJ/mol) is the value of ΔG_{ATP} under standard conditions of molarity, temperature, pH, and [Mg^{2+}], R is the gas constant (8.3 J/molK), and T is temperature in Kelvin. Therefore, at near-maximal work state in the mature heart, a somewhat

lower amount of free energy is made available during the release of a phosphate from ATP at various ATPase sites within the myocyte: ATP → ADP + P_i.

Phosphocreatine provides the major reservoir of high-energy phosphates within the cytosol. In magnetic resonance spectroscopy studies, the phosphocreatine/ATP ratio is considered directly proportional to phosphorylation potential. The creatine kinase equilibrium reaction describes the relationship between phosphocreatine (PCr) and ADP.

$$PCr + ADP + H+ \Leftrightarrow ATP + Cr; \text{ and } K_{eq} = [ATP][Cr]/[PCr][ADP][H+]$$
$$\text{(Eq. 11.2)}$$

In following:

$$[ADP] = [ATP][Cr]/[PCr][H^+] K_{eq}*$$
$$\text{(Eq. 11.3)}$$

*$K_{eq} = 1.66 \times 10^{-9}$, as reported by Veech et al. [8].

Studies in intact animals demonstrated that [ADP] increases and phosphorylation potential declines with more moderate myocardial oxygen consumption ($M\dot{V}O_2$) elevation in the developing heart. The relationship between $M\dot{V}O_2$ and ADP emulates a respiratory control pattern consistent with first-order Michaelis–Menton kinetics, whereby increasing ADP drives $M\dot{V}O_2$. Transition to the mature and less ADP-dependent-type of respiratory control occurs in the first month of development and parallels the accumulation of adenine nucleotide translocator in the mitochondrial membrane. Studies performed in vitro indicated that the degree of respiratory control exerted through the adenine nucleotide translocator decreases with age and depends on the quantity or qualitative function of the adenine nucleotide translocator within the mitochondrial membrane [3]. Thus, phosphorylation potential and $\Delta G^{\circ\prime}$ depend in part on adenine nucleotide translocator function. The ADP/ATP exchange rate must increase in an concert with an increase in ATP hydrolysis at ATPase sites. Any diminution in adenine nucleotide translocator capacity would result in elevated cytosolic ADP concentration with reduced phosphorylation potential and $\Delta G'_{ATP}$ (Eq. 11.1). Qualitative or quantitative deficiencies in the adenine nucleotide translocator and shifts to ADP-dependent respiration occur not only in the developing heart, but also during congestive heart failure in a porcine model in vivo [9]. Qualitative dysfunction can occur through direct allosteric binding of the adenine nucleotide translocator by fatty acyl-coenzyme A derivatives, which accumulate after damage to fatty acid oxidation enzymes.

The efficiency of ATP hydrolysis is markedly diminished at very high work states in the mature heart and at more moderate work states in the developing heart due to the logarithmic nature of the relationship between $\Delta G0'_{ATP}$ and phosphorylation potential. The decrease in efficiency may not be problematic under conditions, where the heart can maintain high levels of ATP synthesis. However, under stress conditions whereby oxygen or substrate supply is limited and/or mitochondrial apparatus is damaged, the decreased efficiency of ATP hydrolysis can limit energy supply to cellular processes including the contractile apparatus.

Thyroid hormone modulates adenine nucleotide translocator function, thereby providing at least one avenue for modulating phosphorylation potential. Sterling identified specific binding for triiodothyronine (T_3) within the inner-mitochondrial membrane and immediate increase in respiration of hepatocyte mitochondria [10]. T_3 also acutely increased ADP/ATP exchange in isolated liver mitochondria, suggesting that T_3 binds directly to the adenine nucleotide translocator [11]. However, similar studies performed in cardiac mitochondria could not confirm these rapid and direct actions on ADP/ATP exchange [12] [13]. Thyroidectomy in newborn sheep did prevent the normal and substantial developmental increase in adenine nucleotide translocator mRNA and protein expression. These abnormalities occurred in parallel with modifications in the relationship between phosphorylation potential and $M\dot{V}O_2$. ADP decreases during increases in cardiac work and oxygen consumption in the thyroidectomized sheep, strongly suggesting that the reduction in adenine nucleotide translocator limits ADP/ATP exchange at the mitochondrial membrane. This finding also conforms to ADP–ATP kinetics in porcine models of heart failure characterized by adenine nucleotide translocator deficiency [9]. Although TH levels have not been evaluated in this model, circulating T_3 decreases in other forms of heart failure, suggesting a cause for reduction in myocardial phosphorylation potential in these states.

Interestingly, the mode of transcriptional regulation of adenine nucleotide translocator by T_3 is not fully clarified. Adenine nucleotide translocator-2 (human) mRNA and mRNA for cytochrome c_1 respond to T_3 [14]. The response depends on the presence of thyroid receptor α_1, though not its typical heterodimeric binding partner, retinoid X receptor (RXR). However, thyroid-receptor-binding half-sites are not apparent within the promoter regions of these genes. The absence of these sites suggests that the thyroid receptor (TR) binds to alternative receptor elements, possibly cross-reacting with peroxisome proliferator activated receptors (PPAR), major modulators of cardiac metabolism, and their DNA binding sites [15].

Creatine kinase (CK) represents another candidate for modulation of phosphorylation potential, as this enzyme is responsible in part for high-energy phosphate transfer within the cardiomyocyte. Mitochondrial CK interacts with adenine nucleotide translocator at the inner, mitochondrial membrane, and activity decreases in heart failure. However, hypothyroid states do not include a diminution in cardiac mitochondrial CK activity [16], reinforcing the importance of TH regulation of the adenine nucleotide translocator in energy transfer.

11.3 Substrate Oxidation

The cardiac energy state can also be modified by adjusting or limiting the carbon substrate or oxygen supply. Several studies in isolated perfused hearts demonstrated that the relationship between ADP and $M\dot{V}O_2$ is highly sensitive to the type of substrate employed. The reversible glycolytic reactions catalyzed by glyceraldehyde-3-phosphate dehydrogenase (GAPDH) and phosphoglycerate kinase (PGK) provide a mechanism for substrate-induced alterations in energy state. These reactions couple the cytosolic NADH redox state with $[ATP]/([ADP] \times [P_i])$ and are purported to be at near-equilibrium in the heart [17]. Cytosolic NADH fluctuates with mitochondrial NADH and increases in parallel during elevations in $M\dot{V}O_2$ in vivo [18]. TH maintains communication between these compartmental NAD pools by regulating enzymes controlling cytosolic-mitochondrial NADH shuttles [19]. ADP levels are lowest with substrates that induce high NADHm (reduced mitochondrial nicotinamide), such as pyruvate or octanoate, and highest with substrates which provide low NADHm, such as glucose or glucose with insulin [20]. For instance, in vivo phosphorylation potential increased in the canine heart during infusion of ketones in the form of β-hydroxybutyrate [21]. Phosphorylation potential decreased during catecholamine infusion in mature porcine right ventricle by blocking fatty acid oxidation with the carnitine palmitoyl transferase inhibitor oxfenecine [22]. Ochiai et al. ameliorated after the dobutamine-dopamine-induced decrease in PCr/ATP and of increase in free ADP in canine myocardium by providing pyruvate to the left ventricle in vivo at maximal work state [4].

Thyroid hormone modifies substrate oxidation through complex integration of transcriptional and post-transcriptional mechanisms [23]. Triiodothyronine rapidly (within 20 min) increases myocardial phosphorylation potential in hypothyroid neonatal sheep [13]. The mechanism does not involve increased rapid activation of the adenine nucleotide translocator. The observed increase in phosphorylation potential, as determined by ^{31}P magnetic resonance spectroscopy, occurred without a change in $M\dot{V}O_2$, suggesting substrate mediation of cytosolic NADH/NAD as the mechanism. This hypothesis is supported by other studies showing that T_3 rapidly modifies substrate oxidation in the isolated rat heart model. Experiments using isolated perfused hearts and employing ^{13}C detection by nuclear magnetic resonance and isotopomer analyses can define the fractional contribution to the citric acid cycle for up to three substrates simultane-

ously [23, 24]. This method has been used to study TH regulation of substrate oxidation in the heart.

A deficit in total substrate oxidation capacity represents the primary abnormality in various hypothyroid states [25, 26]. Though contractile function and citric acid flux are reduced in hypothyroid states, the heart maintains cardiac efficiency, defined as power generated per oxygen molecule consumed. In a transgenic mouse displaying the dominant negative, nonligand binding, and cardioselective thyroid hormone receptor, Δ337T, this adaptation accounts for the increased reliance on glucose and or other glycolytic pathways, such as glycogenolysis, relative to oxidation of fatty acids and ketones. Fatty acid oxidation requires greater oxygen for a given quantity of ATP synthesis than do carbohydrates [27]. For instance, for the fully metabolized molecule of oleate, approximately 2.8 molecules of ATP are produced per oxygen atom utilized as opposed to 3.17 for carbohydrate. Accordingly, although fatty acids or ketone oxidation might enhance NADH redox state and free energy of ATP hydrolysis, they reduce the efficiency of ATP synthesis in respect of oxygen consumed. However, the enhanced cardiac efficiency associated with TR dysfunction is tenuous, existing only during the baseline or resting state. Simple perturbations, such as increasing heart rate through pacing, reduce cardiac systolic function, power generation, and efficiency. The poor response to stress appears to be related to transcriptional mediation of the enzymes controlling glycolytic pathways. These include those regulating glucose transport and phosphorylation, respectively, the glucose transporters, and hexokinase-2, which are down-regulated. Additionally, pyruvate dehydrogenase kinases are increased in expression. These enzymes inhibit pyruvate dehydrogenase, the final step in glucose metabolism prior to substrate entry into the citric acid cycle.

Triiodothyronine modifies substrate oxidation rapidly through mechanisms distinct from transcriptional pathways, thereby explaining in part the rapid alterations in phosphorylation potential mentioned previously. In both the euthyroid and the hypothyroid rat heart, T_3 rapidly alters substrate flux and fractional contribution by shifting utilization patterns away from the pyruvate dehydrogenase pathway [23, 24]. In the euthyroid heart, T_3 acutely increases fatty acid oxidation, while decreasing lactate utilization. In the hypothyroid heart, T_3 rapidly decreases lactate oxidation, with a trend towards increased free fatty acid oxidation.

The molecular basis of this rapid nongenomic action by TH still requires further clarification in the heart. In the following paragraphs we will consider some of the putative controllers of these substrate oxidative pathways and speculate on the impact of TH.

11.3.1 Lactate Oxidation

Lactate supplies approximately 25% of myocardial oxidative substrates, at normal physiological levels [28, 29]. Pyruvate is an oxidized form of lactate, and the two enter the heart cell through the same monocarboxylate transporter (MCT-1) [30]. The compartmentalization and oxidation of lactate by lactate dehydrogenase within the mitochondria explains why the cardiomyocyte can simultaneously oxidize and produce lactate [31]. Several laboratories [23, 24, 32] have shown that, when the heart is provided with lactate, this substrate produces the major flux through pyruvate dehydrogenase, relegating glucose to a minor citric acid cycle contributor. The pyruvate lactate transporter MCT1, the MCT1-chaperone (CD147), and lactate dehydrogenase co-localize within the mitochondrial reticulum of L6 skeletal muscle cells [33]. These transporters show increased protein expression in cardiomyocytes exposed to conditions causing congestive heart failure [34]. The translocation of these proteins to the sarcolemma and, in some cases to the mitochondria likely represents a regulatory mechanism for this complex. T_3 promotes lactate exchange at the skeletal muscle sarcolemma without effecting MCT1 or MCT4 protein expression, instead enhancing activity [35]. The mechanism for the latter still requires elucidation, and specific studies evaluating T_3 promotion of translocation of these protein complexes are needed.

11.3.2 Lipid Kinase Family

The lipid kinase family regulates substrate oxidation in heart and exhibits regulation by TH [36–38]. T_3 and thyroxine (T_4) directly or indirectly activate phosphoinositide-3 kinase (PI3K), which phosphorylates phosphotidylinositols to phosphotidylinositol-3-4-5-phosphate [i.e., PtdIns(3,4,5)P3], PtdIns(3,4)P3, and PtdIns(4,5)P3. The PtdIns regulate downstream kinases such as Akt/PKB, a serine threonine protein kinase with a high sequence homology to protein kinase A. Akt/PKB regulates several downstream kinases, which directly control metabolic pathways. PI3K primarily controls Akt/PKB activity via modulation of PtdIns(3,4,5)P3 levels [39]. These in turn modulate the activity of the phosphoinositide-dependent kinases isoforms 1 and 2, which activate Akt by phosphorylation, respectively, at the threonine residue in the catalytic domain and a serine residue in C-terminal regulatory domain. In addition to phosphorylation by these phosphoinositide-dependent kinases, Akt/PKB activation involves recruitment to the plasma membrane through its PH (plekstrin) domain. Akt/PKB downstream targets involved in metabolism include glycogen synthase kinase-2, AMP-activated protein kinase (AMPK) [40], and mTOR, the mammalian target of rapamycin, which regulates protein synthesis. Additionally, Akt/PKB appears to control translocation of glucose transporter protein 4 (GLUT4). PI3K also regulates insulin-dependent GLUT4 translocation to the cell membrane.

Upstream from Akt/PKB, activation of PI3K by TH involves novel protein-to-protein interaction. Furuya et al. demonstrated that activation of PI3K in thyroid gland extracts occurs through protein-to-protein interaction with TH receptors [37]. They showed TRβ co-localization with PI3K during activation. The level of activation varied according to TH receptor isoform. The TRβPV mutant demonstrated greater binding affinity for PI3K-p85 regulatory subunit and raised PI3K activity more than did the wild-type TRβ. These phenomena suggest an alternate mechanism for changes in glucose transport, as observed by Esaki in heart expressing the PV mutation [41]. The data imply the existence of a novel activation mechanism which does not involve transcriptional regulation. Independently, Cao et al. also showed in skin fibroblasts that PI3K-p85 binds to TRβ1 and requires T_3 binding to this complex in order to activate PI3K [38]. TH stimulation of this regulatory PI3K pathway in cardiomyocytes has, to date, been reported only by two separate laboratories [42]. Kuzman et al. initially reported that T_4 activated Akt signaling. T_3 prevented cardiomyocyte death induced by serum starvation. This protection was inhibited by LY294002, an inhibitor of PI3K [42]. Kenessey and Ojamaa also recently showed direct interaction of the cytosol-localized

TH receptor TRα1 and the p85α subunit of PI3K in cardiomyocytes. T_3 exposure rapidly elevated PI3K activity, resulting in increased phosphorylation of downstream kinases (Akt) and the mammalian target of rapamycin (mTOR) [43]. Thus, these studies indicate that T_3 or T_4 bind to TH receptors, which interact with PI3K, alter the enzyme's conformation, and modify activity.

The direct link between thyroid activation of Akt/PKB on substrate utilization in the heart has not been clearly established. However, Akt/PKB inhibits AMPK, which controls long-chain fatty acid and glucose oxidation in the heart under specific conditions [44]. Long-chain fatty acid oxidation is controlled at the mitochondrial membrane by the activity of carnitine palmitoyl transferase I. Malonyl-CoA, the principal endogenous inhibitor of carnitine palmitoyl transferase I and primary controller of fatty acid oxidation, is rapidly turned over in heart, is produced from acetyl-CoA by acetyl-CoA carboxylase (ACC), and is degraded by malonyl-CoA decarboxylase (MCD). ACC is deactivated via phosphorylation by active AMPK, while regulation of MCD is still controversial. Insulin promoted Akt activity and phosphorylation, while constitutive expression of active Akt in transgenic mice blunted AMPK phosphorylation, thereby inactivating AMPK [40]. A decrease in AMPK activity should activate ACC, increase malonyl-CoA, and inhibit fatty acid oxidation [45, 46]. If THs operated solely along this cascade, inhibition of fatty acid oxidation would occur rather than the observed enhancement. Perfused-heart data regarding AMPK and ACC modulation of fatty acid oxidation have been inconsistent and in fact, fatty acid oxidation regulation may relate more to substrate supply than enzyme activation. While some studies supported the tenet that AMPK directly controls ACC activity, which in turn controls malonyl-CoA, others show that malonyl-CoA level is controlled by MCD [47]. However, both insulin and dobutamine increase Akt/PKB in porcine heart in vivo [48] while neither simultaneously alters AMPK activity. Also, in the porcine heart, acute increases in left ventricular contractile work and oxygen consumption reduce myocardial malonyl-CoA content independently of changes in the activities of MCD, ACC, and AMPK. Thus, TH may interfere with the Akt-PKB modulation of free fatty acid oxidation through an alternate mechanism. Peroxisomal beta-oxidation apparently supplies a portion of the long-chain-fatty-acid-derived cytosolic acetyl-CoA, the chief source of malonyl-CoA [48]. Regulation of this pathway has not been elucidated, but may relate to fatty acid transport and supply to the peroxisomes. Akt appears to enhance translocation of the fatty acid transport protein CD36 to the sarcolemma [49]. Accordingly, CD36 might be an indirect target of TH.

11.3.3 Cardiolipin

Thyroid hormones directly stimulate the activity of cardiolipin synthase and carnitine acylcarnitine translocase (CAT), thereby increasing the content of mitochondrial cardiolipin [50, 52], a key component of the mitochondrial membrane. Although CAT exchanges carnitine for acylcarnitine across the inner mitochondrial membrane, this transporter has not been considered a major regulator of fatty acid oxidation. Other, cardiolipin-dependent mitochondrial enzymes may play a role in controlling substrate oxidation and membrane potential, thus suggesting an important role for THs in remodeling of the mitochondrial membrane.

11.4 Mitochondrial Biogenesis

The failing heart exhibits fragmentation and distortion of mitochondria, suggesting not only damage but failure of mitochondrial biogenesis. A recent review noted that no agent currently exists which promotes mitochondrial biogenesis in the heart [27]. In fact, T_3 has been used as such an agent in a multitude of experimental models, including in cardiomyocytes [52]. Classically, ligand-dependent thyroid receptor actions on DNA occur within the nucleus and result in enhanced transcription of nuclear-encoded mitochondrial components. However, TH receptor interactions with respect to mitochondrial proliferation are quite complex. As noted previously, TH receptors demonstrate crosstalk with other nuclear receptors [15, 53]. PPARs are a subclass within the steroid-nuclear receptor family. They play an important role in regulating myocardial substrate metabolism, and their agonists are currently being evaluated as treatment agents for cardiomyopathies. TH receptors interact with PPARs by sharing binding sites and heterodimeric partners such as the RXR [54–56]. Additionally,

PPARs and TH receptors share co-activation by the PPAR-γ coactivator (PGC-1α). TH promotes the transcription of PGC-1α, which enhances mitochondrial biogenesis through multiple mechanisms. PGC-1 demonstrates a marked increase in proton expression during the TH surge which occurs postnatally. Cross-reactivity between TH receptors and PPARs is demonstrated in mice expressing the cardioselective Δ337T mutation. These mice show an altered cardiac transcriptional response to the PPARα agonist WY14643 [57]. This agonist prompted a robust increase in expression of the reporter gene uncoupling protein 3 (UCP3), which was abrogated in the transgenic mice. Hearts from these mice showed altered responses for multiple genes as determined by polymerase chain reaction and/or gene chip array. The mechanisms for these actions have been shown in studies performed in vitro and in cell culture. Sequestration of RXR, making this heterodimeric binding partner no longer freely available for PPAR, plays an important role in determining cross-talk [55, 58–60].

Thyroid hormone receptor binding and transcriptional activity within the mitochondria represents another mechanism for regulating oxidative metabolism. Mitochondrial biogenesis requires cooperative regulation of protein synthesis by the nuclear and mitochondrial genomes. Encoding occurs in the nucleus for the vast majority of the genes contributing to substrate oxidation, the respiratory chain, and oxidative phosphorylation [61]. The coding capacity of the mammalian mitochondrial genome includes only 13 proteins, representing vital respiratory complex subunits. Thus, any transcriptional activity within the mitochondria itself would not directly alter the synthesis of proteins involved in substrate oxidation. Nevertheless, changes in oxidative capacity could stimulate substrate oxidation pathways. Bigenomic coordination occurs in part through nuclear respiratory factor-1 (NRF-1), which promotes mitochondrial transcription factor A and other nuclear encoded proteins involved in mitochondrial transcription, while simultaneously enhancing synthesis of nuclear-encoded respiratory chain components. The heart, which maintains a high oxidative capacity relative to other organs, must respond rapidly to changing energy requirements encountered physiologically or during stress conditions. T_3 coordinates cardiac mitochondrial and nuclear transcription [52, 62]. Time-course analyses refute the notion that T_3 promotes mitochondrial transcription machinery prior to increasing respiratory complex proteins and/or activity, and suggests that an alternate more direct mechanism promotes mtDNA transcription. Mitochondrial import for various THα1 isoforms has been demonstrated [63–65]. In liver, only truncated versions of these receptors have been identified within mitochondria, although they retain potential for binding and transactivation of the mitochondrial genome. Full length and multiple truncated versions of TRα1 and TRα2 locate within cardiac mitochondria [66]. The TRα2 isoform lacks the ligand-binding domain, but competes for thyroid hormone response elements (TREs) and acts as a dominant negative regulator of T_3 activity [67, 68]. Thus, the stoichiometric relationship between these isoforms may determine mitochondrial transcriptional activity. TRα2 is upregulated in congestive heart failure relative to TRα1, providing a potential mechanism for inhibition of mitochondrial biogenesis in concert with other maladaptive responses.

Key Points

Thyroid hormone regulates numerous metabolic and mitochondrial pathways, which are disrupted in heart failure. Thyroid hormone:

- regulates myocardial oxidative phosphorylation via the adenine nucleotide translocator.
- controls the energy released by ATP hydrolysis.
- controls substrate oxidation through transcriptional and post-transcriptional pathways.
- regulates mitochondrial biogenesis through multiple mechanisms.

References

1. Kinugawa K, Minobe WA, Wood WM et al (2001) Signaling pathways responsible for fetal gene induction in the failing human heart: evidence for altered thyroid hormone receptor gene expression. Circulation 103:1089–1094

2. Kinugawa K, Yonekura K, Ribeiro RC et al (2001) Regulation of thyroid hormone receptor isoforms in physiological and pathological cardiac hypertrophy. Circ Res 89:591–598

3. Portman MA, Xiao Y, Song Y et al (1997) Expression of adenine nucleotide translocator parallels maturation of respiratory control in vivo. Am J Physiol Heart Circ Physiol 273:H1977–1983

4. Ochiai K, Zhang J, Gong G et al (2001) Effects of augmented delivery of pyruvate on myocardial high-energy phosphate metabolism at high workstate. Am J Physiol Heart Circ Physiol 281:H1823–1832

5. Zhang J (2002) Myocardial energetics in cardiac hypertrophy. Clin Exp Pharmacol Physiol 29:351–359

6. Bache RJ, Zhang J, Murakami Y et al (1999) Myocardial oxygenation at high workstates in hearts with left ventricular hypertrophy. Cardiovasc Res 42:616–626

7. Tian R and Ingwall JS (1996) Energetic basis for reduced contractile reserve in isolated rat hearts. Am J Physiol 270:H1207–1216

8. Veech RL, Lawson JWR, Cornell NW et al (1979) Cytosolic phosphorylation potential. J Biol Chem 254:6538–6547

9. Ning X, Zhang J, Liu J et al (2000) Signaling and expression for mitochondrial membrane proteins during left ventricular remodeling and contractile failure after myocardial infarction. J Am Coll Cardiol 36:282–287

10. Sterling K (1987) Direct thyroid hormone activation of mitochondria: identification of adenine nucleotide translocase (AdNT) as the hormone receptor. Trans Assoc Am Phys 100:284–293

11. Sterling K (1986) Direct thyroid hormone activation of mitochondria: the role of adenine nucleotide translocase. Endocrinology 119:292–295

12. Portman MA, Xiao Y, Qian K et al (2000) Thyroid hormone coordinates respiratory control maturation and adenine nucleotide translocator expression in heart in vivo. Circulation 102:1323–1329

13. Portman MA, Qian K, Krueger JJ et al (2005) Direct action of T3 on phosphorylation potential in the sheep heart in vivo. Am J Physiol Heart Circ Physiol 288:2484–2490

14. Li R, Luciakova K, Zaid A et al (1997) Thyroid hormone activates transcription from the promoter regions of some human nuclear-encoded genes of the oxidative phosphorylation system. Mol Cell Endocrinol 128:69–75

15. Hyyti OM, Portman MA (2006) Molecular mechanisms of cross-talk between thyroid hormone and peroxisome proliferator activated receptors: focus on the heart. Cardiovasc Drugs Ther 20:463–469

16. Athea Y, Garnier A, Fortin D et al (2007) Mitochondrial and energetic cardiac phenotype in hypothyroid rat. Relevance to heart failure. Pflugers Arch 455:431–442

17. Heineman FW, Balaban RS (1990) Control of mitochondrial respiration in the heart in vivo. Annu Rev Physiol 52:523–542

18. Zhou L, Cabrera ME, Huang H et al (2007) Parallel activation of mitochondrial oxidative metabolism with increased cardiac energy expenditure is not dependent on fatty acid oxidation in pigs. J Physiol 579:811–821

19. Scholz TD, TenEyck CJ, Schutte BC (2000) Thyroid hormone regulation of the NADH shuttles in liver and cardiac mitochondria. J Mol Cell Cardiol 32:1–10

20. From AH, Zimmer SD, Michurski SP et al (1990) Regulation of the oxidative phosphorylation rate in the intact cell. Biochemistry 29:3731–3743

21. Kim DK, Heineman FW, Balaban RS (1991) Effects of b-hydroxybutyrate on oxidative metabolism and phosphorylation potential in canine heart in vivo. Am J Physiol 260 (Heart Circ Physiol 29):H1767-H1773

22. Schwartz GG, Greyson C, Wisneski JA et al (1994) Inhibition of fatty acid metabolism alters myocardial high-energy phosphates in vivo. Am J Physiol 267:H224–H231

23. Hyyti OM, Ning XH, Buroker NE et al (2006) Thyroid hormone controls myocardial substrate metabolism through nuclear receptor-mediated and rapid posttranscriptional mechanisms. Am J Physiol Endocrinol Metab 290:E372–E379

24. Krueger JJ, Ning XH, Argo BM et al (2001) Triiodothyronine and epinephrine rapidly modify myocardial substrate selection: a (13)C isotopomer analysis. Am J Physiol Endocrinol Metab 281:E983–E990

25. Ning XH, Chen SH, Buroker NE et al (2007) Short-cycle hypoxia in the intact heart: hypoxia-inducible factor 1alpha signaling and the relationship to injury threshold. Am J Physiol Heart Circ Physiol 292:H333–H341

26. Hyyti OM, Olson A, Ge M et al (2008) The cardioselective dominant negative thyroid hormone receptor (D337T) modulates myocardial metabolism and contractile efficiency. Am J Physiol Endocrinol Metab 295:E420–E427

27. Ashrafian H, Frenneaux MP and Opie LH (2007) Metabolic mechanisms in heart failure. Circulation 116:434–448

28. Laughlin MR, Taylor JF, Chesnick AS et al (1992) Regulation of glycogen metabolism in canine myocardium: effects of insulin and epinephrine in vivo. Am J Physiol 262 (Endocrinol Metab 25): E875–E873

29. Drake AJ, Haines JR and Noble MI (1980) Preferential uptake of lactate by the normal myocardium in dogs. Cardiovasc Res 14:65–72

30. Trosper TL, Philipson KD (1987) Lactate transport by cardiac sarcolemmal vesicles. Am J Physiol 252:C483–489

31. Brooks GA (2002) Lactate shuttles in nature. Biochem Soc Trans 30:258–264

32. Lloyd S, Brocks C, Chatham JC (2003) Differential modulation of glucose lactate and pyruvate oxidation by insulin and dichloroacetate in the rat heart. Am J Physiol Heart Circ Physiol 285:H163–H172

33. Hashimoto T, Hussien R, Brooks GA (2006) Co-localization of MCT1, CD147 and LDH in mitochondrial inner membrane of L6 skeletal muscle cells: evidence of a mitochondrial lactate oxidation complex. Am J Physiol Endocrinol Metab 290:E1237–E1244

34. Evans RK, Schwartz DD, Gladden LB (2003) Effect of myocardial volume overload and heart failure on lactate transport into isolated cardiac myocytes. J Appl Physiol 94:1169–1176

35. Wang Y, Tonouchi M, Miskovic D et al (2003) T3 increases lactate transport and the expression of MCT4, but not

MCT1, in rat skeletal muscle. Am J Physiol Endocrinol Metab 285:E622–E628

36. Bergh JJ, Lin HY, Lansing L et al (2005) Integrin alphaV-beta3 contains a cell surface receptor site for thyroid hormone that is linked to activation of mitogen-activated protein kinase and induction of angiogenesis. Endocrinology 146:2864–2871

37. Furuya F, Hanover JA, Cheng SY (2006) Activation of phosphatidylinositol 3-kinase signaling by a mutant thyroid hormone beta receptor. Proc Natl Acad Sci U S A 103:1780–1785

38. Cao X, Kambe F, Moeller LC et al (2005) Thyroid hormone induces rapid activation of Akt/protein kinase B-mammalian target of rapamycin-p70S6K cascade through phosphatidylinositol 3-kinase in human fibroblasts. Mol Endocrinol 19:102–112

39. Oudit GY, Sun H, Kerfant BG et al (2004) The role of phosphoinositide-3 kinase and PTEN in cardiovascular physiology and disease. J Mol Cell Cardiol 37:449–471

40. Kovacic S, Soltys CL, Barr AJ et al (2003) Akt activity negatively regulates phosphorylation of AMP-activated protein kinase in the heart. J Biol Chem 278:39422–39427

41. Esaki T, Suzuki H, Cook M et al (2004) Cardiac glucose utilization in mice with mutated alpha- and beta-thyroid hormone receptors. Am J Physiol Endocrinol Metab 287:E1149–1153

42. Kuzman JA, Gerdes AM, Kobayashi S et al (2005) Thyroid hormone activates Akt and prevents serum starvation-induced cell death in neonatal rat cardiomyocytes. J Mol Cell Cardiol 39:841–844

43. Kenessey A, Ojamaa K (2006) Thyroid hormone stimulates protein synthesis in the cardiomyocyte by activating the Akt-mTOR and p70S6K pathways. J Biol Chem 281:20666–20672

44. Khairallah M, Khairallah R, Young ME et al (2007) Metabolic and signaling alterations in dystrophin-deficient hearts precede overt cardiomyopathy. J Mol Cell Cardiol 43:119–129

45. Gamble J, Lopaschuk GD (1997) Insulin inhibition of 5¢ adenosine monophosphate-activated protein kinase in the heart results in activation of acetyl coenzyme A carboxylase and inhibition of fatty acid oxidation. Metabolism 46:1270–1274

46. Clark H, Carling D, Saggerson D (2004) Covalent activation of heart AMP-activated protein kinase in response to physiological concentrations of long-chain fatty acids. Eur J Biochem 271:2215–2224

47. Goodwin G, Taegtmeyer H (1999) Regulation of fatty acid oxidation of the heart by MCD and ACC during contractile stimulation. Am J Physiol 277:E772–E777

48. King KL, Okere IC, Sharma N et al (2005) Regulation of cardiac malonyl-CoA content and fatty acid oxidation during increased cardiac power. Am J Physiol Heart Circ Physiol 289:H1033–H1037

49. Ouwens DM, Diamant M, Fodor M et al (2007) Cardiac contractile dysfunction in insulin-resistant rats fed a high-fat diet is associated with elevated CD36-mediated fatty acid uptake and esterification. Diabetologia 50:1938–1948

50. Mutter T, Dolinsky VW, Ma BJ et al (2000) Thyroxine regulation of monolysocardiolipin acyltransferase activity in rat heart. Biochem J 346 (Pt 2):403–406

51. Paradies G, Ruggiero FM, Petrosillo G et al (1996) Stimulation of carnitine acylcarnitine translocase activity in heart mitochondria from hyperthyroid rats. FEBS Lett 397:260–262

52. Goldenthal MJ, Weiss HR, Marin-Garcia J (2004) Bioenergetic remodeling of heart mitochondria by thyroid hormone. Mol Cell Biochem 265:97–106

53. McClure TD, Young ME, Taegtmeyer H et al (2005) Thyroid hormone interacts with PPARa and PGC-1 during mitochondrial maturation in sheep heart. Am J Physiol Heart Circ Physiol 289:H2258–H2264

54. Araki O, Ying H, Furuya F et al (2005) Thyroid hormone receptor beta mutants: dominant negative regulators of peroxisome proliferator-activated receptor gamma action. Proc Natl Acad Sci U S A 102:16251–16256

55. Miyamoto T, Kaneko A, Kakizawa T et al (1997) Inhibition of peroxisome proliferator signaling pathways by thyroid hormone receptor. Competitive binding to the response element. J Biol Chem 272:7752–7758.

56. Dillmann WH (2002) Cellular action of thyroid hormone on the heart. Thyroid 12:447–452

57. Buroker NE, Young ME, Wei C et al (2007) The dominant negative thyroid hormone receptor beta-mutant D337T alters PPARa signaling in heart. Am J Physiol Endocrinol Metab 292:E453–E460

58. Hunter J, Kassam A, Winrow CJ et al (1996) Crosstalk between the thyroid hormone and peroxisome proliferator-activated receptors in regulating peroxisome proliferator-responsive genes. Mol Cell Endocrinol 116:213–221

59. Chu R, Madison LD, Lin Y et al (1995) Thyroid hormone (T3) inhibits ciprofibrate-induced transcription of genes encoding beta-oxidation enzymes: cross talk between peroxisome proliferator and T3 signaling pathways. Proc Natl Acad Sci U S A 92:11593–11597

60. Bogazzi F, Hudson LD, Nikodem VM (1994) A novel heterodimerization partner for thyroid hormone receptor. Peroxisome proliferator-activated receptor. J Biol Chem 269:11683–11686

61. Scarpulla RC (2006) Nuclear control of respiratory gene expression in mammalian cells. J Cell Biochem 97:673–683

62. Goldenthal MJ, Ananthakrishnan R, Marin-Garcia J (2005) Nuclear-mitochondrial cross-talk in cardiomyocyte T3 signaling: a time-course analysis. J Mol Cell Cardiol 39:319–326

63. Wrutniak C, Cassar-Malek I, Marchal S et al (1995) A 43-kDa protein related to c-Erb A alpha 1 is located in the mitochondrial matrix of rat liver. J Biol Chem 270:16347–16354

64. Casas F, Daury L, Grandemange S et al (2003) Endocrine regulation of mitochondrial activity: involvement of truncated RXRalpha and c-Erb Aalpha1 proteins. FASEB J 17:426–436

65. Casas F, Rochard P, Rodier A et al (1999) A variant form of the nuclear triiodothyronine receptor c-ErbAalpha1 plays a direct role in regulation of mitochondrial RNA synthesis. Mol Cell Biol 19:7913–7924

66. Morrish F, Buroker NE, Ge M et al (2006) Thyroid hormone receptor isoforms localize to cardiac mitochondrial matrix with potential for binding to receptor elements on mtDNA. Mitochondrion 6:143–148

67. Katz D, Lazar MA (1993) Dominant negative activity of an endogenous thyroid hormone receptor variant (alpha 2) is due to competition for binding sites on target genes. J Biol Chem 268:20904–20910

68. Mitsuhashi T, Tennyson GE, Nikodem VM (1988) Alternative splicing generates messages encoding rat c-erbA proteins that do not bind thyroid hormone. Proc Natl Acad Sci U S A 85:5804–5808

Cardiac Myocyte and Vascular Remodeling in Altered Thyroid Conditions

12

Yuefeng Chen and A. Martin Gerdes

Abstract Ventricular remodeling refers to ventricular morphometric, architectural, and functional changes under different cardiovascular conditions; it consists of cardiomyocyte, coronary vasculature, and collagen network remodeling. Thyroid hormones have important effects on cardiac function and cardiovascular hemodynamics. Altered thyroid conditions can also result in cardiac myocyte and vascular remodeling. Hyperthyroidism causes a proportional increase in myocyte length and cross-sectional area with increased α-MHC expression and decreased β-MHC expression. Hypothyroidism leads to myocyte lengthening and a reduction of myocyte cross-sectional area, with decreased expression of α-MHC and increased expression of β-MHC. Excess thyroid hormones promote growth of coronary arterioles and capillaries, while thyroid hormone deficiency leads to progressive arteriolar loss.

Keywords Ventricular remodeling • Cardiomyocyte • Coronary vasculature • Cardiac hypertrophy

12.1 Concept of Ventricular Remodeling

The term "ventricular remodeling" is now being widely used to describe ventricular morphometric, architectural, and functional changes due to a variety of cardiovascular conditions; it consists of cardiomyocyte, coronary vasculature, and collagen network remodeling. Cardiac hypertrophy is the predominant form of ventricular remodeling and can be classified as either physiological or pathological hypertrophy, each with distinctive characteristics [1–4]. In physiological cardiac hypertrophy, ventricular function is normal and delivery of O_2 to the metabolizing tissue is preserved. The remodeled myocardium can return to normal when abnormal loading conditions are removed. Histologically, cardiomyocytes are surrounded by a fine network of collagen fibers under normal conditions. Usually, there is no re-expression of the fetal gene program. In contrast, in pathological hypertrophy, ventricular function is abnormal, O_2 delivery to the tissue is impaired and myocardial changes are not completely reversible. Cardiac fibroblasts and extracellular matrix proteins accumulate disproportionately and excessively around the cardiomyocytes. Fetal gene expression is often up-regulated, including genes encoding atrial natriuretic peptide (ANP), B-type natriuretic peptide (BNP), α-actin, and β-myosin heavy chain (β-MHC), with down-regulation of α-MHC and sarcoplasmic reticulum Ca^{2+}-ATPase. In adults, physiological hypertrophy occurs in response to regular physical activity, chronic exercise training, or pregnancy, and appears to be regulated by the insulin-like growth factor (IGF)-1–PI3-kinase–Akt signaling pathway. Pathological hypertrophy occurs in response to diverse pathological

A.M. Gerdes (✉)
Cardiovascular Research Center, Sanford Research/University of South Dakota, Sioux Falls, SD, United States

G. Iervasi, A. Pingitore (eds.), *Thyroid and Heart Failure*.

conditions and is often regulated by the $G_{\alpha q}$ pathway [2, 5, 6]. However, other signaling pathways and downstream effectors may also be involved in both types of hypertrophy.

Initial stimuli for cardiac hypertrophy can be classified as pressure overload or volume overload, which lead, respectively, to concentric and eccentric hypertrophy. Concentric hypertrophy is characterized by wall thickening with a normal or reduced chamber cavity. The term "eccentric hypertrophy" was originally used to describe outward displacement of the heart but is now generally used to describe hearts with chamber dilation and a "relative" increase in chamber volume, which is typical of volume-overloading hypertrophy [2, 7, 8] (Fig. 12.1).

12.2 Ventricular Remodeling and Myocardial Infarction

The concept of "ventricular remodeling" was introduced in the 1970s and often referred to the complex alterations in ventricular architecture caused by myocardial infarction, particularly large transmural infarcts, involving the changes in both infarcted and noninfarcted areas [9]. The process of ventricular remodeling in myocardial infarction is mainly caused by volume overload due to the loss of contractile tissue and can be arbitrarily divided into early and later stages. The early stage, termed "infarct expansion," was described in 1978 by Hutchins and Bulkley and defined as "acute

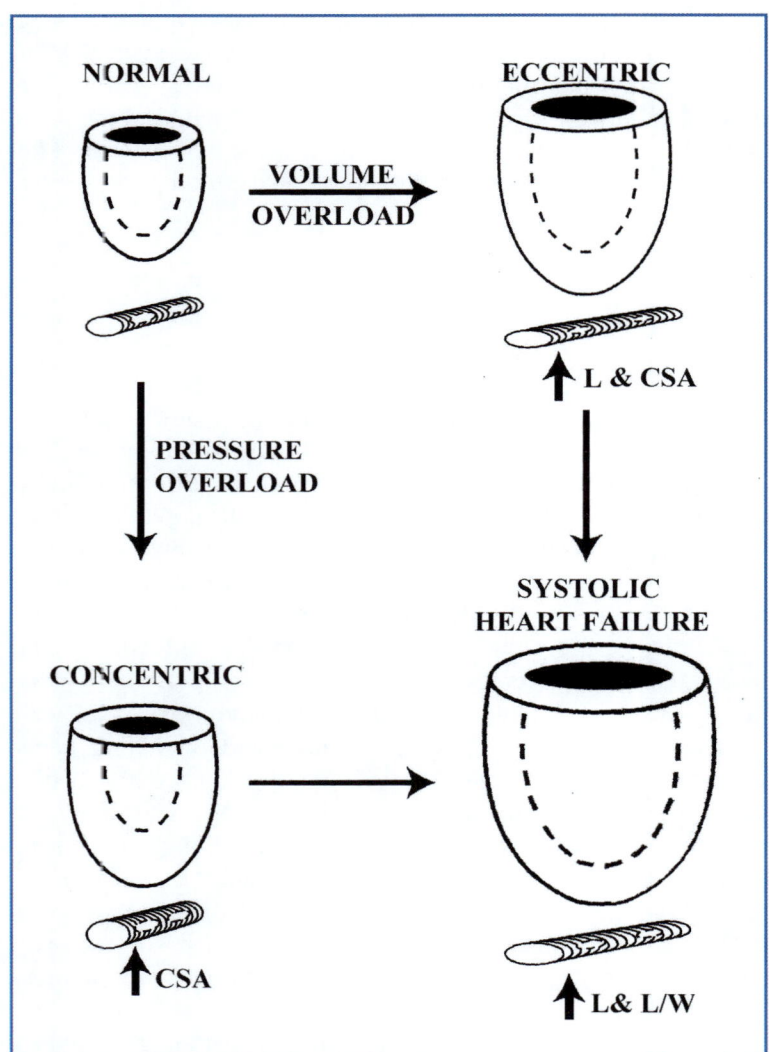

Fig. 12.1 Cardiac hypertrophy and myocyte shape changes with pressure and volume overload and the progression to systolic heart failure. *L* length, *W* width, *L/W* length/width ratio, *CSA* cross-sectional area

dilatation and thinning of the area of infarction not explained by additional myocardial necrosis" [10]. This process of myocyte necrosis, edema, inflammation, and scar formation starts a few hours after myocardial infarction and lasts for weeks or months depending on the species [11, 12]. Histologically, it has been reported that the thinning and lengthening of the infarct area is a consequence of slippage between muscle bundles, resulting in a reduction in the number of myocytes across the infarct region [13]. However, evidence from our lab suggests that myocyte lengthening alone accounts for expansion of the spared myocardium[14]. Infarct expansion is more common in patients with transmural infarctions involving the anterior apical surface than other regions of the left ventricle [15], which may lead to development of congestive heart failure, aneurysm formation, and myocardial rupture. The later stage of ventricular remodeling starts as early as 2 weeks after myocardial infarction [16] and continues after scar formation. This process involves progressive ventricular chamber dilation and eccentric hypertrophy of the noninfarcted area as compensatory responses to the decline in pump function. The acute distension of the noninfarcted myocardium together with other acute compensatory mechanisms can maintain pump function within normal limits. However, long-term dilation would augment diastolic and systolic wall stress and stimulate further ventricular enlargement, creating a vicious cycle as "dilation begets more dilation" [7, 9]. The increase in wall stress of the dilated ventricle can stimulate additional cardiac hypertrophy, which can offset the increased wall stress and reduce the stimulus for further enlargement. However, in severe infarction, the loss of infarcted tissue and volume overloading (chamber dilation) is often out of proportion to the hypertrophic response, resulting in further enlargement and dysfunction [17–19].

12.3 Myocyte Remodeling During Cardiac Hypertrophy

Remodeling during cardiac hypertrophy is often reflected at the myocyte level (Fig. 12.1, Table 12.1). With ventricular pressure overload, myocyte enlargement is due to an increase in cross-sectional area (width) only. In volume overloading, there is an equal increase in length and width, and myocyte length/width ratio is maintained within a normal range (physiological or early, phase pathological). In congestive heart failure, there is a significant increase in myocyte length with limited or no growth in myocyte diameter, leading to an increase in myocyte length/width ratio [14, 20–24]. The increase in myocyte length is due to the addition of new sarcomeres in series, whereas the increase in myocyte width is due to the addition of new sarcomeres in parallel. Myocyte hypertrophy is accompanied by changes in intracellular components, including myofibrils and mitochondria, as well as many cytoskeletal proteins. For example, 10 days after aortic banding there is a significant increase in myofibrillar volume and a significant decrease in mitochondrial volume [25].

Table 12.1 Left ventricular cardiac myocyte shape changes under different conditions [14, 20–24, 40, 45]

	Cell volume (μm^3)	Cell length (μm)	Cross-sectional area (μm^2)	Length/width ratio
Normal	~26,000–35,000	~125–145	~200–260	~8
Volume overload (compensated)	↑	↑	↑	↔
Pressure overload (compensated)	↑	↔	↑	↓
Systolic heart failure	↑	↑↑	↑ or ↔	↑
Hyperthyroidism	↑	↑	↑	↔
Hypothyroidism	↓	↔ or ↑ (long term)	↓	↑

↑increase, ↓decrease, ↔ no change.

Normal values at lower end represent those of females while higher values represent those of males. Values are from rats but most other mammals, including humans, appear to have values in the same range

12.4 Hemodynamic Effects of Thyroid Hormones on Cardiovascular System

The influence of thyroid hormones (THs) on the cardiovascular system has been noted for more than 200 years. THs are important regulators of cardiac function and cardiovascular hemodynamics. Excess THs cause a decrease in peripheral vascular resistance and an increase in venous tone, which leads to augmented blood return to the heart, increased preload, increased blood volume, increased cardiac output, and a hyperdynamic circulatory state [26–30]. THs also cause an increase in systolic and diastolic function [31, 32], although impaired diastolic function has been reported with subclinical hyperthyroidism [33]. The above changes typically cause an increase in systolic arterial pressure and a decrease in diastolic arterial pressure, leading to a wider pulse pressure and a slight decrease in mean arterial pressure [34, 35]. THs also have electrophysiological and pro-angiogenic effects on the heart [36–38].

12.5 Myocyte Remodeling in Hyperthyroidism

The overall hemodynamic effect of THs on the heart is similar to that of volume overload, which can induce physiological and pathological hypertrophy in the heart depending on serum TH levels and duration of hyperthyroidism. Mildly increased serum TH levels may cause concentric physiological cardiac hypertrophy with increased wall thickness but undetectable changes in cavity dimension. It should be pointed out that there is a difference in TH effects on the systemic and pulmonary circulation [39]. While THs decrease systemic peripheral resistance, pulmonary vascular resistance does not change. Consequently, there may be a flow-mediated increase in right ventricular systolic and mean pulmonary artery pressures with minimal changes in left ventricular systolic pressure and mean aortic pressure. As a result, hyperthyroidism typically leads to more pronounced hypertrophy in the right ventricle than in the left ventricle. These changes are reflected at the cellular level by regional differences in myocyte remodeling. After adult rats were treated with a high dose of THs for 10 weeks, myocyte volume was increased in all regions, especially the right ventricle and the epimyocardium of the left ventricle. Cell length was increased in all regions, but about two-thirds of left ventricular hypertrophy was due to increased myocyte cross-sectional area. This translated into an approximately proportional increase in myocyte length and width, suggesting a physiological type of hypertrophy (Table 12.1). There was a more pronounced increase in myocyte cross-sectional area in the right ventricle, reflecting the greater increase in systolic pressure in that chamber [40]. THs can also directly stimulate cardiomyocyte hypertrophy in vitro, suggesting a growth-promoting effect independent of loading [41]. However, higher serum TH may result in pathological hypertrophy and heart failure. BIO F1B hamsters treated with TH for 2 months showed signs of developing heart failure, as reflected in increased chamber diameters, decreased ejection fraction, and positive and negative changes in pressure over time. In this model, myocyte length was increased, with increased α-MHC expression and decreased β-MHC expression [42].

Myocyte ultrastructural alterations caused by TH have been reported and may vary as a result of the duration and degree of hyperthyroidism. McCallister and Page [43] reported an increase in the volume percentage of mitochondria in myocytes in hyperthyroid rats, whereas hypertension led to a reduction. This observation likely reflected the changes in energy needs related to α-myosin (high ATPase activity) and β-myosin (low ATPase activity) isoforms, although this myosin isoform shift was not known at that time. Others have reported pathological alterations in cardiac myocyte ultrastructure in hyperthyroidism, including mitochondrial damage, myofibrillar disarray, and disorganization of intercellular junctions and cytoskeletal proteins such as desmin [44]. In our experience, these changes may result from poor fixation since we observed some of these alterations in unperfused areas but never in areas that were well-perfused with fixative (unpublished observations). This is also a situation in which immersion fixation of tissues from control and hyperthyroid animals may lead to erroneous conclusions based on more rapid breakdown of hypermetabolic cells in hyperthyroid animals during the diffusion time needed for fixation.

12.6 Cardiovascular Hemodynamic Changes and Myocyte Remodeling During Hypothyroidism

The effects of TH deficiency on the cardiovascular system are typically the opposite of those caused by hyperthyroidism but may vary by species. Hypothyroidism leads to increased peripheral vascular resistance and reduced cardiac output. In rodents, this generally is associated with reduced peripheral systolic blood pressure [45, 46]. However, in humans, the increase in peripheral resistance may exceed the decline in cardiac output and this causes systemic hypertension in some patients [34, 47]. Hypothyroidism is also characterized by impaired diastolic function, mildly abnormal systolic function due to decrease in blood volume, reduction of preload, slight depression of myocardial contractility, and bradycardia [48, 49].

Hypothyroidism may cause left ventricular chamber dilatation despite cardiac atrophy. Induction of hypothyroidism in rats by the antithyroid drug propylthiouracil (PTU) for 4 weeks resulted in a 24% heart weight decrease with impaired cardiac function. Myocyte volume was significantly smaller in hypothyroid rats, primarily due to a reduction in myocyte cross-sectional area (Table 12.1). There were no significant differences in the cellular changes in the right and left ventricles in hypothyroidism [45]. Rats treated with PTU for 1 year had severe left ventricular systolic dysfunction, chamber dilation, and cardiac atrophy. Chamber dilation was due to excessive myocyte lengthening from series addition of sarcomeres, a cellular change typical of heart failure [46]. This cellular change is opposite that of cardiac unloading from a left ventricular assist device (LVAD), in which there is series removal of sarcomeres [50]. Chronic hypothyroidism was associated with reduced expression of sarcoplasmic/endoplasmic reticulum Ca^{2+}-ATPase (SERCA)-2a and α-MHC and increased expression of phospholamban and β-MHC [46]. Additionally, in this experiment, serum hormone levels indicated mild hypothyroidism, suggesting that similar changes are present in borderline low thyroid function. Cumulatively, these data provide a convincing case that chronic hypothyroidism alone eventually leads to heart failure.

12.7 Mechanisms of Thyroid Hormone on Myocyte Remodeling

Many mechanisms have been proposed for the effects of THs on myocyte remodeling. THs have both genomic and nongenomic actions. The genomic action is mediated by three TH receptors (TR), $\beta1$, $\alpha1$, and $\alpha2$. TR$\alpha1$ with α-MHC transcription. TR$\beta1$ is associated with β-MHC, SERCA, and TR$\beta1$ transcription [51]. TH-induced cardiac myocyte hypertrophy has been shown to be TR$\alpha1$-specific and involves the transforming growth factor β-activated kinase (TAK1) and p38 [52]. An in vitro study done by Kenessey and Ojamaa [53] showed that triiodothyronine (T_3) stimulates protein synthesis in cardiomyocytes via activation of phosphatidylinositol 3-kinase (PI3K) by cytosolic TR$\alpha1$, with subsequent activation of Akt, mammalian target of rapamycin (mTOR), and p70 (S6K). We found that thyroxine (T_4) activates specific components of the Akt signaling pathway both in vivo and in vitro. T_4-induced cardiac hypertrophy can be completely inhibited by the mTOR inhibitor rapamycin, suggesting that TH-induced cardiac hypertrophy is mediated by AKT/mTOR/S6 kinase signaling [54]. Pantos et al. [55] showed that T_3-induced changes in cardiomyocyte shape and geometry with increased major/minor ratio were accompanied by increased phospho-ERK levels, indicating activation of the ERK signaling pathway. Other neuroendocrinological factors may also be involved in TH-induced cardiac hypertrophy, including the renin–angiotensin system and the sympathetic nervous system [56]. Shohet et al. [57] demonstrated that endothelin 1 (ET-1) produced by cardiac myocytes plays an important role in cardiac hypertrophy from hyperthyroidism. ET-1 acts in a paracrine/autocrine manner, and mice with cardiomyocyte-specific disruption of the ET-1 gene are resistant to TH-induced cardiac hypertrophy. A recent study also showed that T_3-dependent repression of β-MHC is regulated by microRNA-208, which is required for up-regulation of β-MHC in response to PTU [58].

12.8 Coronary Vasculature Changes During Cardiac Hypertrophy

Cardiac hypertrophy is accompanied by growth of the coronary vasculature, which maintains normal coronary flow reserve and oxygen supply. Two levels of the vascular bed are of major importance during the hypertrophic process. First, there may be an increase in the cross-sectional area of precapillary vessels, particularly the arterioles, to maintain sufficient maximal coronary perfusion and adequate coronary reserve. Second, growth of capillaries is important to maintain adequate oxygen diffusion distances [59]. However, vascular changes are variable and dependent on several factors, including age, type of overloading stimulus, and duration of cardiac hypertrophy. In adults, cardiac hypertrophy secondary to pressure overload is often associated with decreased coronary reserve and increased minimal coronary vascular resistance due to inadequate growth of new arterioles and capillaries, or even loss of arterioles. Nonetheless, these changes may become normalized over time by vascular growth after hypertrophy is stabilized [60]. For volume-overload-induced cardiac hypertrophy, studies have shown that arteriolar and capillary growth parallels the magnitude of hypertrophy, leading to normal arteriolar length density (length per unit volume) and capillary density, although some regional variation may occur [61, 62]. Exercise-induced cardiac hypertrophy led to increased capillary density at 3 weeks with return to normal at 16 weeks [63]. There was also an increase in the number of small arterioles and in the diameters of large arteries. The net result per unit mass of myocardium was an unchanged capillary supply but a larger and more profuse arterial supply.

12.9 Coronary Arteriole and Capillary Changes During Thyroid-Hormone-Induced Hypertrophy

Coronary vascular growth during TH-induced cardiac hypertrophy has been well-studied. Marked growth of arterioles and capillaries has been reported in different animal models [37, 64, 65]. However, the temporal angiogenic changes related to thyroid-induced hypertrophy remain controversial. Tomanek et al. [38] reported that the angiogenic effect precedes cardiac enlargement. Administration of thyroxine caused a significant increase in epicardial capillary density by day 5. Heron et al. [66] showed that capillary growth initially exceeds cardiac hypertrophy, with later normalization. Conversely, Anjos-Ramos et al. [67] have shown that 1 week of

treatment with T$_4$ results in a 33% increase in cardiac mass and decreased capillary density. We found that capillary growth does not keep up with myocyte hypertrophy in chronic hyperthyroidism [68]. Obviously, some controversy remains regarding the temporal changes in myocardial vascularization during thyroid-induced cardiac hypertrophy. It is our belief that THs are powerful regulators of vascular growth in low-thyroid conditions, but that vessel "overgrowth" is largely prevented by currently unknown feedback mechanisms during hyperthyroid-induced cardiac hypertrophy.

12.10 Mechanisms of Thyroid-Hormone-Induced Coronary Vascular Remodeling

The regulation of vascular remodeling is complex. Multiple factors and molecular mechanisms have been proposed. Among these, mechanical factors have been suggested as primary stimuli for angiogenesis and are associated with increased blood flow, longitudinal stretch, and prolonged diastole [59]. Coronary blood flow is increased in the hyperthyroid state. There are at least three lines of evidence supporting a role for flow-induced angiogenesis [59]. First, endothelial cells function as mechanoreceptors for shear stress and stretch. Second, DNA synthesis is stimulated by endothelial cell flattening and by increases in flow or turbulence. Third, mechanical stimulation may initiate the synthesis and/or release of growth factors. An increase in longitudinal stretch also occurs in hyperthyroidism due to volume overload and increased diastolic dimensions of the ventricle.

With regard to molecular mechanisms, the angiogenic effects of THs are believed to be due to nongenomic actions and may depend on fibroblast growth factor (FGF). Angiogenesis may involve the cell surface integrin $\alpha_V\beta_3$ receptor and be mediated by a mitogen-activated protein kinase (MAPK; ERK1/2) signaling pathway [69–71]. Vascular endothelial growth factor (VEGF-A) has also been implicated in TH-induced angiogenesis [67]. The Akt1/PKB signaling pathway has been shown to play an important role in cardiac hypertrophy and angiogenesis. Short-term Akt1 activation in the heart induces physiological hypertrophy and angiogenesis, with maintained capillary density and increased myocyte expression of the major angiogenic growth factors VEGF and angiopoietin-2 (Ang-2) in a mTORC1-dependent manner. In contrast, long-term Akt1 activation leads to pathological hypertrophy and decreased capillary density, with down-regulated VEGF and Ang-2 expression [72]. These results also suggest that angiogenesis during cardiac hypertrophy is dependent on paracrine signals from cardiac myocytes. Inhibition of angiogenesis has been shown to impair Akt-mediated or pressure-overload-induced cardiac hypertrophy and cardiac function [72, 73], indicating that cardiac growth is also dependent on coronary angiogenesis. These results implicate the existence of reciprocal cross-talk mechanisms between the coronary vasculature and cardiac myocytes that in coordination regulate myocyte remodeling, heart function, and vascular remodeling. Since THs can

activate Akt signaling in the heart, it is possible that Akt signaling is involved in TH-induced coronary angiogenesis, but this has yet to be demonstrated mechanistically.

12.11 Coronary Arteriolar and Capillary Changes During Hypothyroidism

Hypothyroidism causes progressive arteriolar loss [46] (Fig. 12.2). PTU treatment of rats for 6 weeks led to a dramatic 41% reduction in arteriolar length density and 37% reduction of arteriolar numerical density, with the smallest arterioles (5–15 μm) being affected the most. PTU treatment of rats for 1 year resulted in a 46% reduction in the arteriolar length density and a 53% reduction of arteriolar

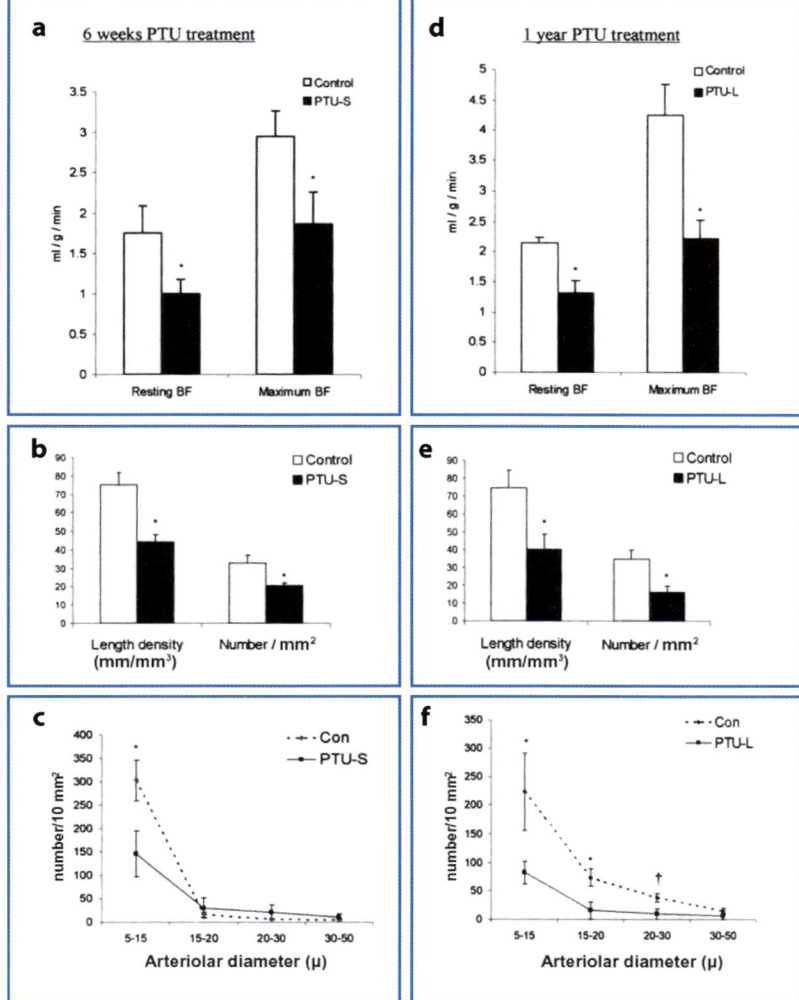

Fig. 12.2 Changes in myocardial blood flow and arterioles in hypothyroid rats. **a-c** Six-week propylthiouracil (*PTU*) treatment: a resting and maximum myocardial blood flow; **b** arteriolar length density and number; **c** size distribution of arterioles. **d-f** One-year PTU treatment: **d** resting and maximum myocardial blood flow; **e** arteriolar length density and number; **f** size distribution of arterioles. *$p < 0.01$ vs. control; $p < 0.05$ vs. control. (Adapted from [46])

numerical density, again primarily affecting the small arterioles. Short-term and chronic hypothyroidism led to impaired myocardial blood flow, which may have contributed to late signs of heart failure. Since the arteriolar density is reduced below normal in hypothyroidism despite myocyte atrophy, the actual loss of arterioles exceeds that suggested by the numerical density reduction. Unlike the situation with arterioles, it has been reported that capillary density increases in hypothyroidism, apparently due to atrophy of myocytes [66, 74].

12.13 Do Serum Thyroid Hormone Levels Accurately Reflect Cardiovascular Tissue Hormone Function?

Thyroid functional changes are typically assessed by measuring the serum levels of T_3, T_4, free T_3 (FT_3), free T_4 (FT_4), and TSH. There is some debate on the threshold level of TSH that should be used to diagnose the presence of subclinical hypothyroidism and hyperthyroidism. Consequently, a narrower TSH reference range has been proposed [75]. A study in our lab recently examined cardiovascular changes in rats with borderline hypothyroidism using surgical thyroidectomy and subcutaneous implantation of slow-release pellets containing T_4 [76]. Cardiac function was assessed by left ventricular catheterization and echocardiography. Serum and cardiac tissue T_3 and T_4

levels were also measured. One of the T_4 doses yielded normalization of serum hormones but not cardiac tissue hormone levels or function. Arteriolar density also remained below normal in this group. These results suggest that serum hormone levels may not accurately reflect tissue hormone function in borderline thyroid conditions. It seems logical that cardiac function would provide a more reliable indicator of TH function at the tissue level than serum hormone levels. Cardiac function reflects the end output of TH action on the heart, including the summation of any abnormalities (changes in membrane transporters, nuclear receptors, deiodinases, etc.). Serum hormones indicate what is available for metabolism.

12.14 Potential Application of Thyroid Hormone in Cardiovascular Diseases

The beneficial effects of THs on cardiac myocyte and arteriolar remodeling suggest potential applications for therapy in heart diseases. In fact, several studies have shown that THs can reduce myocyte apoptosis and improve left ventricular remodeling and function in myocardial infarction and congestive heart failure [77–81] (Fig. 12.3). Treatment of spontaneously hypertensive heart failure (SHHF) rats with desiccated THs led to a reduction in systolic wall stress due to a specific change in myocyte transverse shape [79] (Tables 12.2 and 12.3). The cham-

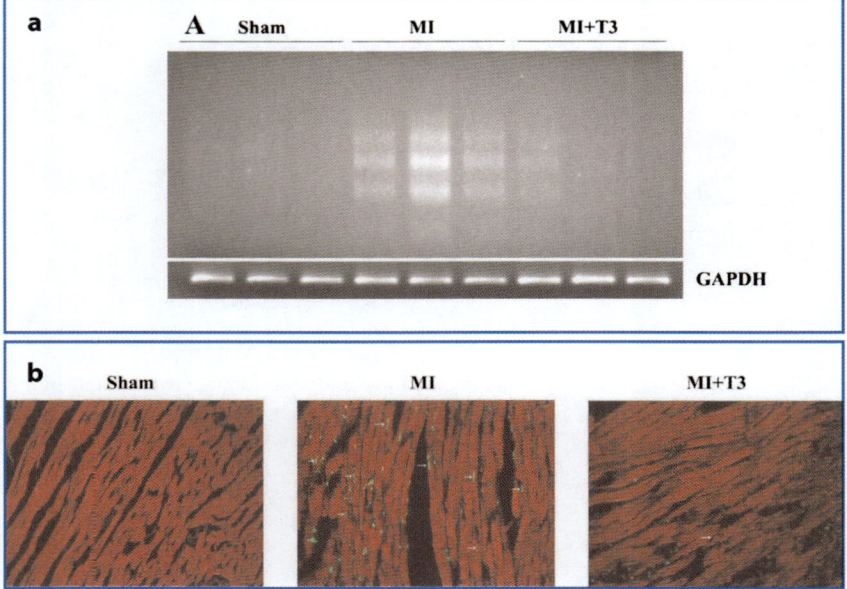

Fig. 12.3 Short-term (3-day) T_3 treatment reduced myocyte apoptosis in border areas of post-myocardial-infarction (post-MI) rat hearts. **a** DNA laddering of post-MI rat hearts. Genomic DNA was extracted from the apex region 72 h after MI for detection of DNA fragmentation using the ligation-mediated polymerase chain reaction (LM-PCR) technique with a LM-PCR DNA ladder assay kit Maxim Biotech, San Francisco, California, USA). Treatment with T_3 significantly decreases the amount of DNA fragments in post-MI rat hearts, indicating inhibition of apoptosis by T_3 treatment. **b** Terminal deoxynucleotidyl transferase dUTP nick end-labeling (TUNEL) of post-MI rat hearts (border area) using APO-BrdU TUNEL Assay Kit (Invitrogen, Carlsbad, California, USA). Treatment with T_3 significantly decreased myocyte apoptosis

Table 12.2 Thyroid hormone treatment improved cardiac function and myocyte remodeling in spontaneously hypertensive heart failure (SHHF) rats: hemodynamic data. Values are means ± SD. (Adapted with permission from [79])

Treatment group	LVP (mmHg)	+dP/dt (mmHg/s)	−dP/dt (mmHg/s)	Wall stress (kdyn/cm^2)	Heart rate (beats/min)
Control rats	162 ± 17	10,374 ± 1,600	9,216 ± 1,538	87 ± 17	376 ± 41
SHHF rats					
Untreated	170 ± 35	8,312 ± 1,798	5,997 ± 1,742[†]	169 ± 65[†]	318 ± 31
0.05% TH	197 ± 31	9,277 ± 1,548	7,302 ± 1,105	157 ± 63[†]	350 ± 12
0.1% TH	220 ± 46*	10,388 ± 2,365	7,999 ± 2,091	105 ± 36*	362 ± 31
0.2% TH	191 ± 31	10,775 ± 2,039*	8,812 ± 1,362*	104 ± 23*	440 ± 74*

LVP left ventricular end-systolic pressure, +dP/dt maximal rate of pressure development, −dP/dt maximal rate of pressure decline
* $p < 0.05$ vs. SHHF untreated rats, [†] $p < 0.05$ vs. control animals

Table 12.3 Thyroid hormone treatment improved cardiac function and myocyte remodeling in spontaneously hypertensive heart failure (SHHF) rats: isolated left ventricular myocyte morphologic data. *A* dimension (major diameter) was determined by tracing isolated myocytes; *B* dimension (minor diameter) was subsequently determined from the formula for volume relative to an elliptical cylinder. Values are means ± SD. (Adapted with permission from [79])

Treatment group	Cell length (μm)	Cell volume (μm^3)	Cross-sectional area (μm^2)	A Dimension (μm)	B Dimension (μm)	A/B Ratio
Control rats	120 ± 9	34,730 ± 4,147	279 ± 27	31 ± 2	12 ± 2	2.7 ± 0.5
SHHF rats						
Untreated	163 ± 9[†]	67,217 ± 9,754[†]	411 ± 51[†]	37 ± 4[†]	14 ± 3	2.7 ± 0.7
0.05% TH	168 ± 4[†]	63,423 ± 1[†]	379 ± 66[†]	35 ± 5	14 ± 2	2.6 ± 0.6
0.1% TH	164 ± 2[†]	77,785 ± 11,366[†]	453 ± 70[†]	33 ± 3	19 ± 3[†]	1.8 ± 0.3
0.2% TH	168 ± 2[†]	77,199 ± 10,593[†]	461 ± 61[†]	30 ± 1*	20 ± 2[†]	1.5 ± 0.1*[†]

* $p < 0.05$ vs. SHHF untreated rats, [†] $p < 0.05$ vs. control animals

ber diameter-to-wall-thickness ratio declined due to a reduction in the ratio of myocyte major to minor transverse diameters. The ratio α-MHC/β-MHC was reduced in untreated SHHF rats and increased in all TH-treated groups, suggesting a reversal of the fetal gene program. However, increased metabolic rate and oxygen consumption may undermine potential benefits in the long run. A TH analogue with more specific effects might be a better choice. More work is clearly needed in humans to determine whether some cardiac patients will benefit from THs or TH analogues.

Key Points

- Ventricular morphometric, architectural, and functional changes, due to a variety of cardiovascular conditions and consisting of cardiomyocyte, coronary vasculature, and collagen network remodeling, are known as ventricular remodeling.

- Thyroid hormones lead to the following changes: an increase in cardiac systolic and diastolic function; a decrease in peripheral vascular resistance; an increase in venous tone; an increase in cardiac output; a hyperdynamic circulatory state; an increase in systolic arterial pressure; a decrease in diastolic arterial pressure; alterations in cardiac electrophysiology; and promotion of angiogenesis.

(Cont. →)

(*cont.*)

- Excess thyroid hormones lead to a proportional increase in myocyte length and cross-sectional area, suggesting a physiological type of hypertrophy, with increased α-MHC expression and decreased β-MHC expression.

- Hypothyroidism causes cardiac atrophy, primarily due to a decrease in myocyte cross-sectional area, with decreased α-MHC expression and increased β-MHC expression. Long-term hypothyroidism also leads to chamber dilatation from series addition of sarcomeres in cardiac myocytes.

- Thyroid hormones promote coronary arteriolar and capillary growth.

- Hypothyroidism causes progressive arteriolar loss and may lead to a slight increase in capillary density due to myocyte atrophy.

- Thyroid hormone supplementation can reduce myocyte apoptosis, improve left ventricular remodeling after myocardial infarction, promote healthy vasculature, and may improve cardiac function in heart failure.

References

1. Weber KT, Clark WA, Janicki JS et al (1987) Physiologic versus pathologic hypertrophy and the pressure-overloaded myocardium. J Cardiovasc Pharmacol 10 Suppl 6:S37–50
2. McMullen JR, Jennings GL (2007) Differences between pathological and physiological cardiac hypertrophy: Novel therapeutic strategies to treat heart failure. Clin Exp Pharmacol Physiol 34(4):255–262
3. Kaplan ML, Cheslow Y, Vikstrom K et al (1994) Cardiac adaptations to chronic exercise in mice. Am J Physiol 267(3 Pt 2):H1167–1173
4. Iemitsu M, Miyauchi T, Maeda S et al (2001) Physiological and pathological cardiac hypertrophy induce different molecular phenotypes in the rat. Am J Physiol Regul Integr Comp Physiol 281(6):R2029–2036
5. Eghbali M, Deva R, Alioua A et al (2005) Molecular and functional signature of heart hypertrophy during pregnancy. Circ Res 96(11):1208–1216
6. McMullen JR, Shioi T, Zhang L et al (2003) Phosphoinositide 3-kinase(p110alpha) plays a critical role for the induction of physiological, but not pathological, cardiac hypertrophy. Proc Natl Acad Sci U S A 100(21):12355–12360
7. Grossman W, Jones D, McLaurin LP (1975) Wall stress and patterns of hypertrophy in the human left ventricle. J Clin Invest 56(1):56–64
8. Pluim BM, Zwinderman AH, van der Laarse A et al (2000) The athlete's heart. A meta-analysis of cardiac structure and function. Circulation 101(3):336–344
9. Pfeffer MA, Braunwald E (1990) Ventricular remodeling after myocardial infarction. Experimental observations and clinical implications. Circulation 81(4):1161–1172
10. Hutchins GM, Bulkley BH (1978) Infarct expansion versus extension: two different complications of acute myocardial infarction. Am J Cardiol 41(7):1127–1132
11. Fishbein MC, Maclean D, Maroko PR (1978) The histopathologic evolution of myocardial infarction. Chest 73(6):843–849
12. Roberts CS, Maclean D, Maroko P et al (1984) Early and late remodeling of the left ventricle after acute myocardial infarction. Am J Cardiol 54(3):407–410
13. Weisman HF, Bush DE, Mannisi JA et al (1988) Cellular mechanisms of myocardial infarct expansion. Circulation 78(1):186–201
14. Zimmer HG, Gerdes AM, Lortet S et al (1990) Changes in heart function and cardiac cell size in rats with chronic myocardial infarction. J Mol Cell Cardiol 22(11):1231–1243
15. Pirolo JS, Hutchins GM, Moore GW (1986) Infarct expansion: pathologic analysis of 204 patients with a single myocardial infarct. J Am Coll Cardiol 7(2):349–354
16. McKay RG, Pfeffer MA, Pasternak RC et al (1986) Left ventricular remodeling after myocardial infarction: a corollary to infarct expansion. Circulation 74(4):693–702
17. Rubin SA, Fishbein MC, Swan HJ (1983) Compensatory hypertrophy in the heart after myocardial infarction in the rat. J Am Coll Cardiol 1(6):1435–1441
18. Fletcher PJ, Pfeffer JM, Pfeffer MA et al (1981) Left ventricular diastolic pressure-volume relations in rats with healed myocardial infarction. Effects on systolic function. Circ Res 49(3):618–626
19. Gould KL, Lipscomb K, Hamilton GW et al (1973) Left ventricular hypertrophy in coronary artery disease. A cardiomyopathy syndrome following myocardial infarction. Am J Med 55(5):595–601
20. Smith SH, McCaslin M, Sreenan C et al (1988) Regional myocyte size in two-kidney, one clip renal hypertension. J Mol Cell Cardiol 20(11):1035–1042
21. Werchan PM, Summer WR, Gerdes AM et al (1989) Right ventricular performance after monocrotaline-induced pulmonary hypertension. Am J Physiol 256(5 Pt 2):H1328–1336
22. Liu Z, Hilbelink DR, Crockett WB et al (1991) Regional changes in hemodynamics and cardiac myocyte size in rats with aortocaval fistulas. 1. Developing and established hypertrophy. Circ Res 69(1):52–58
23. Liu Z, Hilbelink DR, Gerdes AM (1991) Regional changes

in hemodynamics and cardiac myocyte size in rats with aortocaval fistulas. 2. Long-term effects. Circ Res 69(1):59–65

24. Gerdes AM, Kellerman SE, Moore JA et al (1992) Structural remodeling of cardiac myocytes in patients with ischemic cardiomyopathy. Circulation 86(2):426–430

25. Page E, Polimeni PI, Zak R et al (1972) Myofibrillar mass in rat and rabbit heart muscle. Correlation of microchemical and stereological measurements in normal and hypertrophic hearts. Circ Res 30(4):430–439

26. Graettinger JS, Muenster JJ, Selverstone LA et al (1959) A correlation of clinical and hemodynamic studies in patients with hyperthyroidism with and without congestive heart failure. J Clin Invest 38(8):1316–1327

27. Theilen EO, Wilson WR (1967) Hemodynamic effects of peripheral vasoconstriction in normal and thyrotoxic subjects. J Appl Physiol 22(2):207–210

28. DeGroot WJ, Leonard JJ (1970) Hyperthyroidism as a high cardiac output state. Am Heart J 79(2):265–275

29. Goldman S, Olajos M, Morkin E (1984) Control of cardiac output in thyrotoxic calves. Evaluation of changes in the systemic circulation. J Clin Invest 73(2):358–365

30. Napoli R, Biondi B, Guardasole V et al (2001) Impact of hyperthyroidism and its correction on vascular reactivity in humans. Circulation 104(25):3076–3080

31. Biondi B, Palmieri EA, Lombardi G et al (2002) Effects of thyroid hormone on cardiac function: the relative importance of heart rate, loading conditions, and myocardial contractility in the regulation of cardiac performance in human hyperthyroidism. J Clin Endocrinol Metab 87(3):968–974

32. Mintz G, Pizzarello R, Klein I (1991) Enhanced left ventricular diastolic function in hyperthyroidism: noninvasive assessment and response to treatment. J Clin Endocrinol Metab 73(1):146–150

33. Biondi B, Palmieri EA, Lombardi G et al (2002) Effects of subclinical thyroid dysfunction on the heart. Ann Intern Med 137(11):904–914

34. Streeten DH, Anderson GH, Jr., Howland T et al (1988) Effects of thyroid function on blood pressure. Recognition of hypothyroid hypertension. Hypertension 11(1):78–83

35. Fazio S, Palmieri EA, Lombardi G et al (2004) Effects of thyroid hormone on the cardiovascular system. Recent Prog Horm Res 59:31–50

36. Klein I, Ojamaa K (2001) Thyroid hormone and the cardiovascular system. N Engl J Med 344(7):501–509

37. Chilian WM, Wangler RD, Peters KG et al (1985) Thyroxine-induced left ventricular hypertrophy in the rat. Anatomical and physiological evidence for angiogenesis. Circ Res 57(4):591–598

38. Tomanek RJ, Busch TL (1998) Coordinated capillary and myocardial growth in response to thyroxine treatment. Anat Rec 251(1):44–49

39. Zierhut W, Zimmer HG (1989) Differential effects of triiodothyronine on rat left and right ventricular function and the influence of metoprolol. J Mol Cell Cardiol 21(6):617–624

40. Campbell SE, Gerdes AM (1988) Regional changes in myocyte size during the reversal of thyroid-induced cardiac hypertrophy. J Mol Cell Cardiol 20(5):379–387

41. Kuzman JA, Gerdes AM, Kobayashi S et al (2005) Thyroid hormone activates Akt and prevents serum starvation-induced cell death in neonatal rat cardiomyocytes. J Mol

Cell Cardiol 39(5):841–844

42. Kuzman JA, Thomas TA, Vogelsang KA et al (2005) Effects of induced hyperthyroidism in normal and cardiomyopathic hamsters. J Appl Physiol 99(4):1428–1433

43. McCallister LP, Page E (1973) Effects of thyroxin on ultrastructure of rat myocardial cells: A stereological study. J Ultrastruct Res 42(1):136–155

44. Ferreira PJ, L'Abbate C, Abrahamsohn PA et al (2003) Temporal and topographic ultrastructural alterations of rat heart myofibrils caused by thyroid hormone. Microsc Res Tech 62(5):451–459

45. Liu Z, Gerdes AM (1990) Influence of hypothyroidism and the reversal of hypothyroidism on hemodynamics and cell size in the adult rat heart. J Mol Cell Cardiol 22(12):1339–1348

46. Tang YD, Kuzman JA, Said S et al (2005) Low thyroid function leads to cardiac atrophy with chamber dilatation, impaired myocardial blood flow, loss of arterioles, and severe systolic dysfunction. Circulation 112(20):3122–3130

47. Fommei E, Iervasi G (2002) The role of thyroid hormone in blood pressure homeostasis: evidence from short-term hypothyroidism in humans. J Clin Endocrinol Metab 87(5):1996–2000

48. Crowley WF Jr, Ridgway EC, Bough EW et al (1977) Noninvasive evaluation of cardiac function in hypothyroidism. Response to gradual thyroxine replacement. N Engl J Med 296(1):1–6

49. Wieshammer S, Keck FS, Waitzinger J et al (1989) Acute hypothyroidism slows the rate of left ventricular diastolic relaxation. Can J Physiol Pharmacol 67(9):1007–1010

50. Zafeiridis A, Jeevanandam V, Houser SR et al (1998) Regression of cellular hypertrophy after left ventricular assist device support. Circulation 98(7):656–662

51. Kinugawa K, Yonekura K, Ribeiro RC et al (2001) Regulation of thyroid hormone receptor isoforms in physiological and pathological cardiac hypertrophy. Circ Res 89(7):591–598

52. Kinugawa K, Jeong MY, Bristow MR et al (2005) Thyroid hormone induces cardiac myocyte hypertrophy in a thyroid hormone receptor alpha1-specific manner that requires TAK1 and p38 mitogen-activated protein kinase. Mol Endocrinol 19(6):1618–1628

53. Kenessey A, Ojamaa K (2006) Thyroid hormone stimulates protein synthesis in the cardiomyocyte by activating the Akt-mTOR and p70S6K pathways. J Biol Chem 281(30):20666–20672

54. Kuzman JA, O'Connell TD, Gerdes AM (2007) Rapamycin prevents thyroid hormone-induced cardiac hypertrophy. Endocrinology 148(7):3477–3484

55. Pantos C, Xinaris C, Mourouzis I et al (2007) Thyroid hormone changes cardiomyocyte shape and geometry via ERK signaling pathway: potential therapeutic implications in reversing cardiac remodeling? Mol Cell Biochem 297(1–2):65–72

56. Hu LW, Benvenuti LA, Liberti EA et al (2003) Thyroxine-induced cardiac hypertrophy: influence of adrenergic nervous system versus renin-angiotensin system on myocyte remodeling. Am J Physiol Regul Integr Comp Physiol 285(6):R1473–1480

57. Shohet RV, Kisanuki YY, Zhao XS et al (2004) Mice with cardiomyocyte-specific disruption of the endothelin-1 gene are resistant to hyperthyroid cardiac hypertrophy. Proc Natl

Acad Sci U S A 101(7):2088–2093

58. van Rooij E, Sutherland LB, Qi X et al (2007) Control of stress-dependent cardiac growth and gene expression by a microRNA. Science 316(5824):575–579

59. Tomanek RJ, Torry RJ (1994) Growth of the coronary vasculature in hypertrophy: mechanisms and model dependence. Cell Mol Biol Res 40(2):129–136

60. Tomanek RJ (1990) Response of the coronary vasculature to myocardial hypertrophy. J Am Coll Cardiol 15(3):528–533

61. Legault F, Rouleau JL, Juneau C et al (1990) Functional and morphological characteristics of compensated and decompensated cardiac hypertrophy in dogs with chronic infrarenal aorto-caval fistulas. Circ Res 66(3):846–859

62. Chen Y, Torry RJ, Baumbach GL et al (1994) Proportional arteriolar growth accompanies cardiac hypertrophy induced by volume overload. Am J Physiol 267(6 Pt 2): H2132–2137

63. White FC, Bloor CM, McKirnan MD et al (1998) Exercise training in swine promotes growth of arteriolar bed and capillary angiogenesis in heart. J Appl Physiol 85(3):1160–1168

64. Talafih K, Briden KL, Weiss HR (1983) Thyroxine-induced hypertrophy of the rabbit heart. Effect on regional oxygen extraction, flow, and oxygen consumption. Circ Res 52(3):272–279

65. Breisch EA, White FC, Hammond HK et al (1989) Myocardial characteristics of thyroxine stimulated hypertrophy. A structural and functional study. Basic Res Cardiol 84(4):345–358

66. Heron MI, Rakusan K (1994) Geometry of coronary capillaries in hyperthyroid and hypothyroid rat heart. Am J Physiol 267(3 Pt 2):H1024–1031

67. Anjos-Ramos L, Carneiro-Ramos MS, Diniz GP et al (2006) Early cardiac hypertrophy induced by thyroxine is accompanied by an increase in VEGF-a expression but not by an increase in capillary density. Virchows Arch 448(4):472–479

68. Gerdes AM, Callas G, Kasten FH (1979) Differences in regional capillary distribution and myocyte sizes in normal and hypertrophic rat hearts. Am J Anat 156(4):523–531

69. Tomanek RJ, Doty MK, Sandra A (1998) Early coronary angiogenesis in response to thyroxine: growth characteristics and upregulation of basic fibroblast growth factor. Circ Res 82(5):587–593

70. Davis FB, Mousa SA, O'Connor L et al (2004) Proangiogenic action of thyroid hormone is fibroblast growth factor-dependent and is initiated at the cell surface. Circ Res 94(11):1500–1506

71. Mousa SA, Davis FB, Mohamed S et al (2006) Pro-angiogenesis action of thyroid hormone and analogs in a three-dimensional in vitro microvascular endothelial sprouting model. Int Angiol 25(4):407–413

72. Shiojima I, Sato K, Izumiya Y et al (2005) Disruption of coordinated cardiac hypertrophy and angiogenesis contributes to the transition to heart failure. J Clin Invest 115(8):2108–2118

73. Izumiya Y, Shiojima I, Sato K et al (2006) Vascular endothelial growth factor blockade promotes the transition from compensatory cardiac hypertrophy to failure in response to pressure overload. Hypertension 47(5):887–893

74. Tomanek RJ, Barlow PA, Connell PM et al (1993) Effects of hypothyroidism and hypertension on myocardial perfusion and vascularity in rabbits. Am J Physiol 265(5 Pt 2): H1638–1644

75. Wartofsky L, Dickey RA (2005) The evidence for a narrower thyrotropin reference range is compelling. J Clin Endocrinol Metab 90(9):5483–5488

76. Liu Y, Redetzke RA, Said S et al (2008) Serum thyroid hormone levels may not accurately reflect thyroid tissue levels and cardiac function in mild hypothyroidism. Am J Physiol Heart Circ Physiol 294(5):H2137–2143

77. Ojamaa K, Kenessey A, Shenoy R et al (2000) Thyroid hormone metabolism and cardiac gene expression after acute myocardial infarction in the rat. Am J Physiol Endocrinol Metab 279(6):E1319–1324

78. Chen YF, Kobayashi S, Chen J et al (2008) Short term triiodo-l-thyronine treatment inhibits cardiac myocyte apoptosis in border area after myocardial infarction in rats. J Mol Cell Cardiol 44(1):180–187

79. Thomas TA, Kuzman JA, Anderson BE et al (2005) Thyroid hormones induce unique and potentially beneficial changes in cardiac myocyte shape in hypertensive rats near heart failure. Am J Physiol Heart Circ Physiol 288(5):H2118–2122

80. Khalife WI, Tang YD, Kuzman JA et al (2005) Treatment of subclinical hypothyroidism reverses ischemia and prevents myocyte loss and progressive LV dysfunction in hamsters with dilated cardiomyopathy. Am J Physiol Heart Circ Physiol 289(6):H2409–2415

81. Pantos C, Mourouzis I, Markakis K et al (2008) Long-term thyroid hormone administration reshapes left ventricular chamber and improves cardiac function after myocardial infarction in rats. Basic Res Cardiol 103(4):308–318

Thyroid Hormone and Ischemic Myocardium

13

Constantinos Pantos, Iordanis Mourouzis and Dennis V. Cokkinos

Abstract Thyroid hormone (TH) promotes tissue growth and differentiation and as such has pleiotropic actions on the heart: it regulates metabolism, cellular function and morphology, and cellular response to stress. TH increases the tolerance of the heart to ischemia via regulation of cardioprotective intracellular signaling and can improve hemodynamics in the setting of ischemia–reperfusion due to its inotropic and antiapoptotic action. Changes in the thyroid hormone–thyroid hormone receptor (TH–TR) axis occur in the course of postinfarction cardiac remodeling and contribute to fetal cardiac phenotype. A low thyroid hormone state is not uncommon in ischemic myocardial conditions and may be a protective response against ischemic stress, at the expense, though, of impaired cardiac function. In addition TH prevents and/or reverses postinfarction cardiac remodeling by regulating the expression of contractile proteins, inducing novel signaling pathways related to cardiac contractility, and optimizing cardiac chamber geometry. TH or its analogues may be a new therapeutic option for treating ischemic heart disease.

Keywords Thyroid hormone • Thyroid hormone receptors • Hypothyroidism • Myocardial ischemia • Ischemia–reperfusion • Cardiac hypertrophy • Myocardial infarction • Cardiac remodeling • Heart failure • Left ventricular chamber geometry • Neonatal cardiomyocytes • Cell growth • Cell differentiation • Apoptosis • MAPK intracellular signaling pathways • Heat shock proteins • Protein kinase C • Thyroid hormone analogues

13.1 Introduction

Thyroid hormone (TH) appears to have played a critical role in evolution, facilitating adaptation of the organism to the environment and ensuring survival. Important evolutionary events such as "metamorphosis" in amphibians are TH-dependent processes. Furthermore, during development, maturation of all organs and particularly of the myocardium depends on increasing TH signaling after birth, which induces the transcriptional programming leading to the characteristic gene expression profile of the adult. TH, unlike other progrowth stimuli, promotes tissue differentiation and as such critically regulates metabolism (energy supply), contractile and electrical function, and response to stress (hypoxic conditions) and optimizes cellular morphology [1]. These unique properties may be of therapeutic importance in mending the "broken heart." In fact, it is now recognized that the fetal transcriptional profile is reactivated in cardiac diseases, and alterations in thyroid hormone signaling may contribute to this response [2].

C. Pantos (✉)
1 Department of Pharmacology, University of Athens, School of Medicine, Athens, Greece

G. Iervasi, A. Pingitore (eds.), *Thyroid and Heart Failure.*
© Springer-Verlag Italia 2009

However, two dogmas currently dominate the field: that TH is detrimental to ischemic myocardium due to the acceleration of heart rhythm, and that the "low T$_3$ state", which accompanies heart diseases, has a protective role and needs no treatment. These beliefs, though long-standing, are now being challenged by recent experimental and clinical investigations. In fact, low levels of triiodothyronine (T$_3$) in heart failure are associated with increased mortality and morbidity [3–5]. Furthermore, a cardioprotective effect of TH has been demonstrated in cells, animals, and even in humans [6–9] (Table 13.1).

13.2 TH and Ischemia–Reperfusion Injury

13.2.1 TH-Induced "Physiological" Hypertrophy: A Phenotype of Cardioprotection

Buser et al. were the first to observe, in 1990, that isolated rat hearts with "physiological hypertrophy" induced by 10 days of TH treatment could tolerate ischemia–reperfusion injury better than nonhypertrophied hearts or hearts with aortic-constriction-induced cardiac hypertrophy [10]. In 2000, Pantos et al. confirmed this original observation in a similar experimental model and further showed that postischemic recovery of function was enhanced despite the fact that diastolic dysfunction (ischemic contracture) was exacerbated upon ischemia [11] (Fig. 13.1).

13.2.2 The Paradox of Exacerbated Ischemic Contracture: Myocardial Glycogen vs Hypertrophy

Dissociation between ischemic contracture and cardiac function has been observed in isolated rat hearts subjected to ischemic preconditioning (brief episodes of ischemia/reperfusion) prior to long ischemia and reperfusion. This "paradox" appears to correlate strongly with lower preischemic myocardial glycogen content due to the brief ischemia-induced glycogen depletion. Thus, during zero-flow ischemia, the glycogen-dependent supply of energy is limited and marked diastolic dysfunction occurs [12]. This "glycogen hypothesis" seems to explain the effect of TH on ischemic contracture. In fact, changes in TH

are associated with alterations in myocardial glycogen content; myocardial glycogen is lower after TH treatment, while the low TH state increases myocardial glycogen content and depresses and delays ischemic contracture [13, 14] (Fig. 13.1).

A possible role of TH-induced cardiac hypertrophy in the acceleration and intensification of ischemic contracture has also been explored. However, neither propranolol (α- and β-adrenergic antagonist) nor irbesartan (an AT1-receptor antagonist) abolished the paradoxical pattern of ischemic contracture induced by TH, despite the fact that both drugs limited the development of cardiac hypertrophy [11, 15]. Furthermore, a similar response was not observed in hearts with aortic-constriction-induced cardiac hypertrophy [16].

13.2.3 Protein Kinase C: A Potential Key Player in TH-Induced Cardioprotection

Protein kinase C (PKC) has a critical role in protecting of the myocardium against ischemia–reperfusion injury, and certain PKC isoforms have been associated with cardioprotection [17, 18]. Overexpression of PKCδ in cardiomyocytes protects against ischemia by negative regulation of the ischemia-induced activation of proapoptotic p38 MAPK [18]. Furthermore, PKCδ phosphorylates important cardioprotective molecules, such as heat shock protein 27 (HSP27) [19]. TH treatment resulted in increased expression and phosphorylation of PKCδ, and this response was associated with increased phosphorylation of the heat shock protein (HSP) 27 and suppressed activation of ischemia–reperfusion p38 MAPK [7, 20] (Fig. 13.2). Thus, it is likely that PKCδ serves a critical role in TH-mediated cardioprotection.

13.2.4 Heat Shock Proteins: Critical End-Effectors in TH-Mediated Cardioprotection

TH pretreatment results in increased expression of HSP27 (particularly in the cytoskeleton) and HSP70 in the myocardium (Fig. 13.2). TH is a "physiological" regulator of growth and promotes tissue differentiation. Thus, regulation of the cytoskeleton

Table 13.1 Studies demonstrating the effect of TH on the response of the heart to ischemia and reperfusion injury. (Table adapted by permission from [1])

Reference	Model of ischemia–reperfusion	TH treatment	Outcome
Novitzky et al. [27]	Patients undergoing CABG	T_3 treatment at reperfusion (4–10 µg i.v.)	Increase in mean arterial pressure, decrease in left atrial pressure and central venous pressure
Buser et al. [10]	Isolated rat heart – no-flow, global ischemia	T_3 pretreatment for 10 days	Increased recovery of LV function
Dyke et al. [97]	Isolated rabbit heart – no-flow, global ischemia	T_3 treatment at reperfusion	Increased recovery of LV function
Novitzky et al. [98]	In vivo model of regional myocardial ischemia in dog	T_3 treatment at reperfusion (0.2 mg/kg × 6 doses)	Improved LV function
Holland et al. [99]	Isolated working rat heart – hyperkalemic cardioplegic, normothermic ischemia	T_3 treatment at reperfusion (0.06, 0.15, and 0.60 µg/l)	Increased recovery of LV stroke work index
Dyke et al. [100]	Pig model of CABG – global, normothermic ischemia	T_3 treatment at reperfusion (0.1 mg/kg)	Increased recovery of LV function
Kadletz et al. [101]	Isolated rabbit heart – no-flow, global ischemia	T_3 treatment at reperfusion (2.5, 25, and 250 µg/l)	Increased recovery of LV function at 2.5 and 25 but not at 250 µg/l
Klemperer et al. [102]	Patients undergoing CABG	T_3 treatment at reperfusion (0.8 µg/kg followed by 0.113 µg/kg per hour)	Increased cardiac output and lowered systemic vascular resistance
Walker et al. [103]	Healthy and cardiomyopathic porcine myocytes – cardioplegic arrest and rewarming	Acute T_3 pretreatment (80 pmol/l)	Improved myocyte velocity of shortening
Klemperer et al. [104]	Ex vivo canine heart preparation – hypothermic global ischemia	Acute T_3 pretreatment (0.2 µg/kg)	Increased postischemic cardiac work
Liu et al. [105]	Isolated working rat heart – no-flow, global ischemia	Acute T_3 pretreatment (10 nM)	Increased postischemic cardiac work and efficiency
Spinale [106]	Healthy and cardiomyopathic porcine myocytes – cardioplegic arrest and rewarming	Acute T_3 pretreatment (80 pmol/l)	Increased myocyte contractile function and β-adrenergic responsiveness
Pantos et al. [11]	Isolated rat heart – no-flow, global ischemia	T_4 pretreatment for 2 days and 2 weeks (250 µg/kg)	Increased recovery of LV function at 2 weeks but not at 2 days
Lahorra et al. [107]	Isolated rat heart – multidose cardioplegic, hypothermic arrest	T_4 pretreatment, 12 µg/ml in drinking water (~1.2 mg/kg) for 3–5 weeks	No difference in recovery of LV function
Venditti et al. [108]	Isolated rat heart – no-flow, global ischemia	T_3 pretreatment for 10 days (100 µg/kg)	Reduced recovery of LV function
Asahi et al. [109]	Isolated working rat heart – no-flow, global ischemia	T_4 pretreatment for 2 weeks (600 µg/kg)	Reduced recovery of LV pressure–rate product and work
Pantos et al. [7]	Isolated rat heart – no-flow, global ischemia	T_4 pretreatment for 2 weeks (250 µg/kg)	Increased recovery of LV function
Pantos et al. [28]	Isolated rat heart – no-flow, global ischemia	T_4 pretreatment for 2 weeks (250 µg/kg)	Reversed the detrimental effect of dobutamine administration at reperfusion
Pantos et al. [20]	Isolated rat heart – no-flow, global ischemia	T_4 pretreatment for 2 weeks (250 µg/kg)	Increased recovery of LV function and reduced end-diastolic pressure
Kuzman et al. [6]	Neonatal cardiomyocytes – serum starvation	T_3 pretreatment for 4 days	Increased cell viability and reduced apoptosis
Zinman et al. [9]	Neonatal cardiomyocytes – hypoxia	Acute T_3 or T_4 pretreatment (10 and 100 nM)	Reduced LDH release and protection of cytoskeletal filaments
Pantos et al. [24]	Isolated rat heart – no-flow, global ischemia	T_4 pretreatment for 4 days and 2 weeks (250 µg/kg)	Increased recovery of LV function at 2 weeks but not at 4 days
Ranasinghe et al. [8]	Patients undergoing CABG	T_3 treatment at reperfusion (0.8 µg/kg followed by 0.113 µg/kg per hour)	Increased cardiac index and reduced cTnI release

CABG coronary artery bypass graft surgery, *cTnI* cardiac troponin I, *LDH* lactate dehydrogenase, *LV* left ventricular

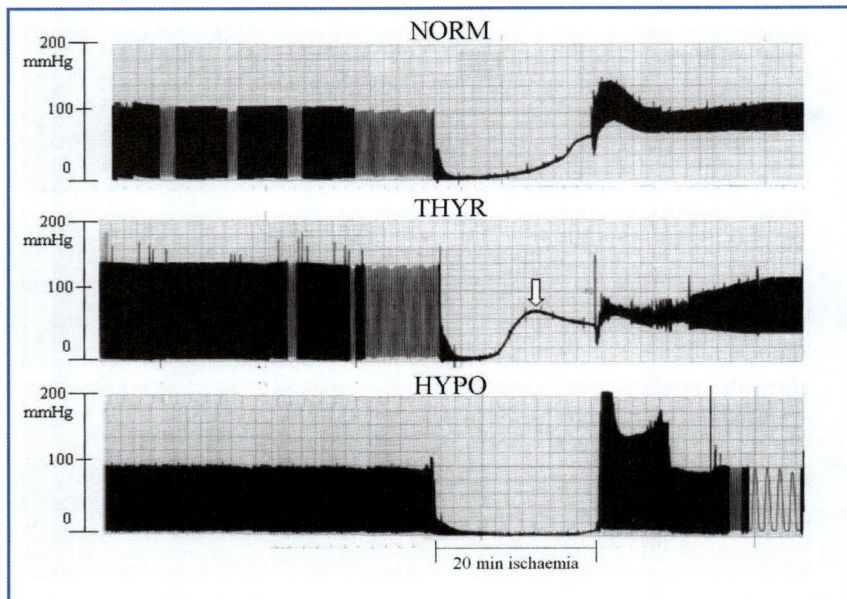

Fig. 13.1 Langendorff recordings of left ventricular pressure from isolated normal (NORM), hyperthyroid (THYR), and hypothyroid rat hearts (HYPO) subjected to 20 min of zero-flow global ischemia and reperfusion. Note the differences and similarities between groups regarding the functional response to ischemia and reperfusion. Hyperthyroid and hypothyroid hearts show increased postischemic recovery of function despite the different patterns of left ventricular dysfunction during the ischemic phase. *Arrow* Peak contracture

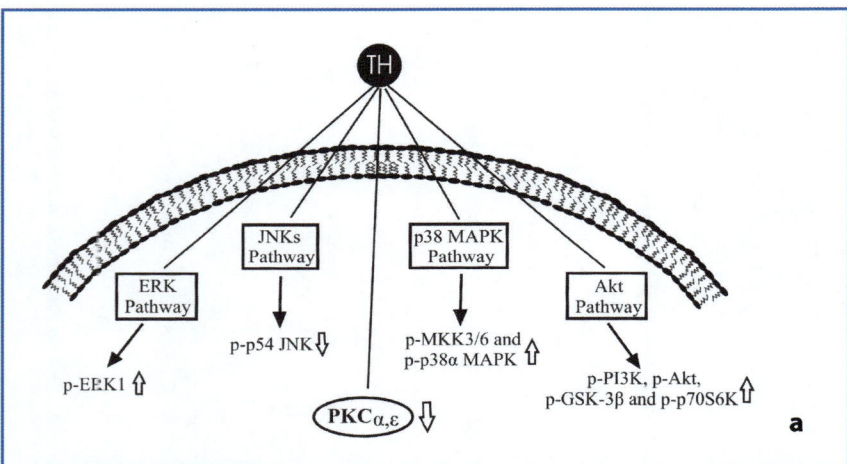

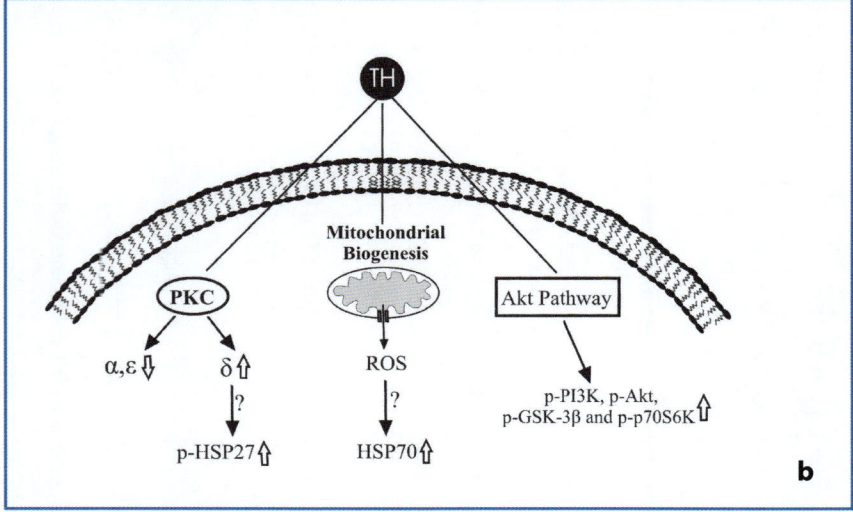

Fig. 13.2 Changes in intracellular signaling pathways induced by thyroid hormone (TH). Data obtained from studies in cardiomyocytes (**a**) and intact heart (**b**). TH appears to up-regulate prosurvival signaling pathways with important physiological consequences for the response to stress and cardiac remodeling. *p* Phosphorylation. (Adapted by permission from [1])

through cytoskeletal proteins such as HSP27 may be critical in this response. Furthermore, proteins such as HSP70 may function as molecular chaperones to prevent proteins from misfolding and aggregation during tissue growth and differentiation. These changes may be of advantage in regard to the response of the myocardium to ischemic stress, since overexpression of these proteins was shown to result in increased tolerance to ischemia [21, 22].

A strong link between HSPs and TH-induced protection was recently demonstrated. TH treatment appears not only to induce the expression of HSP27 in the cytoskeleton of the unstressed myocardium but also to accelerate its translocation and phosphorylation to the cytoskeleton upon subsequent ischemic stress, indicating that TH can increase the tolerance of the heart by preserving cytoskeleton integrity [20]. This has been further documented in studies of neonatal cardiomyocytes exposed to hypoxia [9]. Similarly, apart from the induction of HSP70 in unstressed myocardium, increased expression of HSP70 at the mRNA level was observed in response to ischemia and reperfusion after TH treatment [23]. Furthermore, time course analysis showed that TH-induced cardioprotection coincided with the presence of increased levels of HSP70 expression, while no protection was seen with short-term TH treatment, which failed to upregulate HSP70 [24] (Fig. 13.2).

13.2.5 TH-Induced Oxidative Stress: Bad or Good?

Long-term (14-days) TH treatment in rats was shown to increase oxidative stress, as indicated by increased levels of malondialdehyde (MDA) in the myocardium. This has been suggested to result in myocardial damage [25]. However, this response appears to coincide with increased expression of redox-regulated HSP70 and increased tolerance of the myocardium to ischemia (Fig. 13.2). Thus, it seems likely that oxidative stress, by activating redox-regulating cardioprotective molecules such as HSP70, is a trigger of cardioprotection rather than being detrimental. This is further supported by the fact that short-term TH treatment (4 days) failed to induce cardioprotection, and this response was associated with the absence of increased MDA levels and HSP70 content in the myocardium [24]. It should be noted that mild oxidative stress is the key

mechanism of other paradigms of cardioprotection, such as ischemic preconditioning [26].

13.2.6 TH Administration at Reperfusion: Hemodynamics vs. Apoptosis

In 1989, T_3 treatment at reperfusion was shown to improve cardiac hemodynamics in patients undergoing coronary artery bypass graft [27]. The initial observations were subsequently confirmed by several clinical and experimental studies [1]. More recently, we showed that, unlike dobutamine [28], T_3 not only improves postischemic recovery of function but at the same time limits apoptosis. In fact, in an isolated rat heart model of zero-flow ischemia and reperfusion, T_3 administration at reperfusion limited apoptosis and increased postischemic recovery of function (Fig. 13.3) (unpublished observations). This response, unlike those to other hormones, was shown to be mediated by suppressing of activation of proapoptotic p38 MAPK and not by up-regulation of prosurvival signaling pathways [29]. Furthermore, T_3 administration in rats with myocardial infarction was found to reduce cardiac myocyte apoptosis in the border area of infarction [30]. Thus, T_3 may be considered a suitable therapeutic option for hemodynamic support in the setting of ischemia–reperfusion. This concept is verified by recent data from Ranasinghe et al. showing that T_3 treatment during bypass surgery increases cardiac index while limiting the troponin release [8].

13.2.7 Low TH State: A State of Protection

Low TH state is a common response in several pathological conditions such as myocardial infarction, and heart failure, and is regarded as an energy adaptation to increase protection against stress [31]. In fact, patients with lower circulating TH levels suffer smaller infarctions [32]. Furthermore, tissue hypothyroidism occurs during cardiac remodeling and has been associated with increased tolerance of the postinfarcted heart to ischemia [33].

Hypothyroidism-induced cardioprotection is distinct from that induced by TH and is characterized by suppressed and delayed ischemic contracture (Fig. 13.1). It involves overexpession and activation of PKCε and is mediated by suppressed activation

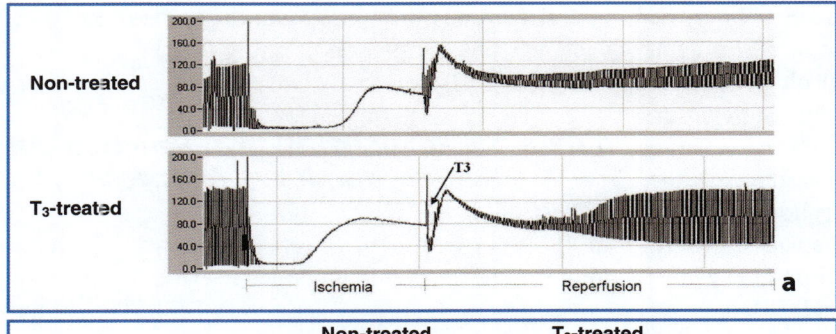

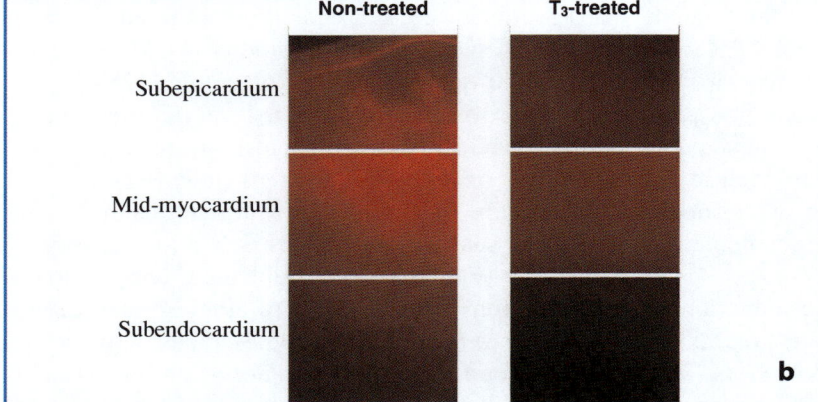

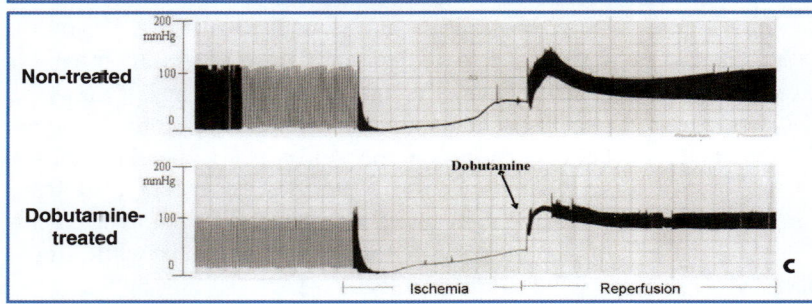

Fig. 13.3 TH improves cardiac hemodynamics while limiting apoptosis in the setting of ischemia–reperfusion. Note the difference in postischemic recovery of function with dobutamine treatment, an inotrope commonly used in clinical practice. **a** Langendorff recordings of left ventricular pressure from isolated rat hearts subjected to ischemia–reperfusion without treatment and with T3 treatment (40 µg/l) at reperfusion. **b** Microscopy images showing caspase-3 activity detected by fluorescent probe in nontreated and T3-treated hearts. The probe was a generous gift from Quidd (Rouen, France). **c** Langendorff recordings of left ventricular pressure from isolated rat hearts subjected to ischemia–reperfusion without treatment and with dobutamine treatment (10 µg/kg per minute) at reperfusion

of the proapoptotic JNK signaling pathway [13].

Here it should be noted that this experimental evidence may provide an explanation for the adverse effects (angina) seen in patients with silent ischemic heart disease and hypothyroidism after TH replacement. This response is probably due to the loss of the cardioprotection conferred by hypothyroidism and not to the effects of thyroid hormone per se.

13.2.8 TH and Ischemic Preconditioning Response

TH status may alter the response of the myocardium to cardioprotective interventions such as ischemic preconditioning. In fact, when TH is in excess, the ischemic preconditioning response is amplified

[14], while the preconditioning effect is lost in low TH state [34]. This is of clinical and therapeutic relevance since hypothyroidism is a common co-morbidity in patients with heart disease [35] and may alter the efficacy of preconditioning mimetic agents used in clinical practice [36].

13.3 TH and Postischemic Cardiac Remodeling

13.3.1 TH Signaling in Postischemic Cardiac Remodeling: "Player" or "Bystander"?

Several changes in the thyroid hormone-thyroid receptor (TH–TR) axis have been identified in the course of cardiac remodeling after myocardial infarction and are thought to contribute to cardiac dysfunction (Table 13.2). In the early study by Ojamaa et al., T_3 levels in plasma were found to be lower within a week and remained abnormal after 4 weeks following coronary ligation, while TH-responsive genes, such as myosin isoforms and SERCA, were altered and nearly normalized by TH administration [37]. Furthermore, D3 activity was shown to be significantly increased in the postinfarcted heart within a week following coronary ligation in rats, contributing to increased TH catabolism [38]. More recently, time-dependent changes in the expression of TRs in the viable nonischemic rat myocardium were observed. At 8 weeks after infarction, TRα1 and TRβ1 protein expression were down-regulated without changes in TH in plasma [33]. This response corresponded to decrease in SERCA expression (which is TH responsive and is shown to be regulated by TRβ1). A different pattern was observed at earlier or later stages; no significant changes were seen either in TR expression or in plasma T_3 during the first 2 weeks after myocardial infarction in rats. However, at 13 weeks, the expression of TRβ1 was decreased while the expression of TRα1 was increased. Furthermore, plasma T_3 was low while T_4 remained unchanged [2]. This response was associated with a shift of myosin isoform expression to the fetal pattern, a decreased ratio of SERCA/PLB, and development of cardiac hypertrophy [2].

This response seems to be of important physiological relevance; overexpression of TRα1 may reflect a compensatory mechanism to enhance TH signaling in the presence of low plasma T_3. However, in a rat model of hypothyroidism, low T_3 was not shown to be accompanied by increased expression of TRα1 (unpublished data). It is therefore likely that overexpressed TRα1, in the presence of low T_3, functions as an apo-receptor (unliganded TRα1) (Fig. 13.4a), thus repression of T_3 positively regulated genes occurs, contributing to the fetal phenotype characteristic of remodeled myocardium. In fact, a similar pattern of TR expression is observed during fetal life, a physiological situation in which TRα1 is overexpressed and TH is low [39, 40].

13.3.2 TRα1 Triggers a Switch to the Fetal Phenotype

The underlying mechanisms of the observed changes in TR expression in the myocardium after infarction remain largely unknown. Neuroendocrine systems and the inflammatory response, both implicated in cardiac remodeling, may be involved. In fact, the proinflammatory response plays a critical

Table 13.2 Changes in thyroid hormone signaling in the course of experimental postinfarction remodeling

Reference	Species model	Changes in TH signaling
Ojamaa et al. [37]	Myocardial infarction in rat (1, 3 and 4 weeks)	Decreased T_3, no change in T_4 in plasma
Pantos et al. [33]	Myocardial infarction in rat (8 weeks)	No change in T_3 and T_4 in plasma. Down-regulation of TRα1 and TRβ1 protein expression in the myocardium
Pantos et al. [49]	Myocardial infarction in rat (2 weeks)	No change in T_3 and T_4 in plasma. No change in TRα1 and TRβ1 protein expression in the myocardium
Pantos et al. [2]	Myocardial infarction in rat (13 weeks)	Decreased T_3, no change in T_4 in plasma. Increased TRα1 and decreased TRβ1 protein expression in the myocardium
Olivares et al. [38]	Myocardial infarction in rat (1 week)	Decreased T_3 and T_4 and increased TSH in plasma. Induction of D3 activity in the myocardium
Chen et al. [30]	Myocardial infarction in rat (3 days)	Decreased T_3 and T_4 in plasma, no change in TSH
Pol et al. [110]	Myocardial infarction in mice (1, 4 and 8 weeks)	Induction of D3 activity in the myocardium

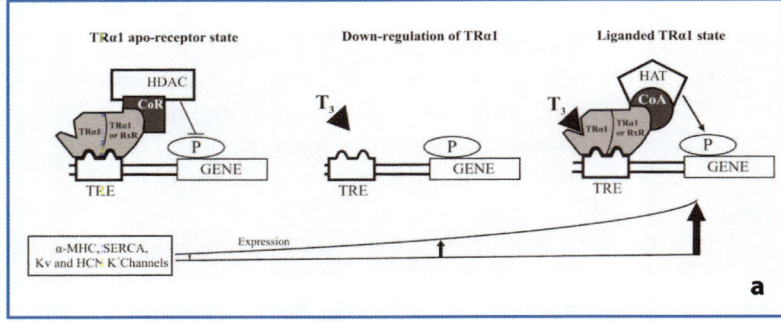

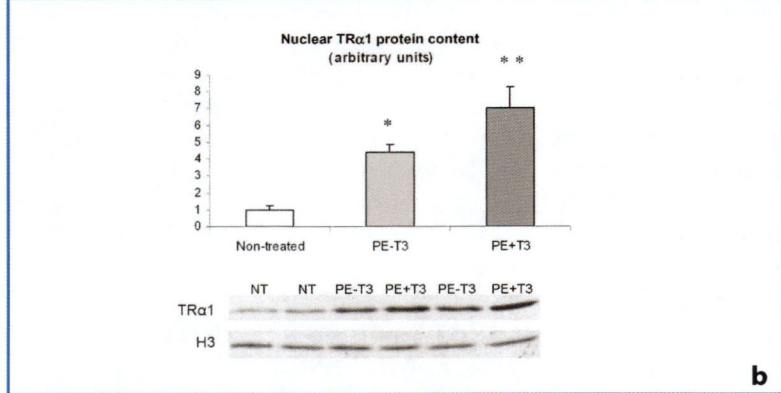

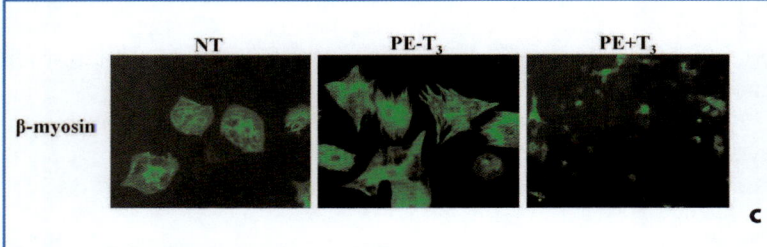

Fig. 13.4 a Molecular model of TRα1-regulated gene expression in three different states: in the absence of ligand (apo-receptor state), in the presence of ligand (holo-receptor state), and in the absence of the receptor. *RxR* Retinoid X receptor, *CoR* co-repressor, *CoA* co-activator, *HDAC* histone deacetylase, *HAT* histone acetyltransferase, *TRE* thyroid-hormone-responsive element, *P* RNA polymerase. **b** Densitometric assessment (in arbitrary units) and representative Western blots of thyroid hormone receptor α1 (TRα1) protein expression in the nucleus. *Columns* are means of optical ratios, *bar* = s.e.m. * $p < 0.05$ vs. NT, ** $p < 0.05$ vs PE-T$_3$. **c** Images of nontreated neonatal cardiomyocytes (NT), cardiomyocytes treated with phenylephrine (20 μM) without T$_3$ (PE–T$_3$), and cardiomyocytes treated with phenylephrine and T$_3$ (PE+T$_3$) for 5 days. Images were obtained from fluorescence microscopy after staining for slow (β)-myosin with specific antibody. TRα1 overexpression in the nucleus after prolonged exposure of cardiomyocytes to phenylephrine corresponds to a differential pattern of myosin isoform expression depending on the presence or absence of TH in the culture medium. TRα1 seems to trigger a switch to the cardiac cell fetal phenotype

role in cardiac remodeling, and cytokines such as tumor necrosis factor (TNF-α) are closely associated with cardiac dysfunction in animals and patients with heart failure [41]. Furthermore, prolonged activation of adrenergic signaling is thought to induce fetal-like changes in the myocardium [42]. Based on this evidence, we explored the possibility of interactions between α$_1$-adrenergic signaling and TRα1 expression in cardiomyocytes exposed to phenylephrine (PE, an α$_1$-adrenergic agonist) in the absence or presence of T$_3$ in the culture medium [43] (Fig. 13.4). PE administration (in the absence of T$_3$ in the culture medium) resulted in differential expression of TRα1 in the nucleus and cytosol; TRα1 expression was increased in the nucleus and decreased in the cytosol. This response was accompanied by a further increase in β-MHC expression in PE-treated cells and was found to

be dependent on the ERK signaling pathway [43]. PE-induced ERK activation was inhibited by the administration of PD98059. As a result, a redistribution of the expression of TRα1 was observed, with a marked decrease in TRα1 expression in the nucleus and increased expression of this receptor in the cytosol. Furthermore, β-MHC expression was significantly reduced [43] (Fig. 13.4c).

In the presence of excess T$_3$ in the medium, a different response to PE was observed: TRα1 was overexpressed in both the nucleus and cytosol and β-MHC expression was decreased, while α-MHC was dominant in PE+T$_3$-treated cells. Thus, TRα1 overexpression in the nucleus appears to correspond to differential myosin isoform expression depending on the availability of TH (liganded vs. unliganded state) (Fig. 13.4). These data suggest that unliganded TRα1 functions as an apo-receptor and induces fetal phenotypic changes in cells exposed to prolonged activation of α_1-adrenergic signaling. This notion is further supported by the fact that overexpression of unliganded TRα1 in neonatal cardiomyocytes resulted in cell growth with a fetal pattern of myosin isoform expression [44], and cardiomyocytes from mice with dominant negative TRα1 displayed impaired calcium handling and contraction [45]. Here, it should be noted that TRα1 appears also to be critical in the differentiation of cardiac embryonic cells [40].

The role of proinflammatory cytokines in TR expression was investigated by the administration of TNF-α in neonatal cardiomyocytes. Interestingly, TNF-α treatment resulted in a differential pattern of TR expression; TRβ1 expression was significantly decreased, while the expression of TRα1 receptor remained unchanged. This response was prevented by high-dose T_3 administration [46]. Taken together, these data indicate that the inflammatory response and the adrenergic system have distinct effects on TH signaling. However, interactions between TH and other signaling pathways known to be involved in cardiac remodeling cannot be excluded. TH treatment in cardiomyocytes was shown to prevent the angiotensin II-induced increased expression of β-MHC and decreased expression of α-MHC, indicating the existence of an interaction of the angiotensin II and TH signaling [47]. Furthermore, PKCα, which is now recognized as a key player in the pathophysiology of heart failure, was shown to alter the expression of TRα1. Overexpression of PKCα in neonatal cardiomyocytes in the absence of TH in the medium resulted in increased TRα1 expression in both cytosol and nucleus. This caused marked expression of the T_3-regulated β-MHC gene, and treatment with T_3 normalized the phenotype [48].

13.3.3 TH Prevents and/or Reverses Contractile Dysfunction After Myocardial Infarction

The important role of TH signaling in the process of cardiac remodeling after myocardial infarction has been further documented by the beneficial effects of TH administration early or late in the course of myocardial infarction [49, 50]. A time course analysis of function showed that left ventricular ejection fraction (EF%) was significantly improved after short- and long-term TH administration beginning immediately after infarction. Furthermore, independent of loading conditions, contractile indices, such as +dp/dt and –dp/dt, were also significantly improved. Similar effects have been demonstrated with TH administration beginning at later stages in the course of infarction (1–3 weeks) [37, 51, 52]. Interestingly, TH improved cardiac contractility even when started 13 weeks after myocardial infarction in rats (unpublished data).

13.3.4 TH Improves Cardiac Function by Regulating the Expression of Contractile Proteins

TH administration early or late after myocardial infarction has been shown to improve contractile function by altering the expression of contractile proteins in the myocardium. Hormone administration immediately after infarction prevented the induction of β-MHC in the viable myocardium of the postinfarcted hearts. Furthermore, the ratio SERCA/PLB, which is reduced in the postinfarcted heart, was significantly increased after TH treatment [49, 50]. Similarly, TH treatment reversed the fetal pattern of myosin isoform expression in hearts from animals with old myocardial infarction (unpublished data).

13.3.5 TH Improves Cardiac Function by Regulating Novel Pathways Related to Cardiac Contractility

It is now recognized that TH regulates cardiac contractility via novel signaling pathways (Fig. 13.2). In fact, TH treatment was shown to reduce the expression of both PKCϵ and PKCα in the postinfarcted rat myocardium [49]. PKC isoforms α and ϵ can control cardiac contractility through myofilament phosphorylation [53, 54]. Pharmacological and gene-therapy-based inhibition of PKCα enhances cardiac contractility and attenuates heart failure [53], while overexpression of PKCϵ results in cardiac dysfunction. Interestingly, the hypocontractile function in hypothyroid hearts was shown to be associated with overexpression of PKCϵ [13, 54].

The beneficial effect of TH on cardiac contractility may also be attributed to its ability to induce the expression of HSP70 in the postinfarcted myocardium, in which HSP70 content is otherwise low [50]. This protein is thought to be crucial for the response to stress and cardiac function, and HSP70 deletion in knockout mice not only reduced tolerance to ischemia but also caused a deterioration in contractile function [21].

13.3.6 TH Optimizes Cardiac Geometry: Contractility vs. Shape

It is now realized that TH, apart from its effect on cardiac contractility, improves cardiac mechanics by altering wall tension and left ventricular geometry (Fig. 13.5). In fact, time course analysis in a rat model of myocardial infarction showed that TH normalized wall stress (as assessed by the ratio of left ventricular diastolic diameter to posterior wall thickness) as early as 2 weeks, due to the development of cardiac hypertrophy early in the course of postinfarction remodeling. Furthermore, TH changed the cardiac geometry at later stages. The left ventricular chamber became progressively more spherical after myocardial infarction, as indicated by the progressive decrease of the sphericity index (the ratio between the long and short axes). With TH treatment, the sphericity index, although not changed in the first 2 weeks, was significantly increased after 13 weeks of treatment [50] (Fig. 13.5a). Thus, it appears that TH improves cardiac mechanics at early stages due to the development of hypertrophy

and at later stages by ellipsoidal reshaping of the left ventricular chamber [50]. The latter effect is probably due to the unique changes induced in cell shape and geometry by TH [55]. Taken together, TH seems to adapt the postinfarcted heart to unfavorable hemodynamics by inducing "physiological" hypertrophy and changing the cardiac geometry. This effect may be of therapeutic relevance and constitutes a different approach from simply inhibiting the hypertrophic response. It should be noted that left ventricular geometry is an independent predictor of mortality after acute myocardial infarction [56] and interventions aiming to preserve cardiac geometry are sought. So far, cardiac support devices that ensure passive epicardial constraint seem to confer some benefit [57].

13.3.7 TH Promotes Cardiac Cell Plasticity: Growth vs. Shape

13.3.7.1 TH Induces Physiological Growth

TH promotes cardiac growth through mechanisms that are not fully understood. This response initially was thought to be secondary to the increased workload induced by TH, since T_4 treatment failed to increase cardiac mass in heterotopic transplanted rat hearts [58]. Subsequent studies investigated possible involvement of the adrenergic and/or

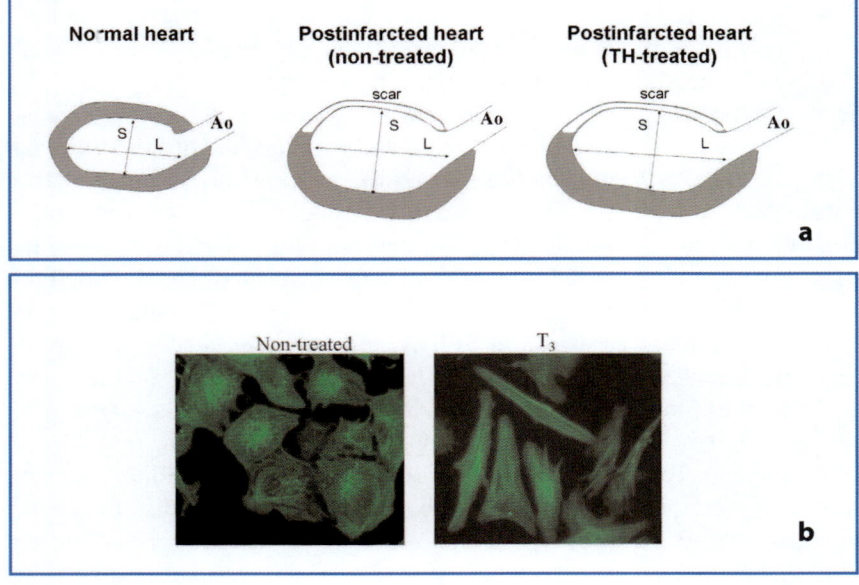

Fig. 13.5 a Changes in left ventricular shape after myocardial infarction in TH-treated and nontreated hearts. The left ventricular chamber is more spherical in shape in nontreated postinfarcted hearts. The ratio of the maximum long axis (*L*) to the maximum short axis (*S*) of the left ventricle is reduced and the viable segment becomes hypertrophied (with a shift of myosin isoform expression to the fetal pattern). TH reshapes the left ventricular chamber towards a more ellipsoidal shape. Hypertrophy also develops with myosin isoform expression of an adult phenotype. This effect may be due to the unique changes induced in cell shape by TH (**b**). *Ao* Aorta

renin–angiotensin system (both are activated in hyperthyroidism) in TH-mediated hypertrophy. In fact, pharmacological inhibition of β-adrenergic signaling induced by propranolol or angiotensin II at the level of the AT1 receptor diminished the development of cardiac hypertrophy [11, 15]. More recently, a direct effect of TH on cardiac growth was demonstrated. Overexpression of TRα1 in neonatal cardiomyocytes resulted in the activation of p38 MAPK and cell growth in the presence of TH. This response was abrogated by SB203580 (an inhibitor of p38 MAPK) [44]. Here, it is interesting to note that overexpression of TRα1 receptor in the absence of ligand can also result in cell growth, although with pathological characteristics; myosin isoform expression shifts to the fetal pattern [44]. TH appears also to induce cellular growth by activating the PI3K/Akt/mTOR signaling pathway via cytosolic TRα1 [59] (Fig. 13.2).

TH-mediated cardiac hypertrophy is not accompanied by cardiac fibrosis [60]. TH inhibits the pro-α1 collagen promoter activity and downregulates the collagen type I biosynthesis. Interestingly, in a genetic model of cardiac fibrosis, TH normalized the increased collagen type I gene expression in ventricular tissue and prevented fibrosis after induction of cardiac hypertrophy in rats with aortic constriction [61, 62].

13.3.7.2 TH Induces Unique Changes in Cardiac Cell Shape

TH, unlike other pro-growth stimuli, induces unique changes in cardiomyocyte morphology; neonatal cardiac cells become elongated, with well-oriented myofibrils when exposed to T_3. This was in contrast to the irregular cell shape and myofibril disorganization observed after cell exposure to phenylephrine (PE) [55] (Fig. 13.6). Furthermore, although both TH and PE increased cell area and protein synthesis, TH, in contrast to PE, enhanced α-MHC and repressed β-MHC expression. Interestingly, this response was associated with a differential pattern of intracellular kinase signaling activation, which may account for the two distinct types of hypertrophy induced by PE and TH administration [55, 63] (Fig. 13.6). PE induced an early and sustained activation of ERK (p44 and p42), which was accompanied by increased phosphorylation of p38 MAPK, JNK, and Akt. In contrast, with TH, a different pat-

tern of activation was seen; activation of ERK (only the p44 isoform, ERK1) occurred early and was non-sustained. In addition, ERK was translocated to the nucleus. Phospho-JNK levels were found to be decreased and no changes in the expression of phospho-Akt and phospho-p38 MAPK were observed (Fig. 13.6c). The effect of TH on cell morphology was shown to be abolished by PD98059, an ERK inhibitor, while the hypertrophic effect of TH (as determined by increased cell size and/or protein synthesis) was prevented by the administration of rapamycin, an mTOR inhibitor [55, 64]. Taken together, these data strongly indicate that TH induces changes in cell growth and geometry through activation of distinct pathways, and that the ERK cascade is critical in TH-induced cardiomyocyte plasticity. This may be of physiological and therapeutic importance: changes in cell shape may be translated into alterations in cardiac chamber geometry [50].

13.3.8 TH and Tissue Engineering

Wheter TH improves cardiac remodeling by increasing the endogenous regenerative capacity of the myocardium is an issue that remains largely unresolved. Although this hypothesis is of important therapeutic relevance, it has not yet been tested in models of myocardial infarction. There is now some evidence that T_3 administration in rats is associated with re-entry of cardiomyocytes into the cell cycle, with increased cyclin D1 protein synthesis and nuclear translocation. Interestingly, cardiomyocyte DNA synthesis increased after T_3 treatment, with the absence of tissue injury [65]. Along this line, T_3 has been further shown to promote differentiation of embryonic cardiomyoblasts via activation of TRα1 [43] and to enhance contractility in cardioids (contractile tissue constructed from self-organized neonatal cardiac cells) [66]. The latter may be of therapeutic importance since tissue-engineered heart muscle may provide an alternative treatment modality for end-stage heart failure.

13.4 TH and Arrhythmia: Proarrhythmic vs. Antiarrhythmic Effect

The arrhythmogenic effects of TH remain a poorly explored controversial issue. The effects of acute and long-term action of TH on cardiac susceptibili-

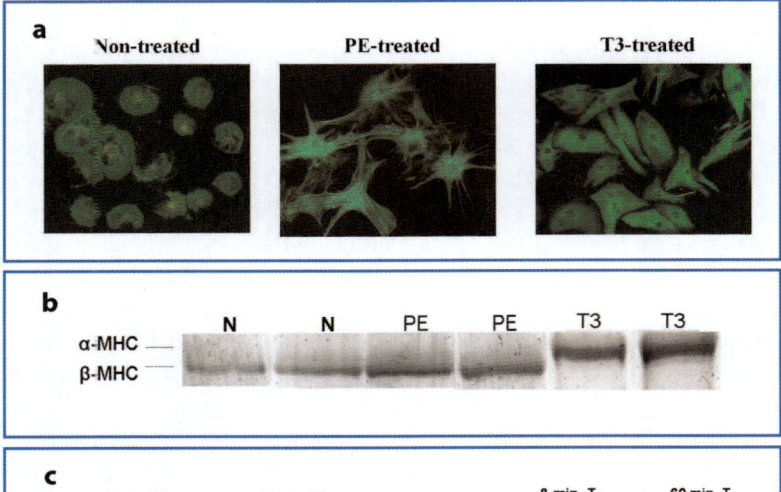

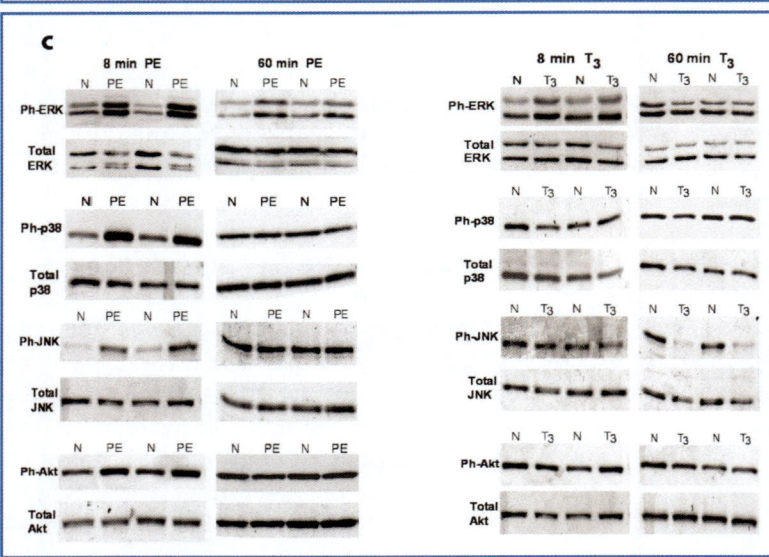

Fig. 13.6 TH and PE induce distinct changes in cell morphology corresponding to a differential pattern of myosin isoform expression. This response involves a differential pattern of activation of kinase-mediated intracellular signaling pathways and may account for TH-induced "physiological" and PE-induced "pathological" hypertrophy. **a** Fluorescence microscopy of nontreated, PE-treated and T_3-treated neonatal cardiomyocytes after 5 days of treatment. Actin myofilaments were stained with phalloidin. **b** Representative image showing α and β myosin isoform expression in nontreated, PE-treated, and T_3-treated neonatal cardiomyocytes after 5 days of treatment. **c** Representative Western blot showing phosphorylated ERKs, p38, JNKs, and Akt levels in nontreated, PE-treated, and T_3-treated (T_3) neonatal cardiomyocytes at 8 min and 60 min, respectively

ty to hypokalemia-induced ventricular fibrillation and the heart's ability to terminate ventricular fibrillation and restore sinus rhythm have been recently investigated in guinea pig hearts [67]. These studies clearly showed that TH has an anti- or proarrhythmic potential, depending on animal age and on the dose of TH used. It is interesting to note that episodes of torsades de pointes in patients with cardiomyopathy may be due to hypothyroidism-induced prolongation of the QT interval, a situation that could be reversed by TH treatment [68].

13.5 Clinical Implications: Protection vs. Function

Several studies have provided evidence that TH metabolism is altered during cardiac and noncardiac illnesses and after cardiac surgery [31]. The cause of low T_3 state seems to be multifactorial and cytokines have been implicated [69]. Interferon-α and interleukin-6 (IL-6) cause a response similar to "low T_3 syndrome," and in patients with acute myocardial infarction a negative correlation between IL-6 or C-reactive protein (CRP) and T_3 levels has been observed [70].

T_3 levels in serum decline within 48 h after acute myocardial infarction [71] or within 6–24 h after cardiac surgery [72]. This response is thought to contribute to energy preservation and, thus, to protection under stress. Patients with low TH levels at the onset of infarction to have smaller infarctions [32]. Furthermore, tissue hypothyroidism during cardiac remodeling increases tolerance of the postischemic myocardium to ischemia [33]. However, this is achieved at the expense of impaired cardiac function. Low T_3 levels were shown to be correlated with the severity of the clinical assessment of heart dysfunction in patients with congestive heart failure, and to be the only predictor of NYHA class in a multivariate analysis that included several neurohormonal parameters that change in heart failure [4, 73]. Along these lines, we recently found that total T_3 in plasma correlated strongly with maximum oxygen consumption (peak V_{O_2}) in patients with dilated cardiomyopathy, as assessed by cardiorespiratory stress testing [3]. Furthermore, low T_3 plasma levels appear to be an independent risk factor for increased mortality and morbidity in patients with heart failure [73], and low TH levels after infarction increase mortality in patients with acute myocardial infarction [32].

13.6 Therapeutic Implications

13.6.1 Selective Hypothyroidism and Cardioprotection

Antiarrhythmic compounds like amiodarone and its metabolite desethylamiodarone (DEA) are noncompetitive inhibitors of $TR\beta1$ and competitive inhibitors of $TR\alpha1$. Furthermore, dronedarone, a noniodinated amiodarone-like agent, and particularly its metabolite debutyldronedarone are selective $TR\alpha1$ antagonists [74]. The latter may be of therapeutic relevance in treating ischemia. The beneficial effects of hypothyroidism on cardiac protection may be elicited without the adverse effects of hypothyroidism, particularly those related to lipid metabolism ($TR\beta1$-mediated effects). Indeed, administration of dronedarone (at high doses), by inhibiting $TR\alpha1$ while sparing $TR\beta1$, resulted in an increase in myocardial glycogen levels, delayed ischemic contracture, and increased tolerance to ischemia–reperfusion [75].

13.6.2 TH: An Inotrope with Antiapoptotic Action

Several effects of TH on the cardiovascular system could be therapeutically exploited. So far, the clinical application of TH has been mainly due to its positive inotropic and vasodilatory effect [31, 76]. However, the beneficial effects of TH on the response of the heart to ischemia also may be of

therapeutic importance [77–79]. In fact, T_3 administration to patients undergoing bypass surgery increased cardiac index and reduced tissue injury [8]. However, in adult patients undergoing routine cardiac surgery, whilst some studies report improved hemodynamic parameters in the immediate postbypass period, there is no evidence that its use influences postoperative morbidity, mortality, or length of stay in the elective patient [80].

13.6.3 Rescue Treatments

TH may also have a role as rescue therapy in supporting some high-risk patients during weaning from bypass surgery or bridging left ventricular assist device or transplant [81, 82]. A recent experimental study showed that the depressed contractile reserve and impaired calcium handling of cardiac myocytes from chronically unloaded rat hearts were ameliorated with administration of a physiological dose of T_3 [83, 84].

13.6.4 Thyroid Analogues

The use of TH in clinical practice may be limited due to its undesirable side effects [85]. However, several pharmacological agents have been developed that can specifically activate or antagonize TRs or influence their binding with co-regulators. Selective $TR\beta1$ and $TR\alpha1$ agonists and antagonists have been synthesized that have fewer side effects [86, 87]. Interestingly, GC-1, a $TR\beta1$ agonist with no effect on cardiac rhythm, has been shown to have a proangiogenic action that is initiated at the plasma membrane and requires the activation of MAPK signaling [88]. However, GC-1 exhibits relatively decreased uptake by the heart compared to the liver, and GC-1 appears mainly to lower plasma cholesterol and to reduce body weight [86]. KB-141 is another $TR\beta1$ agonist thought to be suitable for treating obesity, hyperlipidemia, and diabetes [89]. More recently, $TR\alpha1$ agonists have also been synthesized [87] and await testing. 3,5-Diiodothyropropionic acid (DITPA) is the most well-studied thyroid analogue in relation to heart failure. It displays a positive inotropic effect without chronotropic action. Because of its minimal effect on heart rate, the efficacy of DITPA was tested in postinfarction cardiac remodeling in rats and rabbits [90–95]. DITPA administration immediately after infarction was shown to improve cardiac hemo-dynamics and induce angiogenesis [90–92, 94]. It is currently under clinical investigation [96].

13.7 Conclusions

TH is critical in tissue growth and differentiation and as such has pleiotropic cellular actions through its regulation of important regulatory and structural genes related to metabolism, cell function and mor-phology, and cellular response to stress.

TH appears to increase the resistance of the myocardium to ischemic stress. This response involves suppression of the proapoptotic p38 MAPK signaling pathway and the up-regulation of cardiopro-tective end-effectors, such as HSP27 and HSP70.

Hypothyroidism can also induce cardioprotec-tion that is distinct from that mediated by TH. Ischemic contracture is suppressed and delayed, and the proapoptotic JNK signaling pathway seems to be critical in hypothyroidism-induced protection. A low thyroid state is common in myocardial infarc-tion and heart failure patients, and this may be a protective adaptive response with respect to ischemic stress but a maladaptive response in terms of cardiac function. As proof of concept, patients with low plasma TH have smaller infarctions but a worse prognosis.

Time-dependent changes in the TH–TR axis occur in the course of postischemic cardiac remod-eling and may be involved in the progression of car-diac dysfunction after acute myocardial infarction.

Adrenergic signaling (α_1-adrenergic) and inflammatory factors (TNF-α) appear to interact with TH signaling at the level of TRs, with impor-tant physiological consequences. The α_1-adrenergic stimulation redistributes the TRα1 in the nucleus which, in the absence of TH, acts as an apo-receptor and induces fetal-like myosin expression.

TH administration early or late after acute myocardial infarction has been shown to prevent and/or reverse cardiac remodeling. TH improves contractile function via its classical effect on the expression of contractile proteins and/or via its effect on novel signaling pathways related to car-diac contractility (PKC, HSP70). More importantly, TH appears to improve hemodynamics by optimiz-ing cardiac geometry. This effect is likely due to the unique changes in cell shape induced by TH. Interestingly, TH effects on cell growth and cell shape seem to be mediated by distinct signaling pathways. TH changes in cell geometry appear to involve transient activation of the ERK signaling pathway, while TH induces cell growth through activation of mTOR.

The unique TH effects on cardiac cell plasticity and cell response to ischemic insults may be of ther-apeutic relevance in treating ischemic heart disease. TH as an inotrope possessing antiapoptotic proper-ties may be an optional treatment for supporting hemodynamics in the setting of ischemia–reperfu-sion. As proof of concept, TH improved hemody-namics while reducing troponin release in patients undergoing bypass surgery.

The antiapoptotic effect of TH and its potential to change cardiac geometry have aroused interest in TH as a new therapeutic modality to support hemo-dynamics in the setting of ischemia–reperfusion and in postischemic remodeling. TH analogues have already been synthesized, and clinical trials are needed to test the efficacy of TH in patients.

Key Points

- Thyroid hormone promotes tissue growth and differentiation and as such has pleiotropic actions on the heart: it regulates metabolism, cellular function and morphology, and the cellular response to stress.

- Thyroid hormone increases the tolerance of the heart to ischemia via regulation of cardioprotective intracellular signaling.

- Thyroid hormone can improve hemodynamics in the setting of ischemia-reperfusion due to its inotropic and antiapoptotic action.

(Cont. →)

(*cont.*)

- Changes in the thyroid hormone–thyroid hormone receptor axis occur in the course of postinfarction cardiac remodeling and contribute to the fetal cardiac phenotype. TRα1 appears to be critical in this response.

- A low thyroid hormone state is not uncommon in ischemic myocardial conditions and may be a protective response against ischemic stress, at the expense, however, of impaired cardiac function.

- Thyroid hormone prevents/reverses postinfarction cardiac remodeling.

- Thyroid hormone improves postinfarction cardiac function by regulating the expression of contractile proteins, regulating novel signaling pathways related to cardiac contractility, and optimizing cardiac chamber geometry.

- Thyroid hormone or thyroid hormone analogues may be a new therapeutic option for treating ischemic heart disease.

References

1. Pantos C, Mourouzis I, Xinaris C et al (2008) Thyroid hormone and "cardiac metamorphosis": potential therapeutic implications. Pharmacol Ther 118:277–294
2. Pantos C, Mourouzis I, Xinaris C et al (2007) Time-dependent changes in the expression of thyroid hormone receptor a1 in the myocardium after acute myocardial infarction: possible implications in cardiac remodelling. Eur J Endocrinol 156:415–424
3. Pantos C, Dritsas A, Mourouzis I et al (2007) Thyroid hormone is a critical determinant of myocardial performance in patients with heart failure: potential therapeutic implications. Eur J Endocrinol 157:515–520
4. Pingitore A, Iervasi G, Barison A et al (2006) Early activation of an altered thyroid hormone profile in asymptomatic or mildly symptomatic idiopathic left ventricular dysfunction. J Card Fail 12:520–526
5. Pingitore A, Landi P, Taddei MC et al (2005) Triiodothyronine levels for risk stratification of patients with chronic heart failure. Am J Med 118:132–136
6. Kuzman JA, Gerdes AM, Kobayashi S et al (2005) Thyroid hormone activates Akt and prevents serum starvation-induced cell death in neonatal rat cardiomyocytes. J Mol Cell Cardiol 39:841–844
7. Pantos CI, Malliopoulou VA, Mourouzis IS et al (2002) Long-term thyroxine administration protects the heart in a pattern similar to ischemic preconditioning. Thyroid 12:325–329
8. Ranasinghe AM, Quinn DW, Pagano D et al (2006) Glucose-insulin-potassium and tri-iodothyronine individually improve hemodynamic performance and are associated with reduced troponin I release after on-pump coronary artery bypass grafting. Circulation 114:I245–250
9. Zinman T, Shneyvays V, Tribulova N et al (2006) Acute, nongenomic effect of thyroid hormones in preventing calcium overload in newborn rat cardiocytes. J Cell Physiol 207:220–231
10. Buser PT, Wikman-Coffelt J, Wu ST et al (1990) Postischemic recovery of mechanical performance and energy metabolism in the presence of left ventricular hypertrophy. A 31P-MRS study. Circ Res 66:735–746
11. Pantos CI, Mourouzis IS, Tzeis SM et al (2000) Propranolol diminishes cardiac hypertrophy but does not abolish acceleration of the ischemic contracture in hyperthyroid hearts. J Cardiovasc Pharmacol 36:384–389
12. Kolocassides KG, Galinanes M, Hearse DJ (1996) Dichotomy of ischemic preconditioning: improved postischemic contractile function despite intensification of ischemic contracture. Circulation 93:1725–1733
13. Pantos C, Malliopoulou V, Mourouzis I et al (2003) Propylthiouracil-induced hypothyroidism is associated with increased tolerance of the isolated rat heart to ischaemia-reperfusion. J Endocrinol 178:427–435
14. Pantos CI, Cokkinos DD, Tzeis SM et al (1999) Hyperthyroidism is associated with preserved preconditioning capacity but intensified and accelerated ischaemic contracture in rat heart. Basic Res Cardiol 94:254–260
15. Pantos C, Paizis I, Mourouzis I et al (2005) Blockade of angiotensin II type 1 receptor diminishes cardiac hypertrophy, but does not abolish thyroxin-induced preconditioning. Horm Metab Res 37:500–504
16. Pantos CI, Davos CH, Carageorgiou HC et al (1996) Ischaemic preconditioning protects against myocardial dysfunction caused by ischaemia in isolated hypertrophied rat hearts. Basic Res Cardiol 91:444–449
17. Speechly-Dick ME, Mocanu MM, Yellon DM (1994) Protein kinase C. Its role in ischemic preconditioning in the rat. Circ Res 75:586–590
18. Zhao J, Renner O, Wightman L et al (1998) The expression of constitutively active isotypes of protein kinase C to investigate preconditioning. J Biol Chem 273:23072–23079
19. Maizels ET, Peters CA, Kline M et al (1998) Heat-shock protein-25/27 phosphorylation by the delta isoform of protein kinase C. Biochem J 332 (Pt 3):703–712
20. Pantos C, Malliopoulou V, Mourouzis I et al (2003) Thyroxine pretreatment increases basal myocardial heat-shock protein 27 expression and accelerates translocation and phosphorylation of this protein upon ischaemia. Eur J Pharmacol 478:53–60
21. Kim YK, Suarez J, Hu Y et al (2006) Deletion of the in-

ducible 70-kDa heat shock protein genes in mice impairs cardiac contractile function and calcium handling associated with hypertrophy. Circulation 113:2589–2597

22. Martin JL, Mestril R, Hilal-Dandan R et al (1997) Small heat shock proteins and protection against ischemic injury in cardiac myocytes. Circulation 96:4343–4348

23. Pantos CI, Malliopoulou VA, Mourouzis IS et al (2001) Long-term thyroxine administration increases heat stress protein-70 mRNA expression and attenuates p38 MAP kinase activity in response to ischaemia. J Endocrinol 170:207–2015

24. Pantos C, Malliopoulou V, Mourouzis I et al (2006) Hyperthyroid hearts display a phenotype of cardioprotection against ischemic stress: a possible involvement of heat shock protein 70. Horm Metab Res 38:308–313

25. Venditti P, Di Meo S (2006) Thyroid hormone-induced oxidative stress. Cell Mol Life Sci 63:414–434

26. Downey JM, Davis AM, Cohen MV (2007) Signaling pathways in ischemic preconditioning. Heart Fail Rev 12:181–188

27. Novitzky D, Cooper DK, Swanepoel A (1989) Inotropic effect of triiodothyronine (T3) in low cardiac output following cardioplegic arrest and cardiopulmonary bypass: an initial experience in patients undergoing open heart surgery. Eur J Cardiothorac Surg 3:140–145

28. Pantos C, Mourouzis I, Tzeis S et al (2003) Dobutamine administration exacerbates postischaemic myocardial dysfunction in isolated rat hearts: an effect reversed by thyroxine pretreatment. Eur J Pharmacol 460:155–161

29. Pantos C, Cokkinos DV (2006) Hormones signaling and myocardial ischemia. In: Cokkinos DV, Pantos C, Heusch G, Taegtmeyer H (eds) Myocardial ischemia: from mechanisms to theurapeutic potentials. Springer, New York, pp 11–77

30. Chen YF, Kobayashi S, Chen J et al (2008) Short term triiodo-l-thyronine treatment inhibits cardiac myocyte apoptosis in border area after myocardial infarction in rats. J Mol Cell Cardiol 44:180–187

31. Klein I, Ojamaa K (2001) Thyroid hormone and the cardiovascular system. N Engl J Med 344:501–509

32. Friberg L, Werner S, Eggertsen G et al (2002) Rapid downregulation of thyroid hormones in acute myocardial infarction: is it cardioprotective in patients with angina? Arch Intern Med 162:1388–1394

33. Pantos C, Mourouzis I, Saranteas T et al (2005) Thyroid hormone receptors alpha1 and beta1 are downregulated in the post-infarcted rat heart: consequences on the response to ischaemia-reperfusion. Basic Res Cardiol 100:422–432

34. Mourouzis I, Dimopoulos A, Saranteas T et al (2008) Ischemic preconditioning fails to confer additional protection against ischemia-reperfusion injury in the hypothyroid rat heart. Physiol Res. Epub ahead of print: http://www.bio-med.cas.cz/physiolres/pdf/prepress/1387.pdf

35. Biondi B, Klein I (2004) Hypothyroidism as a risk factor for cardiovascular disease. Endocrine 24:1–13

36. Ferdinandy P, Schulz R, Baxter GF (2007) Interaction of cardiovascular risk factors with myocardial ischemia/reperfusion injury, preconditioning, and postconditioning. Pharmacol Rev 59:418–458

37. Ojamaa K, Kenessey A, Shenoy R et al (2000) Thyroid hormone metabolism and cardiac gene expression after acute myocardial infarction in the rat. Am J Physiol Endocrinol Metab 279:E1319–324

38. Olivares EL, Marassi MP, Fortunato RS et al (2007) Thyroid function disturbance and type 3 iodothyronine deiodinase induction after myocardial infarction in rats: a time course study. Endocrinology 148:4786–4792

39. Mai W, Janier MF, Allioli N et al (2004) Thyroid hormone receptor alpha is a molecular switch of cardiac function between fetal and postnatal life. Proc Natl Acad Sci U S A 101:10332–10337

40. White P, Burton KA, Fowden AL et al (2001) Developmental expression analysis of thyroid hormone receptor isoforms reveals new insights into their essential functions in cardiac and skeletal muscles. FASEB J 15:1367–1376

41. Torre-Amione G (2005) Immune activation in chronic heart failure. Am J Cardiol 95:3C–8C; discussion 38C–40C

42. Barron AJ, Finn SG, Fuller SJ (2003) Chronic activation of extracellular-signal-regulated protein kinases by phenylephrine is required to elicit a hypertrophic response in cardiac myocytes. Biochem J 371:71–79

43. Pantos C, Xinaris C, Mourouzis I et al (2008) Thyroid hormone receptor a1 : a switch to cardiac cell "metamorphosis" ? J Physiol Pharmacol 59:253–269

44. Kinugawa K, Jeong MY, Bristow MR et al (2005) Thyroid hormone induces cardiac myocyte hypertrophy in a thyroid hormone receptor alpha1-specific manner that requires TAK1 and p38 mitogen-activated protein kinase. Mol Endocrinol 19:1618–1628

45. Tavi P, Sjogren M, Lunde PK et al (2005) Impaired Ca2+ handling and contraction in cardiomyocytes from mice with a dominant negative thyroid hormone receptor alpha1. J Mol Cell Cardiol 38:655–663

46. Pantos C, Xinaris C, Mourouzis I et al (2008) TNF-a administration in neonatal cardiomyocytes is associated with differential expression of thyroid hormone receptors: a response prevented by T3. Horm Metab Res 40:731–734

47. Wang B, Ouyang J, Xia Z (2006) Effects of triiodo-thyronine on angiotensin-induced cardiomyocyte hypertrophy: reversal of increased beta-myosin heavy chain gene expression. Can J Physiol Pharmacol 84:935–941

48. Kenessey A, Sullivan EA, Ojamaa K (2006) Nuclear localization of protein kinase C-alpha induces thyroid hormone receptor-alpha1 expression in the cardiomyocyte. Am J Physiol Heart Circ Physiol 290:H381–389

49. Pantos C, Mourouzis I, Markakis K et al (2007) Thyroid hormone attenuates cardiac remodeling and improves hemodynamics early after acute myocardial infarction in rats. Eur J Cardiothorac Surg 32:333–339

50. Pantos C, Mourouzis I, Markakis K et al (2008) Long-term thyroid hormone administration re-shapes left ventricular chamber and improves cardiac function after myocardial infarction in rats. Basic Res Cardiol 103:308–318

51. Gay R, Gustafson TA, Goldman S et al (1987) Effects of l-thyroxine in rats with chronic heart failure after myocardial infarction. Am J Physiol 253:H341–346

52. Gay RG, Graham S, Aguirre M et al (1988) Effects of 10- to 12-day treatment with l-thyroxine in rats with myocardial infarction. Am J Physiol 255:H801–806

53. Hambleton M, Hahn H, Pleger ST et al (2006) Pharmacological- and gene therapy-based inhibition of protein kinase Calpha/beta enhances cardiac contractility and attenuates heart failure. Circulation 114:574–582

54. Scruggs SB, Walker LA, Lyu T et al (2006) Partial re-

placement of cardiac troponin I with a non-phosphorylatable mutant at serines 43/45 attenuates the contractile dysfunction associated with PKCe phosphorylation. J Mol Cell Cardiol 40:465–473

55. Pantos C, Xinaris C, Mourouzis I et al (2007) Thyroid hormone changes cardiomyocyte shape and geometry via ERK signaling pathway: potential therapeutic implications in reversing cardiac remodeling? Mol Cell Biochem 297:65–72

56. Wong SP, French JK, Lydon AM et al (2004) Relation of left ventricular sphericity to 10-year survival after acute myocardial infarction. Am J Cardiol 94:1270–1275

57. Lembcke A, Dushe S, Dohmen PM et al (2006) Early and late effects of passive epicardial constraint on left ventricular geometry: ellipsoidal re-shaping confirmed by electron-beam computed tomography. J Heart Lung Transplant 25:90–98

58. Klein I, Hong C (1986) Effects of thyroid hormone on cardiac size and myosin content of the heterotopically transplanted rat heart. J Clin Invest 77:1694–1698

59. Kenessey A, Ojamaa K (2006) Thyroid hormone stimulates protein synthesis in the cardiomyocyte by activating the Akt-mTOR and p70S6K pathways. J Biol Chem 281:20666–20672

60. Ziegelhoffer-Mihalovicova B, Briest W, Baba HA et al (2003) The expression of mRNA of cytokines and of extracellular matrix proteins in triiodothyronine-treated rat hearts. Mol Cell Biochem 247:61–68

61. Wong K, Boheler KR, Petrou M et al (1997) Pharmacological modulation of pressure-overload cardiac hypertrophy: changes in ventricular function, extracellular matrix, and gene expression. Circulation 96:2239–2246

62. Yao J, Eghbali M (1992) Decreased collagen gene expression and absence of fibrosis in thyroid hormone-induced myocardial hypertrophy. Response of cardiac fibroblasts to thyroid hormone in vitro. Circ Res 71:831–839

63. Xinaris C, Mourouzis I, Carageorgiou H et al (2006) Differential activation of stress kinase signaling by phenylephrine and thyroid hormone in neonatal cardiomyocytes. J Mol Cell Cardiol 40:999

64. Xinaris C, Mourouzis I, Pantos C et al (2006) Thyroid hormone promotes cardiac myocyte plasticity via activation of stress kinase signalling [abstract]. J Mol Cell Cardiol 40:218 (Abstract)

65. Columbano A, Pibiri M, Deidda M et al (2006) The thyroid hormone receptor-beta agonist GC-1 induces cell proliferation in rat liver and pancreas. Endocrinology 147:3211–3218

66. Khait L, Birla RK (2008) Effect of thyroid hormone on the contractility of self-organized heart muscle. In Vitro Cell Dev Biol Anim 44:204–213

67. Knezl V, Soukup T, Okruhlicova L et al (2008) Thyroid hormones modulate occurrence and termination of ventricular fibrillation by both long-term and acute actions. Physiol Res 57(Suppl 2):S91–96

68. Ellis CR, Murray KT (2008) When an ICD is not the answer... Hypothyroidism-induced cardiomyopathy and torsades de pointes. J Cardiovasc Electrophysiol 19:1105–1107

69. Abo-Zenah HA, Shoeb SA, Sabry AA et al (2008) Relating circulating thyroid hormone concentrations to serum interleukins-6 and 10 in association with non-thyroidal illnesses including chronic renal insufficiency.

BMC Endocr Disord 8:1

70. Kimura T, Kanda T, Kotajima N et al (2000) Involvement of circulating interleukin-6 and its receptor in the development of euthyroid sick syndrome in patients with acute myocardial infarction. Eur J Endocrinol 143:179–184

71. Eber B, Schumacher M, Langsteger W et al (1995) Changes in thyroid hormone parameters after acute myocardial infarction. Cardiology 86:152–156

72. Holland FW 2nd, Brown PS Jr, Weintraub BD et al (1991) Cardiopulmonary bypass and thyroid function: a "euthyroid sick syndrome". Ann Thorac Surg 52:46–50

73. Iervasi G, Pingitore A, Landi P et al (2003) Low-T3 syndrome: a strong prognostic predictor of death in patients with heart disease. Circulation 107:708–713

74. Van Beeren HC, Jong WM, Kaptein E et al (2003) Dronerarone acts as a selective inhibitor of 3,5,3?-triiodothyronine binding to thyroid hormone receptor-alpha1: in vitro and in vivo evidence. Endocrinology 144:552–558

75. Pantos C, Mourouzis I, Malliopoulou V et al (2005) Dronedarone administration prevents body weight gain and increases tolerance of the heart to ischemic stress: a possible involvement of thyroid hormone receptor alpha1. Thyroid 15:16–23

76. Klein I (2003) Thyroid hormone and cardiac contractility. Am J Cardiol 91:1331–1332

77. Naito H, Melnychenko I, Didie M et al (2006) Optimizing engineered heart tissue for therapeutic applications as surrogate heart muscle. Circulation 114:I72–728

78. Pantos C, Malliopoulou V, Varonos DD et al (2004) Thyroid hormone and phenotypes of cardioprotection. Basic Res Cardiol 99:101–120

79. Tomanek RJ, Doty MK, Sandra A (1998) Early coronary angiogenesis in response to thyroxine: growth characteristics and upregulation of basic fibroblast growth factor. Circ Res 82:587–593

80. Ronald A, Dunning J (2006) Does perioperative thyroxine have a role during adult cardiac surgery? Interact Cardiovasc Thorac Surg 5:166–178

81. Novitzky D, Fontanet H, Snyder M et al (1996) Impact of triiodothyronine on the survival of high-risk patients undergoing open heart surgery. Cardiology 87:509–515

82. Malik FS, Mehra MR, Uber PA et al (1999) Intravenous thyroid hormone supplementation in heart failure with cardiogenic shock. J Card Fail 5:31–37

83. Minatoya Y, Ito K, Kagaya Y et al (2007) Depressed contractile reserve and impaired calcium handling of cardiac myocytes from chronically unloaded hearts are ameliorated with the administration of physiological treatment dose of T3 in rats. Acta Physiol (Oxf) 189:221–231

84. Pantos C (2007) Thyroid hormone at physiological doses restores depressed contractile reserve and impaired calcium handling of cardiac myocytes from chronically unloaded hearts. Acta Physiol (Oxf) 189:219

85. Sawin CT (2002) Subclinical hyperthyroidism and atrial fibrillation. Thyroid 12:501–503

86. Trost SU, Swanson E, Gloss B et al (2000) The thyroid hormone receptor-beta-selective agonist GC-1 differentially affects plasma lipids and cardiac activity. Endocrinology 141:3057–3064

87. Ocasio CA, Scanlan TS (2006) Design and characterization of a thyroid hormone receptor alpha (TRa)-specific agonist. ACS Chem Biol 1:585–593

88. Mousa SA, O'Connor LJ, Bergh JJ et al (2005) The proangiogenic action of thyroid hormone analogue GC-1 is initiated at an integrin. J Cardiovasc Pharmacol 46:356–360

89. Grover GJ, Mellstrom K, Malm J (2007) Therapeutic potential for thyroid hormone receptor-beta selective agonists for treating obesity, hyperlipidemia and diabetes. Curr Vasc Pharmacol 5:141–154

90. Litwin SE, Zhang D, Roberge P et al (2000) DITPA prevents the blunted contraction-frequency relationship in myocytes from infarcted hearts. Am J Physiol Heart Circ Physiol 278:H862–870

91. Mahaffey KW, Raya TE, Pennock GD et al (1995) Left ventricular performance and remodeling in rabbits after myocardial infarction. Effects of a thyroid hormone analogue. Circulation 91:794–801

92. Pennock GD, Spooner PH, Summers CE et al (2000) Prevention of abnormal sarcoplasmic reticulum calcium transport and protein expression in post-infarction heart failure using 3,5-diiodothyropropionic acid (DITPA). J Mol Cell Cardiol 32:1939–1953

93. Spooner PH, Thai HM, Goldman S et al (2004) Thyroid hormone analog, DITPA, improves endothelial nitric oxide and beta-adrenergic mediated vasorelaxation after myocardial infarction. J Cardiovasc Pharmacol 44:453–459

94. Tomanek RJ, Zimmerman MB, Suvarna PR et al (1998) A thyroid hormone analog stimulates angiogenesis in the post-infarcted rat heart. J Mol Cell Cardiol 30:923–932

95. Zheng W, Weiss RM, Wang X et al (2004) DITPA stimulates arteriolar growth and modifies myocardial postinfarction remodeling. Am J Physiol Heart Circ Physiol 286:H1994–2000

96. Morkin E, Pennock GD, Spooner PH et al (2002) Clinical and experimental studies on the use of 3,5-diiodothyropropionic acid, a thyroid hormone analogue, in heart failure. Thyroid 12:527–533

97. Dyke CM, Yeh T, Jr., Lehman JD et al (1991) Triiodothyronine-enhanced left ventricular function after ischemic injury. Ann Thorac Surg 52:14–19

98. Novitzky D, Matthews N, Shawley D et al (1991) Triiodothyronine in the recovery of stunned myocardium in dogs. Ann Thorac Surg 51:10–16; discussion 16–17

99. Holland FW 2nd, Brown PS Jr, Clark RE (1992) Acute severe postischemic myocardial depression reversed by triiodothyronine. Ann Thorac Surg 54:301–305

100. Dyke CM, Ding M, Abd-Elfattah AS et al (1993) Effects of triiodothyronine supplementation after myocardial ischemia. Ann Thorac Surg 56:215–222

101. Kadletz M, Mullen PG, Ding M et al (1994) Effect of triiodothyronine on postischemic myocardial function in the isolated heart. Ann Thorac Surg 57:657–662

102. Klemperer JD, Klein I, Gomez M et al (1995) Thyroid hormone treatment after coronary-artery bypass surgery. N Engl J Med 333:1522–1527

103. Walker JD, Crawford FA, Jr., Spinale FG (1995) 3,5,3?-Triiodo-l-thyronine pretreatment with cardioplegic arrest and chronic left ventricular dysfunction. Ann Thorac Surg 60:292–299

104. Klemperer JD, Zelano J, Helm RE et al (1995) Triiodothyronine improves left ventricular function without oxygen wasting effects after global hypothermic ischemia. J Thorac Cardiovasc Surg 109:457–465

105. Liu Q, Clanachan AS, Lopaschuk GD (1998) Acute effects of triiodothyronine on glucose and fatty acid metabolism during reperfusion of ischemic rat hearts. Am J Physiol 275:E392–399

106. Spinale FG (1999) Cellular and molecular therapeutic targets for treatment of contractile dysfunction after cardioplegic arrest. Ann Thorac Surg 68:1934–1941

107. Lahorra JA, Torchiana DF, Hahn C et al (2000) Recovery after cardioplegia in the hypertrophic rat heart. J Surg Res 88:88–96

108. Venditti P, Masullo P, Agnisola C et al (2000) Effect of vitamin E on the response to ischemia-reperfusion of Langendorff heart preparations from hyperthyroid rats. Life Sci 66:697–708

109. Asahi T, Shimabukuro M, Oshiro Y et al (2001) Cilazapril prevents cardiac hypertrophy and postischemic myocardial dysfunction in hyperthyroid rats. Thyroid 11:1009–1015

110. Pol CJ, van Deel ED, Muller A et al (2008) Left ventricular myocardial infarction in mice induces sustained cardiac deiodinase type III activity. J Mol Cell Cardiol 44:722–723

Thyroid and Cardiovascular Risk

14

Avantika C. Waring and Anne R. Cappola

Abstract Here we present data on the clinical effects of alterations in thyroid hormone levels, with a focus on the cardiovascular risk associated with subclinical thyroid dysfunction. Observational studies and small randomized trials have suggested that subclinical hypothyroidism causes reversible alterations in traditional cardiovascular risk factors and surrogate markers of cardiovascular disease. The data supporting the assumption of such cardiovascular risk from subclinical hypothyroidism are inconsistent, but patients less than 65 years of age or those with a TSH concentration of 10 mU/l or higher may be at increased risk of coronary heart disease and cardiac death. Subclinical hyperthyroidism is a risk factor for atrial fibrillation. Large, randomized clinical trials are needed to identify the populations of individuals with subclinical thyroid dysfunction whose cardiovascular risk would improve with treatment.

Keywords Lipids • Total cholesterol • LDL cholesterol • Triglycerides • HDL cholesterol • Lp(a) cholesterol • Levothyroxine replacement • C-reactive protein • Homocysteine • Hemostatic factors • Fibrinogen • Arterial stiffness • Central pulse wave velocity • Aortic augmentation index • Brachial-artery flow-mediated dilation • Carotid intima–media thickness • Prevalence of coronary heart disease • Cardiovascular mortality • Atrial fibrillation

14.1 Introduction

The preceding chapters have presented compelling mechanistic data regarding the actions of thyroid hormone on the myocardium. In this chapter, we present data on the clinical effects of alterations in thyroid hormone levels, focusing on human studies that have examined how abnormalities in thyroid function affect cardiovascular risk. After a brief historical overview of overt hypothyroidism and cardiovascular disease, we discuss studies of subclinical thyroid dysfunction, defined as an abnormal thyroid-stimulating hormone (TSH) level with a normal free thyroxine (T$_4$) level, since subclinical thyroid dysfunction represents an area whose management is debated. For subclinical hypothyroidism, data are presented on cardiovascular risk factors (both traditional and potential), surrogate markers of coronary heart disease (CHD), and CHD events. For each outcome, we present the findings from observational studies first, followed by the results from clinical trials of levothyroxine therapy. For overt and subclinical hyperthyroidism, data are presented on the risk of atrial fibrillation.

A.R. Cappola (✉)
Division of Endocrinology, Diabetes and Metabolism,
University of Pennsylvania School of Medicine,
Philadelphia, PA, United States

G. Iervasi, A. Pingitore (eds.), *Thyroid and Heart Failure*.
© Springer-Verlag Italia 2009

14.2　Overt Hypothyroidism and Cardiovascular Disease

Untreated overt hypothyroidism can result in profound cardiac consequences, notably pericardial effusions and congestive heart failure. Fortunately, these clinical sequelae are rare in the modern era of thyroid function testing and early intervention. Because overt hypothyroidism affects only 0.3% of the population [1] and immediate treatment is indicated, the majority of published studies of overt hypothyroidism have employed small study samples and were cross-sectional in design. Autopsy studies have suggested that there is more atherosclerosis in patients with overt hypothyroidism than in healthy controls [2]. Additional case–control studies have demonstrated a greater prevalence of circulatory dysfunction and atherosclerotic risk factors (higher cholesterol levels, increased diastolic hypertension, and adversely altered coagulability) in patients with overt hypothyroidism, with improvement upon treatment with levothyroxine therapy [2, 3]. However, the actual cardiovascular risk of overt hypothyroidism has never been quantified and is unlikely to be, as treatment of overt hypothyroidism is without question. Instead where the field is still in need of guidance is in the management of subclinical hypothyroidism.

14.3　Subclinical Hypothyroidism

Subclinical hypothyroidism, defined as an elevated TSH with a normal free thyroxine level, is a relatively common condition, affecting anywhere from 4 to 20% of the general population [1, 4–7]. The prevalence also tends to increase with increasing age of the population sampled, with rates in the elderly ranging from 10 to 20% [4, 5, 7–9].

The clinical cardiovascular effects of the mild thyroid abnormalities found in subclinical hypothyroidism are unknown. There are many mechanisms by which subclinical hypothyroidism might increase the risk of cardiovascular disease. As mentioned above, atherosclerosis has been documented by autopsy studies to be more severe in patients with overt hypothyroidism than in matched euthyroid patients [2], and increased atherosclerosis as measured by surrogate markers has been observed in patients with subclinical hypothyroidism [10]. Alterations in lipid profiles in these patients, partic-

ularly elevated total cholesterol and low-density lipoprotein (LDL) levels, have been invoked as a potentially reversible cause of cardiovascular risk [10–12]. Newer biomarkers and surrogate markers for cardiovascular risk, such as C-reactive protein (CRP), arterial stiffness, and brachial artery reactivity, may also be altered in patients with subclinical hypothyroidism compared to the euthyroid population [13, 14].

Associations between subclinical hypothyroidism and increased prevalence and incidence of cardiovascular disease have also been observed; however, these results are heterogeneous across studies. Furthermore, interventional trials aimed at correcting the TSH to within a normal range also revealed conflicting evidence on the cardiovascular benefits of such treatment. How do we reconcile the seemingly contradictory data from these studies? Recent meta-analyses of the observational studies suggested that the relationship is in part dependent upon the age of the patient and the level of TSH elevation [15, 16]. Thus, the cardiovascular risk may not be uniform across all ages and all degrees of subclinical hypothyroidism. Instead, these analyses suggest that there are subpopulations of patients with subclinical hypothyroidism who would derive the most benefit from treatment with levothyroxine therapy.

14.3.1　Subclinical Hypothyroidism and Lipids

14.3.1.1　Observed Associations Between Subclinical Hypothyroidism and Lipid Parameters

A dose–response pattern is apparent in studies that have examined lipid profiles across the spectrum of thyroid function, with the highest levels in overt hypothyroidism and the lowest in overt hyperthyroidism [4, 6, 17]. When the category of subclinical hypothyroidism is examined separately, several observational studies have found an association between subclinical hypothyroidism and alterations in lipid profiles [17–19]. It is widely accepted that an elevated LDL cholesterol level is associated with increased cardiovascular events and cardiovascular mortality [20]; therefore, it is reasonable to presume that the elevations of LDL cholesterol found in subclinical hypothyroidism would confer a similar degree of risk. In addition, two other lipid measures that may be adversely altered in subclinical hypothyroidism, high-density lipoprotein (HDL) cholesterol and lipoprotein (a) [Lp(a)], have been associated with poor cardiovascular outcomes [20, 21].

Total and LDL cholesterol have been observed in several studies to be elevated in people with subclinical hypothyroidism versus their euthyroid counterparts. In the Colorado Thyroid Disease Prevalence Study, participants with subclinical hypothyroidism had significantly higher total cholesterol and LDL levels than did those with normal TSH, and use of lipid-lowering medications did not differ between the two groups [6]. Kanaya et al. also noted an association between subclinical hypothyroidism and elevated total cholesterol levels, but this association was only statistically significant among African-American women [17]. In a cohort of 85-year-olds, rising TSH was associated with a statistically significant trend toward higher total cholesterol and triglyceride levels [22].

Caron et al. noted lower HDL levels in 29 premenopausal women with subclinical hypothyroidism versus matched controls, with no difference in total cholesterol or triglyceride levels [23]. In a small study of younger participants with a mean age of 41 years, elevated Lp(a) levels were observed in patients with subclinical hypothyroidism compared with matched controls [19].

These associations, however, have not been consistently seen. Several large, population-based studies found no significant association between subclinical hypothyroidism and unfavorable lipid profiles. In the Whickham Survey, a cross-sectional analysis revealed no relationship between elevated TSH and total cholesterol or triglyceride levels [24]. Several recent large cohort studies also supported the lack of association between subclinical hypothyroidism and elevated LDL, total cholesterol, or triglycerides, or low HDL [4, 7, 25].

One reason for the variability among studies may be related to the age of the participants. For example, studies including older participants, such as the Rotterdam Study and the Cardiovascular Health Study, in which the mean age, was 69 and 73 years, respectively, found no association between subclinical hypothyroidism and elevated serum lipids [4, 7]. This stands in contrast with studies with a younger mean age of participants that showed a positive association between subclinical hypothyroidism and elevated total cholesterol, LDL,

or Lp(a), or low HDL [6, 19, 23]. Another confounder that may be contributing to such conflicting results is the variability between studies regarding the use of lipid-lowering medications. In the 2006 study by Cappola et al., analysis after exclusion of patients taking lipid-lowering medications showed no significant difference between groups [4]. In a similar elderly cohort, Gussekloo et al. did find a positive trend toward elevated total cholesterol and triglycerides; however, use of these medications was not described in the analysis [22]. Furthermore, the association between elevated total cholesterol and subclinical hypothyroidism seen by Kanaya et al. was significant only among African-American women, after excluding participants on lipid-lowering medications [17]. Differences in mean TSH between studies may also contribute to the variable association between subclinical hypothyroidism and lipid abnormalities. For example, in several studies reporting a mean TSH of less than 10 mU/l, no association was seen [4, 24–26]. Many of the studies reporting elevated total or LDL cholesterol, low HDL, or elevated Lp(a) associated with subclinical hypothyroidism studied subjects whose mean TSH level was greater than 10 mU/l [19, 23, 27].

14.3.1.2 Effect of Levothyroxine Replacement on Lipid Profiles in Subclinical Hypothyroidism

Interventional trials aimed at treating subclinical hypothyroidism have shown mixed benefit on serum lipids and lipoproteins. Few were randomized controlled trials, and even among the well-designed trials, results varied. A randomized, double-blind placebo-controlled trial by Cooper et al. showed no significant difference in total cholesterol or triglycerides after 1 year of levothyroxine (L-T4) or placebo, even in patients with baseline total cholesterol of greater than 200 mg/dl [28]. Interestingly, all but one of the 33 patients enrolled had subclinical hypothyroidism as a result of treatment for Graves' disease, and none were undertreated for overt hypothyroidism. Kong et al. randomized 40 women with subclinical hypothyroidism but no prior history of thyroid disease to receive L-T4 or placebo for 6 months, also with no significant change in total cholesterol, LDL, HDL, or Lp(a) [26].

In the Basel Thyroid Study, 66 women with a mean age of 57 years were randomized to receive either placebo or L-T$_4$ [27]. Treatment for 48 weeks was associated with a significant although modest decrease in total (−3.8%) and LDL (−8.2%) cholesterol that was more remarkable in patients with a baseline TSH greater than 12 mU/l. Treatment was not associated with changes in HDL, triglycerides, or Lp(a). Another trial randomized 49 young patients with subclinical hypothyroidism (mean age 35 years) to L-T$_4$ or placebo until 6 months of euthyroidism was established [12]. A significant decrease in total cholesterol and LDL of close to 10% was noted in the treatment group. Lp(a) levels did not change. Finally, Monzani et al. randomized 45 young Italian patients (mean age 35 years) with subclinical hypothyroidism to receive placebo or L-T$_4$ for 6 months [10]. At baseline, the subclinical hypothyroidism group had higher LDL and total cholesterol than matched controls, and after 6 months the treatment group had a statistically significant mean decrease in total cholesterol of 10%, or 22.6 mg/dl, and in LDL of 13%, or 19.7 mg/dl. Given the evidence that a 20% reduction in total cholesterol with statin use can reduce the risk of coronary events by 30%, a reduction of 10% as seen in two of the above-mentioned trials is relatively small but could represent a meaningful reduction in adverse cardiovascular outcomes [29].

Meta-analyses and systematic reviews have attempted to synthesize the conflicting data from interventional trials. In a meta-analysis by Danese et al. [30], 13 trials were reviewed; overall, there was a modest but significant decrease in total and LDL cholesterol, with mean decreases of 7.9 and 10 mg/dl, respectively. However, there was significant heterogeneity among the studies examined. Furthermore, only three of the trials reviewed were randomized controlled trials, and when subgroup analysis was done of studies meeting at least four of the eight internal validity criteria, there was no significant difference in the change in lipid profiles between treatment and placebo groups. Interestingly, patients with undertreated overt hypothyroidism and a baseline total cholesterol > 240 mg/dL had the greatest decrease in total cholesterol and LDL with L-T$_4$ treatment. In contrast, in patients with mild (subclinical) hypothyroidism or a baseline total cholesterol level of less than 240 mg/dl, treatment with L-T$_4$ did not provide significant benefit.

A Cochrane review similarly found a trend toward decreased total cholesterol with L-T$_4$ treatment, but no statistically significant change in total cholesterol, LDL, HDL, triglycerides, or Lp(a) [31]. A subgroup analysis of patients with baseline LDL above 155 mg/dl showed a significant decrease with treatment, further supporting the theory that patients with subclinical hypothyroidism and higher baseline total cholesterol or LDL are more likely to benefit from L-T$_4$. This review only included randomized trials, most of which were double-blinded and therefore of higher quality than the studies included in the meta-analysis by Danese et al.

In summary, there appears to be a trend toward increasing total cholesterol and LDL with rising TSH, and a dose–response effect between the degree of hypothyroidism and the magnitude of cholesterol elevation. The effects of L-T$_4$ therapy on lipids vary widely across studies, all of which have been of relatively small sample size and many of which were not placebo-controlled. However, careful examination of these trials suggests that treatment with L-T$_4$ with normalization of TSH causes significant, albeit modest, decreases in total cholesterol and LDL, particularly in patients with higher baseline total cholesterol and LDL, higher baseline TSH values, or subclinical hypothyroidism as a result of undertreated overt hypothyroidism (Table 14.1). Similar effects are not consistently seen with respect to HDL, triglycerides, or Lp(a).

14.3.2 Nontraditional Biomarkers of Cardiovascular Risk in Subclinical Hypothyroidism

14.3.2.1 C-reactive Protein

Several serum biomarkers have been associated with cardiovascular risk in the general population. Of these, CRP is one of the most validated. Observational data from the National Health and Nutrition Examination Survey (NHANES), the Framingham Heart Study, the Cardiovascular Health Study, and the Physician's Health Study showed a positive association between serum CRP and cardiovascular events and stroke, although the addition of this biomarker to traditional risk factors results in a relatively small improvement in prediction models [32–34]. CRP has also been associated with increased cardiovascular events in women [35]. Whether or not CRP levels are higher at baseline in patients with subclinical hypothyroidism versus their euthyroid counterparts is not clear. Several large, population-based cohorts showed no association between subclinical hypothyroidism and elevated levels of CRP, including data from NHANES and the Cardiovascular Health Study [4, 22, 36]. In two relatively small, nonrandomized interventional trials, subclinical hypothyroidism was associated with elevated serum levels of CRP [14, 37]. However, only in the trial by Ozcan et al. [37] did treatment with L-T$_4$ result in normalization of CRP levels, and neither of these studies were adequately powered to examine cardiovascular events (Table 14.1).

14.3.2.2 Homocysteine

Homocysteine has also been associated in several epidemiological studies with atherosclerosis, CHD, peripheral vascular disease, and stroke [38, 39]. While prospective trials aimed at lowering serum homocysteine levels with folic acid, vitamin B$_6$, and vitamin B$_{12}$ have shown no significant reduction in cardiovascular events, the epidemiological association remains [39]. Therefore, hyperhomocysteinemia has also been invoked as a possible cardiovascular risk marker in the subclinical hypothyroidism population. While an inverse relationship between free T$_4$ levels and homocysteine has been observed in overt hypothyroidism, to date a significant association between homocysteine and subclinical hypothyroidism has not been established [5, 14, 36, 37]. Likewise, in a small prospective trial, L-T$_4$ replacement normalized baseline elevated homocysteine levels in overtly hypothyroid patients [40], whereas in two interventional trials conducted in subclinical

hypothyroid patients L-T$_4$ had no effect on serum homocysteine levels [14, 37]. Thus, in contrast to overt hypothyroidism, homocysteine levels are not elevated in subclinical hypothyroidism compared with the euthyroid population and are not improved with normalization of TSH (Table 14.1).

14.3.2.3 Hemostatic Factors

Hemostatic factors, such as von Willebrand factor, factor VII, and fibrinogen, may contribute to the atherogenesis and thrombogenesis involved in acute coronary syndromes [41]. Fibrinogen increases platelet aggregation, fibrin formation, and plasma viscosity and is thought to be the most important hemostatic risk factor for cardiovascular disease [42]. In the Framingham Heart Study, fibrinogen levels were significantly higher in people with prevalent cardiovascular disease, even after adjustment for traditional risk factors [43]. Alterations in these hemostatic factors have been examined in the subclinical hypothyroidism population as potential causes of increased thromboembolic disease and increased cardiovascular risk. In a study by Chadarevian et al. [44], low fibrinogen levels (consistent with increased fibrinolysis) were observed in severely hypothyroid patients. Interestingly, as the TSH normalized with L-T$_4$ therapy, patients with moderate hypothyroidism had elevated fibrinogen levels (consistent with decreased fibrinolytic activity), which ultimately normalized when euthyroidism was achieved, suggesting that milder elevations in TSH, as seen in subclinical hypothyroidism, are associated with an increase in thrombogenesis

Table 14.1 Association of serum biomarkers with subclinical hypothyroidism

Cardiovascular risk factor	Association with subclinical hypothyroidism	References
Total cholesterol	+	[6, 10, 12, 17, 22]
LDL	+	[6, 10, 12]
HDL	−	[4, 10, 26]
Triglycerides	−	[10, 24, 26, 57]
Lipoprotein (a)	−	[4, 19, 26]
C-reactive protein	±	[14, 37]
Homocysteine	−	[10, 36]

+ Several studies showed a positive association
± A few small studies showed positive association, larger studies did not
− Several studies showed no association

[44]. This study, however, did not define "moderate hypothyroidism" with reference to TSH and free T$_4$ levels; therefore, it is not clear how to interpret these findings using current definitions of subclinical hypothyroidism. In one small, nonrandomized trial evaluating hemostatic factors in subclinical hypothyroidism patients before and after L-T$_4$ treatment, fibrinogen levels were found to be elevated at baseline versus healthy controls, but did not normalize after euthyroidism was achieved [45]. In contrast, an observational study of a small Turkish cohort found no difference in levels of fibrinogen, von Willebrand factor, or factor VIII between subclinical hypothyroidism patients and euthyroid controls [46]. In general, there are limited data regarding the association between fibrinolytic activity and cardiovascular risk in subclinical hypothyroidism, although this is also true of the general population. More investigation needs to be done before these hemostatic factors become validated screening tools for cardiovascular risk assessment.

14.3.3 Vascular Risk Factors and Subclinical Hypothyroidism

14.3.3.1 Arterial Stiffness

Arterial stiffness, as measured by central (or aortic) pulse wave velocity and aortic augmentation index, is increasingly recognized as an important contributor to cardiovascular risk. Central pulse wave velocity is essentially a measure of how quickly an aortic pulse wave travels a specified distance in the vascular bed. This velocity is in part affected by the elasticity of the vessel and the degree of vascular calcification. Central pulse wave velocity can be measured by a variety of different methods, mainly distinguished by the device used and the vessels evaluated. Distance is measured by recording the pulse wave at two different sites (typically the carotid and femoral arteries), while time is measured using an event, such as the QRS complex on an electrocardiogram. Pulse wave velocity can also be measured in the brachial arteries and ankles (the brachial–ankle pulse wave velocity). However, in this case, peripheral muscular arteries are examined, and therefore central pulse wave velocity is inferred. The aortic augmentation index (AIx), another measure of arterial stiffness, is calculated from a measured pulse waveform at the radial artery

[47]. Increased central pulse wave velocity and AIx have been associated with cardiovascular and all-cause mortality in the end-stage renal disease population, and in healthy adults increased central pulse wave velocity is an independent predictor of CHD and stroke [47, 48].

Several small studies have evaluated pulse wave velocity and AIx in subclinical hypothyroidism, in an effort to further clarify cardiovascular risk in these patients. Nagasaki et al. noted increased brachial–ankle pulse wave velocity (baPWV) in subclinically hypothyroid patients versus controls [49]. This finding was independent of the degree of TSH elevation. The same investigators also examined the effect of L-T$_4$ treatment on brachial–ankle pulse wave velocity in individuals with subclinical hypothyroidism [50]. They found a significant decrease in pulse wave velocity with normalization of TSH only in patients with baseline elevated baPWV. In another observational study of 19 female subclinical hypothyroidism patients, AIx and central pulse wave velocity were higher in subclinically hypothyroid patients than in matched controls. Both parameters significantly decreased to control levels after 6 months of L-T$_4$ treatment and normalization of TSH [51].

14.3.3.2 Brachial Artery Flow-Mediated Dilation

Brachial artery flow-mediated dilation (FMD) is measured by transiently occluding the brachial artery with a blood pressure cuff, then comparing the maximum diameter after deflation of the cuff with the baseline diameter of the vessel. Impaired brachial artery FMD is thought to be a marker of endothelial dysfunction. In the Cardiovascular Health Study, impaired brachial FMD was found to be an independent predictor of cardiovascular events after adjustment for traditional cardiovascular risk factors [52]. A recent randomized, double-blind, cross-over study in 100 patients with subclinical hypothyroidism demonstrated an increase in FMD with L-T$_4$ therapy [13].

14.3.3.3 Other Measures of Endothelial Dysfunction

The vasodilatory response of the brachial artery to acetylcholine (Ach) infusion is another indicator of endothelial function. A prospective study has shown that impaired response to Ach infusion, indicative of endothelial dysfunction, predicted cardiovascular events in a cohort of patients with documented coronary artery disease [53]. In a nonrandomized trial, Taddei et al. evaluated endothelium-dependent vasodilation as response to Ach infusion in 14 patients with subclinical hypothyroidism and then re-evaluated these patients after treatment with L-T_4. After 6 months of euthyroidism, the patients showed a statistically significant increase in vasodilation in response to Ach infusion, suggesting improved endothelial function [54].

In summary, newer surrogate markers for cardiovascular risk, such as the aortic augmentation index, central pulse wave velocity, brachial artery FMD, and endothelium-dependent vasodilation, may be altered in patients with subclinical hypothyroidism. In a small number of trials (only one of which was randomized and placebo-controlled), treatment with L-T_4 appeared to be beneficial. However, these methods of predicting cardiovascular risk are not yet standard risk assessment tools, and their utility remains to be seen in the general and in the subclinically hypothyroid populations.

14.3.4 Surrogate Markers of Cardiovascular Disease in Subclinical Hypothyroidism

14.3.4.1 Carotid Intima–Media Thickness

Accelerated atherosclerosis is thought to be one of the means by which thyroid dysfunction increases cardiovascular risk. A reliable and noninvasive measure of atherosclerosis is the carotid intima-media thickness (IMT). Several observational studies have shown an association between carotid IMT and risk of CHD and all-cause mortality independent of traditional risk factors [33, 55]. A case–control study of 35 patients with overt hypothyroidism documented increased carotid IMT and higher cholesterol levels at baseline compared to age- and sex-matched controls [56]. Treatment with L-T_4 for 1 year with normalization of TSH resulted in a significant decrease in carotid IMT. This decrease showed a trend toward a positive association with total cholesterol levels, suggesting that the primary mediator of increased atherosclerosis in patients with thyroid dysfunction is the lipid abnormalities. A double-

blind, placebo-controlled trial by Monzani et al. showed significantly increased carotid IMT in patients with subclinical hypothyroidism at baseline versus controls [10]. This association was similar in patients with mild (TSH < 10 mg/dl) and moderate (TSH > 10 mg/dl) subclinical hypothyroidism. Treatment with L-T_4 resulted in a significant mean decrease in IMT of 10%, again independent of the degree of TSH elevation. Reduction in mean IMT was directly related to the absolute reduction in total cholesterol, providing additional support for a strong link between atherosclerosis and serum lipid abnormalities in subclinical hypothyroidism.

14.3.5 Prevalence and Incidence of CHD in Subclinical Hypothyroidism

While studies looking specifically at the prevalence of risk factors in subclinical hypothyroidism provide insight into possible mechanisms of cardiovascular disease in this patient population, they do not ultimately clarify whether or not this translates into increased incidence of cardiovascular events. Several large, population-based cohort studies have examined the prevalence and incidence of cardiovascular disease, specifically coronary heart disease (CHD) and related mortality, in an effort to determine whether or not individuals with untreated endogenous subclinical hypothyroidism are at increased cardiovascular risk.

14.3.5.1 Prevalence of CHD in Subclinical Hypothyroidism

The prevalence of CHD in patients with subclinical hypothyroidism compared with euthyroid individuals varies among cross-sectional studies. In the original Whickham cohort, Tunbridge et al. found no association between prevalent CHD and subclinical hypothyroidism [24]. Subsequent cross-sectional analyses in cohorts whose average age was in the 50s have not reliably reproduced this finding. A Japanese study of atomic bomb survivors and the Busselton Health Study both reported a positive association between prevalent CHD and subclinical hypothyroidism [25, 57]. In contrast, two studies in elderly cohorts did not show this association [4, 11].

A recent meta-analysis of 12 studies found a higher prevalence of CHD in people with subclinical hypothyroidism than in euthyroid controls [odds ratio (OR) 1.23; 95% confidence interval (95% CI) 1.02–1.48], but with significant statistical heterogeneity among these studies [15]. When age-stratified analyses were performed (age greater than or less than 65 years), the statistical heterogeneity resolved, and CHD was only more prevalent in studies whose mean subject age was less than 65 years (OR 1.57; 95% CI 1.19–2.06) [15]. Thus, the relationship between prevalent CHD and subclinical hypothyroidism may depend upon the age of the patient in question.

14.3.5.2 Incidence of Cardiovascular Disease and Cardiovascular Mortality in Subclinical Hypothyroidism

Longitudinal studies assessing the incidence of cardiovascular disease and mortality have also produced mixed results (Table 14.2). Vanderpump et al. found no increased incidence of CHD or mortality among patients with subclinical hypothyroidism in 20 years of follow-up [58]. Similarly, longitudinal

studies by Cappola et al., Rodondi et al., and Parle et al. found no increase in the development of CHD, or cardiovascular or total mortality [4, 11, 60]. One study of 85-year-old men and women found decreased mortality from cardiovascular and non-cardiovascular causes in the subclinical hypothyroidism group [22]. Conversely, in a 10-year follow-up study by Imaizumi et al., subclinical hypothyroidism was associated with increased total mortality in men, and there was a suggestive, but not statistically significant, increase in the incidence of CHD in male subjects [25]. In the Rotterdam Study, Hak et al. found a higher incidence of myocardial infarction in elderly women with subclinical hypothyroidism, but this increase was not statistically significant and was based on only 16 events (OR 2.5; 95% CI 0.7–9.1) [7].

There are several possible explanations for the conflicting results obtained from these longitudinal studies. In an analogous situation to prevalent disease, the age of the cohort may play a role in the association between subclinical hypothyroidism and incident disease. In the meta-analysis by Razvi et al., the incidence of CHD increased significantly in

Table 14.2 Observational studies of the incidence of cardiovascular disease or mortality in subclinical hypothyroidism

Study	No. of patients, sex	Mean patient age (years)	Mean duration of follow-up (years)	Findings compared to euthyroid control
Rotterdam Study [7]	957 F	69	4.6	↑ MI HR 2.5 (95% CI 0.7–9.1)
Nagasaki [25]	2,443 F+M	59	10	↑ Total death HR 1.2 (95% CI 0.8–1.6)
Busselton Health Study [57]	1,926 F+M	50	20	↑ CHD events HR 1.8 (95% CI 1.2–2.7)
Whickham Survey [58]	2,122 F+M	44	20	No difference CHD
Birmingham [60]	1,191 F+M	70	10	No difference CV death
Health ABC Study [11]	2,730 F+M	75	4	No difference CV disease
Cardiovascular Health Study [4]	3,135 F+M	73	13	No difference CHD, CV death
Leiden 85+ Study [22]	558 F+M	85	3.7	CV death with increasing TSH

MI myocardial infarction, *HR* hazard ratio, *CI* confidence interval, *CHD* coronary heart disease, *CV* cardiovascular the group whose mean age was less than 65 years (OR 1.68; 95% CI 1.27–2.23), but not in the group whose study subjects were all 65 years or older (OR 1.02; 95% CI 0.85–1.22) [15]. Similarly, in the meta-analyses conducted by Ochs et al., a significantly increased risk of CHD was found when patients less than 65 years of age were analyzed [relative risk (RR) 1.51; 95% CI 1.09–2.09], which was not reproduced in the 65 and over group (RR 1.05; 95% CI 0.90–1.31) [16] (Table 14.3). The association between subclinical hypothyroidism and incident CHD may also be determined by the degree of TSH elevation. Those studies that reported CHD risk separately by severity of subclinical hypothyroidism demonstrated an increased, albeit nonstatistically significant, risk in partecipants with TSH levels of 10 mU/l or higher (RR 1.69; 95% CI 0.64–4.45), whereas study that only reported the standard definition of subclinical hypothyroidism of TSH ≥ 4.5 mU/L did not (RR 1.06; 95% CI 0.91–1.25) (Table 14.3).

Differences across studies in the quality of study design provide another possible explanation for inconsistent results. Cardiovascular events in some studies were adjudicated and in others were not, exclusion of study participants on medications affecting thyroid hormone was not consistent, and adjustment for confounders varied significantly between studies. For example, the Busselton Health Study, Whickham Survey, Health ABC Study, and Leiden 85+ study did not exclude patients who were taking thyroid hormone prepa-

rations. While several other studies did exclude patients on thyroxine replacement at baseline, only two accounted for L-T$_4$ use at follow-up [4, 25]. If L-T$_4$ replacement attenuates cardiovascular risk, then failure to account for its initiation could have resulted in an underestimate of the impact of untreated, endogenous subclinical hypothyroidism. In addition, methods used to define outcomes differed significantly between studies. In the Whickham Survey, Vanderpump et al. used multiple criteria to confirm incident cases of CHD, including physician records, patient reports, and major and minor electrocardiographic criteria [58]. More recent studies similarly used multiple criteria to ascertain cardiovascular events, including patient report, hospital discharge records, electrocardiograms, and review of cases by a committee [4, 11, 25]. This contrasts with studies in which events were determined by record linkage or ICD-9 codes without confirmation by another method [57, 60]. In two recent meta-analyses, subgroup analyses were done for study quality. Ochs et al. found that when data were pooled from higher-quality studies (based on blinded adjudication of outcomes and degree of loss to follow-up), a lower risk of incident disease and cardiovascular and total mortality was seen [16] (Table 14.3). Razvi et al. similarly stratified studies based on quality criteria, and an increased incidence of ischemic heart disease events was still seen among studies with subjects less than 65 years old; however, cardiovascular mortality became nonsignificant [15].

Table 14.3 Stratified meta-analysis of the association of subclinical hypothyroidism with the risk of coronary heart disease or cardiovascular mortality. (Adapted from [16])

Characteristic	Coronary heart disease Summary RR (95% CI)	Studies, n	CV mortality Summary RR (95% CI)	Studies, n
Stratified by mean age				
< 65 years	1.51 (1.09–2.09)	4	1.50 (0.97–2.30)	3
≥ 65 years	1.05 (0.90–1.22)	6	1.12 (0.91–1.37)	5
Definition of subclinical hypothyroidism				
TSH ≥ 4.5 mU/l	1.06 (0.91–1.25)	7	1.13 (0.92–1.39)	6
TSH ≥ 10.0 mU/l	1.69 (0.64–4.45)	2	2.26 (0.54–9.45)	1
Study quality				
Formal adjudication	1.02 (0.86–1.22)	5	1.09 (0.88–1.35)	4
Adjudication without knowledge of thyroid status	1.08 (0.90–1.31)	8	1.13 (0.92–1.39)	6

CV cardiovascular, *RR* relative risk

Other limitations of many of these longitudinal studies include the relatively short duration of follow-up, and, for all of these studies, use of only a single set of thyroid function tests to define subclinical hypothyroidism. TSH elevations can be transient, as was seen in the Leiden 85-Plus study, where almost half the participants with subclinical hypothyroidism at baseline were euthyroid when the TSH level was repeated 3 years later [22]. If many of the patients designated at baseline as subclinically hypothyroid ultimately reverted to euthyroidism during the course of follow-up, this could bias studies towards the null and decrease the incidence of subclinical-hypothyroidism-related cardiovascular disease.

Similar issues arise when examining cardiovascular mortality outcomes, with the suggestion of an increased cardiovascular mortality when all studies are included [hazard ratio (HR) 1.19; 95% CI 0.81–1.76), but larger risk estimates in those with partecipants age younger than 65 or with TSH levels of 10 mU/l or higher [16] (Table 14.3). In distinction to the studies that focused on populations without pre-existing cardiovascular disease, Iervasi et al. conducted a study in cardiac patients. They found greater cardiovascular mortality in patients with subclinical hypothyroidism than in euthyroid patients (HR 2.40; 95% CI 1.36–4.21) [61]. Furthermore, the risk appeared to be highest in patients with ischemic heart disease (HR 3.1; 95% CI 1.6–5.9), suggesting that the consequences of untreated subclinical hypothyroidism may be more severe in those with pre-existing cardiovascular disease.

Overall, a trend toward increased prevalence and incidence of cardiovascular disease and cardiovascular mortality is seen in a subgroup of younger patients with subclinical hypothyroidism, particularly in those less than 65 years old. In elderly cohorts, this association is found inconsistently and is particularly absent in higher-quality studies with more rigorous inclusion/exclusion criteria and ascertainment of outcomes. The discrepancy between results in younger versus older populations could be secondary to the high prevalence of conventional cardiovascular risk factors in older populations, minimizing the impact of any single risk factor. It is also possible that the traditional cardiovascular risk factors identified in middle-aged populations are less relevant in those who have survived to old age. For example, in older adults, serum lipids are only weakly associated with risk of developing cardiovascular disease [62]. Therefore, if cardiovascular risk in subclinical hypothyroidism is mediated by elevated serum lipids (particularly LDL and total cholesterol), subclinical hypothyroidism may be a less important contributor to the development of cardiovascular disease in older populations.

Importantly, there are no prospective, randomized controlled trials of treatment of subclinical hypothyroidism with a primary endpoint of cardiovascular events and mortality, rather than a surrogate outcome such as carotid IMT or arterial stiffness. Although the observational data suggest appropriate target groups for therapy, based on age and degree of TSH elevation, the degree to which the cardiovascular risk is reversible in these subpopulations is unknown. Accordingly, data from an appropriately powered, randomized, controlled trial looking at clinically meaningful cardiovascular outcomes are needed to inform practicing clinicians about the need for treatment of subclinical hypothyroidism.

14.4 Overt Hyperthyroidism and Cardiovascular Disease

Untreated overt hyperthyroidism induces significant cardiac effects, including tachycardia, exercise intolerance, dyspnea on exertion, widened pulse pressure, and atrial fibrillation [63]. Recent data suggested that these are common effects, although they are not reversed in all overtly hyperthyroid subjects after therapy to normalize thyroid function tests, but instead depend on the underlying health status of the study subject [64]. As with overt hypothyroidism, immediate treatment is indicated once overt hyperthyroidism is detected. However, the field continues to require guidance in defining the management of subclinical hyperthyroidism.

14.5 Subclinical Hyperthyroidism

Subclinical hyperthyroidism, defined by a low TSH with a normal free thyroxine level, affects anywhere from 1 to 6% of the US population [1, 4, 6, 59, 65], although the prevalence is as high as 11% in areas of iodine insufficiency [66].

The clinical cardiovascular effects of subclinical hyperthyroidism appear to parallel those of overt hyperthyroidism, but are of decreased frequency and severity. The most clinically significant cardiovascular risk from subclinical hyperthyroidism is atrial fibrillation, which has been demonstrated in several studies, as outlined below. In addition, several studies have examined CHD and cardiovascular mortality in individuals with subclinical hyperthyroidism.

14.5.1 Subclinical Hyperthyroidism and Atrial Fibrillation

In 1994, Sawin et al., using data from the Framingham Heart Study, reported an increased risk of atrial fibrillation in subjects with subclinical hyperthyroidism compared to the euthyroid state [67]. They found that individuals with TSH values of 0.1 mU/l or less who were not receiving thyroid hormone therapy had an adjusted relative risk of 3.8 (95% CI 1.7–8.3) for developing atrial fibrillation and those with TSH values between 0.1 and 0.4 mU/l had an adjusted relative risk of 1.6 (95% CI 1.0–2.5). The lack of a statistically significant difference in the 0.1–0.4 mU/l group led to lingering questions about the risks of endogenous mild subclinical hyperthyroidism, which is more commonly found than a TSH level below 0.1 mU/l. Furthermore, individuals with elevated thyroxine levels, indicating overt hyperthyroidism, were included in the category of TSH values of 0.1 mU/l or less, which could have led to an overestimate of the effect of subclinical hyperthyroidism. An analysis by Cappola et al. of data from the Cardiovascular Health Study, in which subjects with elevated free thyroxine levels were excluded, also showed an increased risk of atrial fibrillation in those with subclinical hyperthyroidism (HR 1.98; 95% CI 1.29–3.03) [4]. Furthermore, the adjusted hazard ratio was 1.85 (95% CI 1.1–3.0) in the subgroup of those with a TSH of 0.1–0.44 mU/l, showing a statistically significant increase in risk in this subgroup. The analyses of the seven individuals with subclinical hyperthyroidism and a TSH of less than 0.1 mU/l were not published with these data due to the small number of subjects, but they are displayed in Fig. 14.1, in order to demonstrate the dose-response relationship between the degree of subclinical hyperthyroidism and the risk of atrial fibrillation.

Both of these studies were conducted in individuals age 65 and over. Their findings are supported in younger populations by an increased prevalence of atrial fibrillation in a cross-sectional study of people age 45 and older who were referred to a single institution for thyroid function testing [68]. Another cross-sectional study in people 65 and older confirmed a higher prevalence of atrial fibrillation in those with subclinical hyperthyroidism [59]. Interestingly, in an analysis limit-

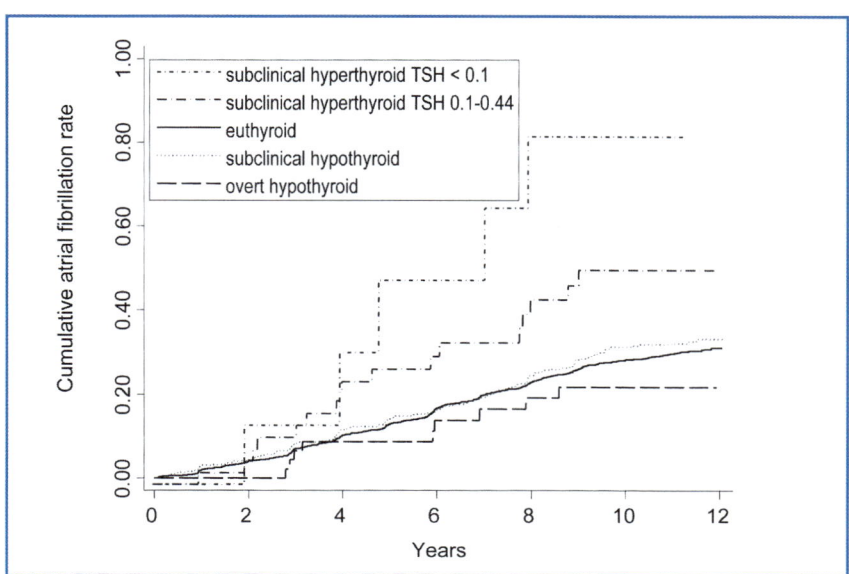

Fig. 14.1 Incidence of atrial fibrillation by thyroid group in the Cardiovascular Health Study. (Adapted with permission from [4]. Copyright© (2006) American Medical Association. All rights reserved)

ed to subjects with TSH levels in the euthyroid range, increasing free T$_4$ level was also independently associated with atrial fibrillation, supporting a dose-dependent effect of free thyroxine on the promotion of atrial fibrillation, even the presence of TSH levels that are considered to be normal.

14.5.2 Subclinical Hyperthyroidism and CHD and Cardiovascular Mortality

Two studies have examined the risk of CHD [4, 57] and five have studied cardiovascular mortality in individuals with subclinical hyperthyroidism [4, 22, 57, 60, 69]. In the Cardiovascular Health Study, there was no relationship between subclinical hyperthyroidism and incident CHD, compared to euthyroid individuals (HR 1.04; 95% CI 0.64–1.69) [4]. Likewise, in the Busselton Health Study, there was no statistically significant increase in CHD (HR 1.30; 95% CI 0.60–3.30), although with only five cardiovascular events in the subclinical hyperthyroid group, these data should be interpreted with caution.

Two studies [22, 60] reported a slight risk of increased cardiovascular mortality in the subclinically hyperthyroid state, whereas three did not [4, 57, 69]. None of these studies found statistically significant results, consistent with the small sample sizes of individuals with subclinical hyperthyroidism and the resultant low power of the study. In the meta-analysis by Ochs et al., the overall hazard ratio of cardiovascular mortality was 1.19, which was not statistically significant (95% CI 0.81–1.76). Several of these studies were also plagued by the same design issues as the observational studies of subclinical hypothyroidism, including a lack of adjudicated outcomes, inclusion of study participants who were taking thyroid hormone, and, in all of these studies, measurement of thyroid function tests at a single baseline timepoint.

Cardiovascular mortality was greater in patients with subclinical hyperthyroidism than in euthyroid patients in the study conducted in cardiac patients by Iervasi et al., with a hazard ratio of 2.32 (95% CI 1.11–4.85) [61]. Furthermore, the risk appeared to be exclusively limited to those with ischemic heart disease (HR 3.5; 95% CI 1.2–7.9), suggesting that the consequences of untreated subclinical hyperthyroidism are more severe in patients with pre-existing cardiac conditions.

There are no prospective, randomized controlled trials of treatment of subclinical hyperthyroidism with a primary endpoint of cardiovascular events and mortality. Although the observational data strongly support the treatment of subclinical hyperthyroidism to prevent atrial fibrillation, particularly in those age 65 years and older, the degree to which the cardiovascular risk is reversible is unknown. In the absence of data from an appropriately powered, randomized, controlled trial to examine the impact of therapy on the incidence of atrial fibrillation, treatment of subclinical hyperthyroidism should be considered, particularly in patients 65 years and older and those with pre-existing ischemic heart disease.

Key Points

- Small case–control studies and autopsy data have suggested an association between overt hypothyroidism and atherosclerotic cardiovascular disease.

- Overt hypothyroidism should always be treated as soon as it is detected. The major clinical controversy is the cardiovascular risk from subclinical hypothyroidism.

- Some observational studies and small randomized clinical trials have suggested that subclinical hypothyroidism causes reversible alterations in traditional cardiovascular risk factors and surrogate markers of cardiovascular disease.

(Cont. →)

(*cont.*)

- Data about the cardiovascular risk of subclinical hypothyroidism are inconsistent, though meta-analyses suggest increased cardiovascular risk in those age less than 65 years or with a TSH concentration of 10 mU/l or higher.

- Both overt and subclinical hyperthyroidism are risk factors for atrial fibrillation.

- Large, randomized clinical trials are needed to identify the target populations of individuals with subclinical thyroid dysfunction whose cardiovascular risk would improve with treatment.

References

1. Hollowell JG, Staehling NW, Flanders WD et al (2002) Serum TSH, T(4), and thyroid antibodies in the United States population (1988 to 1994): National Health and Nutrition Examination Survey (NHANES III). J Clin Endocrinol Metab 87:489–499

2. Cappola AR, Ladenson PW (2003) Hypothyroidism and atherosclerosis. J Clin Endocrinol Metab 88:2438–2444

3. Mariotti S, Cambuli VM (2007) Cardiovascular risk in elderly hypothyroid patients. Thyroid 17:1067–1073

4. Cappola AR, Fried LP, Arnold AM et al (2006) Thyroid status, cardiovascular risk, and mortality in older adults. JAMA 295:1033–1041

5. Lindeman RD, Romero LJ, Schade DS et al (2003) Impact of subclinical hypothyroidism on serum total homocysteine concentrations, the prevalence of coronary heart disease (CHD), and CHD risk factors in the New Mexico Elder Health Survey. Thyroid 13:595–600

6. Canaris GJ, Manowitz NR, Mayor G, Ridgway EC (2000) The Colorado thyroid disease prevalence study. Arch Intern Med 160:526–534

7. Hak AE, Pols HA, Visser TJ et al (2000) Subclinical hypothyroidism is an independent risk factor for atherosclerosis and myocardial infarction in elderly women: the Rotterdam Study. Ann Intern Med 132:270–278

8. Surks MI, Hollowell JG (2007) Age-specific distribution of serum thyrotropin and antithyroid antibodies in the US population: implications for the prevalence of subclinical hypothyroidism. J Clin Endocrinol Metab 92:4575–4582

9. Sawin CT, Chopra D, Azizi F et al (1979) The aging thyroid. Increased prevalence of elevated serum thyrotropin levels in the elderly. JAMA 242:247–250

10. Monzani F, Caraccio N, Kozakowa M et al (2004) Effect of levothyroxine replacement on lipid profile and intima-media thickness in subclinical hypothyroidism: a double-blind, placebo- controlled study. J Clin Endocrinol Metab 89:2099–2106

11. Rodondi N, Newman AB, Vittinghoff E et al (2005) Subclinical hypothyroidism and the risk of heart failure, other cardiovascular events, and death. Arch Intern Med 165:2460–2466

12. Caraccio N, Ferrannini E, Monzani F (2002) Lipoprotein profile in subclinical hypothyroidism: response to levothyroxine replacement, a randomized placebo-controlled study. J Clin Endocrinol Metab 87:1533–1538

13. Razvi S, Ingoe L, Keeka G et al (2007) The beneficial effect of L-thyroxine on cardiovascular risk factors, endothelial function, and quality of life in subclinical hypothyroidism: randomized, crossover trial. J Clin Endocrinol Metab 92:1715–1723

14. Christ-Crain M, Meier C, Guglielmetti M et al (2003) Elevated C-reactive protein and homocysteine values: cardiovascular risk factors in hypothyroidism? A cross-sectional and a double-blind, placebo-controlled trial. Atherosclerosis 166:379–386

15. Razvi S, Shakoor A, Vanderpump M et al (2008) The influence of age on the relationship between subclinical hypothyroidism and ischemic heart disease: a metaanalysis. J Clin Endocrinol Metab 93:2998–3007

16. Ochs N, Auer R, Bauer DC et al (2008) Meta-analysis: subclinical thyroid dysfunction and the risk for coronary heart disease and mortality. Ann Intern Med 148:832–845

17. Kanaya AM, Harris F, Volpato S et al (2002) Association between thyroid dysfunction and total cholesterol level in an older biracial population: the health, aging and body composition study. Arch Intern Med 162:773–779

18. Bauer DC, Ettinger B, Browner WS (1998) Thyroid functions and serum lipids in older women: a population-based study. Am J Med 104:546–551

19. Yildirimkaya M, Ozata M, Yilmaz K et al (1996) Lipoprotein(a) concentration in subclinical hypothyroidism before and after levo-thyroxine therapy. Endocr J 43:731–736

20. Grundy SM, Cleeman JI, Merz CN et al (2004) Implications of recent clinical trials for the National Cholesterol Education Program Adult Treatment Panel III guidelines. Arterioscler Thromb Vasc Biol 24:e149-e161

21. Danesh J, Collins R, Peto R (2000) Lipoprotein(a) and coronary heart disease. Meta-analysis of prospective studies. Circulation 102:1082–1085

22. Gussekloo J, van EE, de Craen AJ et al (2004) Thyroid status, disability and cognitive function, and survival in old age. JAMA 292:2591–2599

23. Caron P, Calazel C, Parra HJ et al (1990) Decreased HDL cholesterol in subclinical hypothyroidism: the effect of L-thyroxine therapy. Clin Endocrinol (Oxf) 33:519–523

24. Tunbridge WM, Evered DC, Hall R et al (1977) Lipid profiles and cardiovascular disease in the Whickham area with particular reference to thyroid failure. Clin Endocrinol (Oxf) 7:495–508

25. Imaizumi M, Akahoshi M, Ichimaru S et al (2004) Risk for ischemic heart disease and all-cause mortality in subclin-

ical hypothyroidism. J Clin Endocrinol Metab 89:3365–3370

26. Kong WM, Sheikh MH, Lumb PJ et al (2002) A 6-month randomized trial of thyroxine treatment in women with mild subclinical hypothyroidism. Am J Med 112:348–354

27. Meier C, Staub JJ, Roth CB et al (2001) TSH-controlled L-thyroxine therapy reduces cholesterol levels and clinical symptoms in subclinical hypothyroidism: a double blind, placebo-controlled trial (Basel Thyroid Study). J Clin Endocrinol Metab 86:4860–4866

28. Cooper DS, Halpern R, Wood LC et al (1984) L-Thyroxine therapy in subclinical hypothyroidism. A double-blind, placebo-controlled trial. Ann Intern Med 101:18–24

29. LaRosa JC, He J, Vupputuri S (1999) Effect of statins on risk of coronary disease: a meta-analysis of randomized controlled trials. JAMA 282:2340–2346

30. Danese MD, Ladenson PW, Meinert CL, Powe NR (2000) Clinical review 115: effect of thyroxine therapy on serum lipoproteins in patients with mild thyroid failure: a quantitative review of the literature. J Clin Endocrinol Metab 85:2993–3001

31. Villar HC, Saconato H, Valente O, Atallah AN (2007) Thyroid hormone replacement for subclinical hypothyroidism. Cochrane Database Syst Rev 3:CD003419

32. Wang TJ, Gona P, Larson MG et al (2006) Multiple biomarkers for the prediction of first major cardiovascular events and death. N Engl J Med 355:2631–2639

33. Cao JJ, Arnold AM, Manolio TA et al (2007) Association of carotid artery intima-media thickness, plaques, and C-reactive protein with future cardiovascular disease and all-cause mortality: the Cardiovascular Health Study. Circulation 116:32–38

34. Ridker PM, Cushman M, Stampfer MJ, Tracy RP, Hennekens CH (1997) Inflammation, aspirin, and the risk of cardiovascular disease in apparently healthy men. N Engl J Med 336:973–979

35. Ridker PM, Hennekens CH, Buring JE, Rifai N (2000) C-reactive protein and other markers of inflammation in the prediction of cardiovascular disease in women. N Engl J Med 342:836–843

36. Hueston WJ, King DE, Geesey ME (2005) Serum biomarkers for cardiovascular inflammation in subclinical hypothyroidism. Clin Endocrinol (Oxf) 63:582–587

37. Ozcan O, Cakir E, Yaman H et al (2005) The effects of thyroxine replacement on the levels of serum asymmetric dimethylarginine (ADMA) and other biochemical cardiovascular risk markers in patients with subclinical hypothyroidism. Clin Endocrinol (Oxf) 63:203–206

38. Clarke R, Daly L, Robinson K et al (1991) Hyperhomocysteinemia: an independent risk factor for vascular disease. N Engl J Med 324:1149–1155

39. Loscalzo J (2006) Homocysteine trials – clear outcomes for complex reasons. N Engl J Med 354:1629–1632

40. Hussein WI, Green R, Jacobsen DW, Faiman C (1999) Normalization of hyperhomocysteinemia with L-thyroxine in hypothyroidism. Ann Intern Med 131:348–351

41. Folsom AR, Wu KK, Rosamond WD et al (1997) Prospective study of hemostatic factors and incidence of coronary heart disease: the Atherosclerosis Risk in Communities (ARIC) Study. Circulation 96:1102–1108

42. Kannel WB (2005) Overview of hemostatic factors involved in atherosclerotic cardiovascular disease. Lipids 40:1215–1220

43. Stec JJ, Silbershatz H, Tofler GH et al (2000) Association of fibrinogen with cardiovascular risk factors and cardiovascular disease in the Framingham Offspring Population. Circulation 102:1634–1638

44. Chadarevian R, Jublanc C, Bruckert E et al (2005) Effect of levothyroxine replacement therapy on coagulation and fibrinolysis in severe hypothyroidism. J Endocrinol Invest 28:398–404

45. Canturk Z, Cetinarslan B, Tarkun I et al (2003) Hemostatic system as a risk factor for cardiovascular disease in women with subclinical hypothyroidism. Thyroid 13:971–977

46. Erem C (2006) Blood coagulation, fibrinolytic activity and lipid profile in subclinical thyroid disease: subclinical hyperthyroidism increases plasma factor X activity. Clin Endocrinol (Oxf) 64:323–329

47. DeLoach SS, Townsend RR (2008) Vascular stiffness: its measurement and significance for epidemiologic and outcome studies. Clin J Am Soc Nephrol 3:184–192

48. Mattace-Raso FU, van der Cammen TJ, Hofman A et al (2006) Arterial stiffness and risk of coronary heart disease and stroke: the Rotterdam Study. Circulation 113:657–663

49. Nagasaki T, Inaba M, Kumeda Y et al (2006) Increased pulse wave velocity in subclinical hypothyroidism. J Clin Endocrinol Metab 91:154–158

50. Nagasaki T, Inaba M, Yamada S et al (2007) Changes in brachial-ankle pulse wave velocity in subclinical hypothyroidism during normalization of thyroid function. Biomed Pharmacother 61:482–487

51. Owen PJ, Rajiv C, Vinereanu D et al (2006) Subclinical hypothyroidism, arterial stiffness, and myocardial reserve. J Clin Endocrinol Metab 91:2126–2132

52. Yeboah J, Sutton-Tyrrell K, Mcburnie MA et al (2008) Association between brachial artery reactivity and cardiovascular disease status in an elderly cohort: the cardiovascular health study. Atherosclerosis 197:768–776

53. Heitzer T, Schlinzig T, Krohn K et al (2001) Endothelial dysfunction, oxidative stress, and risk of cardiovascular events in patients with coronary artery disease. Circulation 104:2673–2678

54. Taddei S, Caraccio N, Virdis A et al (2003) Impaired endothelium-dependent vasodilatation in subclinical hypothyroidism: beneficial effect of levothyroxine therapy. J Clin Endocrinol Metab 88:3731–3737

55. O'Leary DH, Polak JF, Kronmal RA et al (1999) Carotid-artery intima and media thickness as a risk factor for myocardial infarction and stroke in older adults. Cardiovascular Health Study Collaborative Research Group. N Engl J Med 340:14–22

56. Nagasaki T, Inaba M, Henmi Y et al (2003) Decrease in carotid intima-media thickness in hypothyroid patients after normalization of thyroid function. Clin Endocrinol (Oxf) 59:607–612

57. Walsh JP, Bremner AP, Bulsara MK et al (2005) Subclinical thyroid dysfunction as a risk factor for cardiovascular disease. Arch Intern Med 165:2467–2472

58. Vanderpump MP, Tunbridge WM, French JM et al (1996) The development of ischemic heart disease in relation to autoimmune thyroid disease in a 20-year follow-up study of an English community. Thyroid 6:155–160

59. Gammage MD, Parle JV, Holder RL et al (2007) Associa-

tion between serum free thyroxine concentration and atrial fibrillation. Arch Intern Med 167:928–934

60. Parle JV, Maisonneuve P, Sheppard MC et al (2001) Prediction of all-cause and cardiovascular mortality in elderly people from one low serum thyrotropin result: a 10-year cohort study. Lancet 358:861–865

61. Iervasi G, Molinaro S, Landi P et al (2007) Association between increased mortality and mild thyroid dysfunction in cardiac patients. Arch Intern Med 167:1526–1532

62. Psaty BM, Anderson M, Kronmal RA et al (2004) The association between lipid levels and the risks of incident myocardial infarction, stroke, and total mortality: The Cardiovascular Health Study. J Am Geriatr Soc 52:1639–1647

63. Klein I, Danzi S (2007) Thyroid disease and the heart. Circulation 116:1725–1735

64. Osman F, Franklyn JA, Holder RL et al (2007) Cardiovascular manifestations of hyperthyroidism before and after antithyroid therapy: a matched case-control study. J Am Coll Cardiol 49:71–81

65. Parle JV, Franklyn JA, Cross KW et al (1991) Prevalence and follow-up of abnormal thyrotrophin (TSH) concentrations in the elderly in the United Kingdom. Clin Endocrinol (Oxf) 34:77–83

66. Volzke H, Ludemann J, Robinson DM et al (2003) The prevalence of undiagnosed thyroid disorders in a previously iodine-deficient area. Thyroid 13:803–810

67. Sawin CT, Geller A, Wolf PA et al (1994) Low serum thyrotropin concentrations as a risk factor for atrial fibrillation in older persons. N Engl J Med 331:1249–1252

68. Auer J, Scheibner P, Mische T et al (2001) Subclinical hyperthyroidism as a risk factor for atrial fibrillation. Am Heart J 142:838–842

69. Bauer DC, Rodondi N, Stone KL, Hillier TA (2007) Thyroid hormone use, hyperthyroidism and mortality in older women. Am J Med 120:343–349

Relationship Between Subclinical Thyroid Dysfunction and Heart Failure and Mortality

Reto Auer and Nicolas Rodondi

Abstract This chapter reviews the data on subclinical thyroid dysfunction and heart failure and mortality. Observational studies have suggested that subclinical hypothyroidism is associated with a moderately elevated risk of heart failure events among older adults with a thyrotropin level higher than 7–10 mU/L. Such data are lacking for middle-aged adults. Subclinical thyroid dysfunction might also represent a potentially modifiable risk factor for mortality. In a recent systematic review and meta-analysis of prospective cohorts, adults less than 65 years of age with subclinical hypothyroidism were found to be at increased risk of all-cause and cardiovascular mortality. The situation might be reversed in the elderly. Data are more limited for subclinical hyperthyroidism. Large, randomized clinical trials are needed to assess the efficacy of thyroxine replacement or antithyroid medications on clinical outcomes such as cardiovascular disease (coronary heart disease, heart failure, cardiovascular mortality) in adults with subclinical thyroid dysfunction.

Keywords Subclinical hypothyroidism • Subclinical hyperthyroidism • Heart failure • Mortality • Prospective studies

15.1 Introduction

"Subclinical thyroid dysfunction" refers to a condition in which patients have an abnormal thyrotropin (thyroid-stimulating hormone, TSH) level and a normal free thyroxine (T_4) level [1]. Several reviews have suggested a TSH upper-limit cut-off of 4.5–5.0 mU/l [1, 2], but some authors concluded that the upper limit of the TSH range should be lowered to 2.5–3.0 mU/l [3, 4]. Based on these reference ranges, the prevalence of subclinical hypothyroidism (SHypo) is about 4% in adults, and that of subclinical hyperthyroidism (SHyper) 1%, with higher prevalences in older adults and in women [2, 5–7]. Controversy persists as to whether screening and treatment of subclinical thyroid dysfunction is warranted [1, 2, 8, 9], as current evidence about the risks is limited [1, 2] and randomized controlled trials on relevant clinical outcomes have not yet been performed [2, 10]. Here we review the evidence regarding the relationship between subclinical thyroid dysfunction and heart failure and mortality.

15.2 Subclinical Hypothyroidism and the Risk of Heart Failure Events

Heart failure (HF) is the leading cause of hospitalization in persons older than 65 years [11]. Recognizing and treating risk factors for HF events is important for prevention. SHypo seems to be

N. Rodondi (✉)
Department of Ambulatory Care and Community Medicine,
University of Lausanne, Lausanne, Switzerland

G. Iervasi, A. Pingitore (eds.), *Thyroid and Heart Failure*.
© Springer-Verlag Italia 2009

associated with diastolic and systolic cardiac dysfunction, and thyroxine replacement improves cardiac function in patients with SHypo [12]. However, only a few studies have directly addressed the relationship between SHypo and HF.

The Health, Aging, and Body Composition study is a population-based study of a cohort of elderly men and women (age 70–79) that began in 1997 in the areas surrounding Pittsburgh, Pennsylvania, and Memphis, Tennessee, USA. Among the 2,730 black and white adults who were followed for 4 years [13], participants with a TSH level greater than 0.1 mU/l but less than 4.5 mU/l were considered euthyroid. Free T$_4$ was measured in all participants with a TSH level of 7.0 mU/l or greater. Hypothyroidism was further classified according to TSH levels: mild elevation (4.5–6.9 mU/l), moderate elevation (7.0–9.9 mU/l), and marked elevation (10.0 mU/l or greater). Participants with overt thyroid disease under amiodarone or thyroid hormone therapy were excluded. Rodondi et al. found that participants with a TSH of 7.0 mU/l or greater had a higher rate of HF events than euthyroid subjects (35.0 vs. 16.5/1,000 person-years, $p = 0.006$; (Fig. 15.1 and Table 15.1) [13]. In multivariate analysis, including adjustment for prevalent cardiovascular disease and HF, the risk of HF was about three times as high among those with high TSH levels. In those with a TSH level of 7.0–9.9 mU/l, the hazard ratio (HR) was 2.58 (95% CI 1.19–5.60), and it was 3.26 (95% CI 1.37–7.77) for those with a TSH of 10.0 mU/l or greater. After exclusion of 175 participants with prevalent HF, there were 127 who

had incident HF events. The adjusted HR for incident HF events was 2.33 (95% CI 1.10–4.96; $p = 0.03$) in those with a TSH level of 7.0 mU/l or greater. Among the participants with prevalent HF, 51 had recurrent HF events; the adjusted HR was 7.62 (95% CI 2.25–25.77; $p = 0.001$) in those with a TSH level of 7.0 mU/l or greater. Results were similar after excluding thyroid hormone users, and there was no interaction with race or sex ($p > 0.20$ for each interaction). However these results were limited by the lack of routine echocardiography, which limited the identification of HF and the type of cardiac dysfunction involved.

This issue was also examined among 3,065 adults over 65 years of age in the Cardiovascular Health Study, who underwent echocardiography at baseline and at follow-up [14]. The definition of SHypo was the same as in the study described above. The authors compared adjudicated incident HF events over 12 years of follow-up and changes in cardiac function over 6 years between participants with SHypo, SHyper, and euthyroidism. They found a greater incidence of HF events among participants with a TSH level above 10 mU/l than among euthyroid participants (45.2 vs. 22.2/100 person-years, $p = 0.003$), but not among those with TSH between 4.5 and 9.9 mU/l or among those with SHyper. Compared to euthyroid participants, most baseline echocardiographic parameters did not differ by thyroid status; participants with TSH of 10.0 mU/l or greater had a higher peak E velocity (0.80 vs. 0.72 m/s, $p = 0.002$), and this difference persisted after adjustment for age, gender, heart rate, and

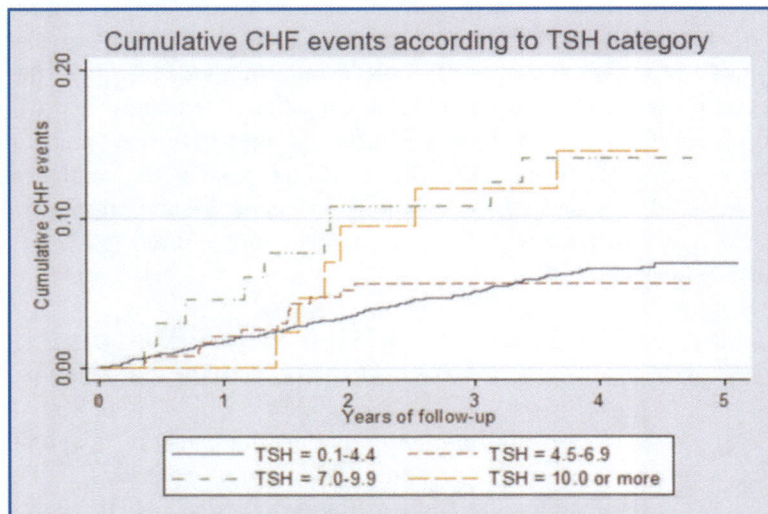

Fig. 15.1 Cumulative congestive heart failure (*CHF*) events in older subjects in relation to thyrotropin (*TSH*) levels. The rate of CHF events increased with higher TSH levels ($p = 0.03$ for trend). Participants with a TSH level of 7.0 mU/l or greater had a higher rate of CHF events than did euthyroid participants ($p = 0.006$); this was not the case for those with a TSH level between 4.5 and 6.9 mU/l. (Reproduced with permission from [13]. Copyright© American Medical Association. All rights reserved)

Table 15.1 Subclinical hypothyroidism and the risk of heart failure events

Study	Population studied	Age, years (range or mean age)	Percentage of women in the study	Follow-up duration, years	TSH cut-off mU/l (no. of participants with abnormal TSH)	Description and no. of CHF events or cardiac abnormalities	Adjusted HR (95% CI)	Adjustments
Cross-sectional studies								
Manovitz et al. 1996 [15]	31 participants with left ventricular ejection fraction assessed by echocardiography of ≤ 35%	57.5	24	–	> 3.6 mU/l	8 out of 31 had subclinical hypothyroidism	–	–
Fruhwald et al. 1997 [16]	61 participants with invasively diagnosed idiopathic dilated cardiomyopathy according to WHO criteria	21–73	18	–	0.1–5 mU/l	Morphologic or functional thyroid abnormality in 59/61 patients	–	–
Cohort studies								
Rodondi et al. [13] 2005 Health, Aging, and Body Composition Study	2730 community-dwelling adults in areas surrounding Pittsburgh, PA and Memphis, TN	70–79	51	4	Euthyroid subjects (2392) ≥ 4.5–6.9 mU/l (230) 7.0–9.9 mU/l (64) ≥ 10 mU/l (44)	CHF events 151 13 8 6	1.00 1.07 (0.57–2.01) 2.58 (1.19–5.60) 3.26 (1.37–7.77)	Age, sex, race, smoking, diabetes, prevalent CVD, poor/fair health, BP, total cholesterol, creatinine, education, income, thyroid hormone and ACE inhibitors use
Rodondi et al. 2008 [14] Cardiovascular Health Study	3065 community-dwelling adults in Sacramento County, CA; Washington County, MD; Forsyth County, NC; and Allegheny County (Pittsburgh), PA, USA	2.6 7	60	12	Euthyroid subjects ≥ 4.5–9.9 mU/l ≥ 10 mU/l < 0.45 mU/l	CHF events 621 89 16 10	1.00 0.92 (0.73–1.17) 1.88 (1.05–3.34) 0.94 (0.48–1.83)	Age, sex, race, prevalent CVD, atrial fibrillation, alcohol, smoking, diabetes mellitus, hypertension, body mass index, LDL-cholesterol, HDL-cholesterol and creatinine

TSH thyroid-stimulating hormone, *HR* hazard ratio, *CI* 95% confidence interval, *CVD* cardiovascular disease, *BP* blood pressure, *ACE* angiotensin-converting enzyme systolic blood pressure. Peak E velocity, a sign of decreased left ventricular compliance, was associated with incident HF in the overall study sample (HR 1.14 for each 0.1 m/s increment, 95% CI 1.09–1.18, $p < 0.001$) and in those with TSH of 10.0 mU/l or greater (HR 1.45, 95% CI 1.20–1.76, $p < 0.001$) after adjustment for age, gender, and systolic blood pressure. Over 5 years, most changes in echocardiographic parameters did not significantly differ by thyroid status, except that participants with TSH of 10.0 mU/l or greater had a larger increase in left ventricular mass (+21 vs. +4 g, $p = 0.04$) and a greater proportion of HF events associated with low ejection fraction than did euthyroid participants (80% vs. 45%, $p = 0.08$).

Two small cross-sectional studies also evaluated the association between thyroid hormones and HF. One small cross-sectional study found that 8 of 31 patients (26%) with HF had a TSH level greater than 3.6 mU/l, with normal T_4 levels [15]. Fruhwald et al. found either functional or morphological thyroid disorder in 59 of 61 patients with invasively diagnosed idiopathic dilated cardiomyopathy [16]. However, neither study was prospective or included a control group without HF.

In conclusion, SHypo is associated with a moderately elevated risk of HF among older adults with a TSH greater than 10 mU/l. This issue has not been examined in cohorts of younger adults. To date, there is no evidence that SHyper is associated with clinical HF events, but only one study has examined this issue [14].

15.3 Subclinical Thyroid Dysfunction and the Risk of Mortality

SHypo is associated with elevated cholesterol levels and increased risk of atherosclerosis [17–21]. Yet, data on the relationship between SHypo and cardiovascular and total mortality are conflicting [13, 22–24]. In this section, we present the results of seven prospective studies with total or cardiovascular mortality outcomes that followed participants with SHypo or SHyper, based on a meta-analysis [25].

Atomic bomb survivors from Nagasaki have had a biannual health examination since 1958. Between 1984 and 1987, 2,856 subjects agreed to participate in a thyroid disease screening program and were followed for 10 years [26]. Mean age at baseline was 58.5 years and levels of TSH of 0.6–5.0 mU/l and free T_4 levels of 0.8–2.5 ng/dl (10.3–32.3 pmol/l) were considered normal (see Table 15.2). Participants with a history of thyroid hormone treatment and those with subsequent thyroid hormone treatment were excluded. The analysis made adjustments for age, systolic blood pressure, smoking status, erythrocyte sedimentation rate, and the presence of diabetes mellitus. Among the 2,550 participants included in the analysis, 11% had SHypo. After 6 years, all-cause mortality and, particularly cardiovascular mortality, was increased in men with SHypo. After 10 years, however, there was no significant association between the presence of SHypo at baseline and an increase in all-cause mortality in both sexes (HR 1.2; 95% CI 0.8–1.6). The authors did not report data on participants with SHyper.

In the Busselton Health Study, 3,447 people on an electoral roll in 1981 responded to a health survey (65% response rate; mean age 49.8 years) [24]. Twenty years later, Walsh et al. measured thyroid hormone levels in the blood samples of 2,108 participants that were frozen in a blood bank [24]. After the exclusion of subjects with coronary heart disease at baseline, they linked the thyroid data with administrative mortality data, adjusting their analysis for major cardiovascular risk factors among other factors. SHypo was defined as a TSH level higher than 4.0 mU/l, with normal free T_4. The SHypo group was further divided into subjects with a serum TSH level of 10 mU/l or less and those with serum TSH level of more than 10 mU/l. SHyper was defined as a TSH level of less than 0.4 mU/l, with normal free T_4. These authors found a pattern of increased cardiovascular mortality among subjects with SHypo (HR 1.5, 95% CI 0.9–2.5). Participants with SHyper had no increased cardiovascular mortality (HR 1.0, 95% CI 0.2–4.3). One strength of this study is the retrospective thyroid hormone measurement, as participants were unaware of their thyroid status during follow-up. However, data on subsequent thyroid hormone use were lacking and could therefore not be included in the model. Similarly, only total cholesterol and HDL cholesterol level were measured at baseline, and data on LDL cholesterol, a potentially important covariate, could not be included in the model [24].

The 1.5-point estimate found in the Busselton study contrasts with prospective studies that enrolled older participants.

Table 15.2 Subclinical hypothyroidism and the risk of mortality. (Adapted from [25], with permission from Annals of Internal Medicine)

Study	Population studied	Age, years (range or age ± SD)	Percentage of women in the study	Follow-up starting, year	Follow-up duration years	TSH cut-off mU/l (no. of participants with abnormal TSH)	Exclusion of thyroid hormone/antithyroid drug users	Type of outcomes (no. of outcomes in euthyroid/subclinical hypothyroid participants)	HR (95% CI)	Adjustments
Imaizumi et al. Nagasaki 2004 [26] Adult Health Study	999 atomic bomb survivors in Nagasaki, Japan	58 (58±10)	0	1984–1987	6	> 5.0 (96)	Yes/NA	CHD mortality (3/2)	4.8 (0.8–29.3)	Age, sex, and smoking
	2550	58 (58±10)	60.8	1984–1987	10	> 5.0 (257)	Yes/NA	Total mortality (268/42)	1.2 (0.8–1.6)	
	999	58 (58±10)	0	1984–1987	6	> 5.0 (96)	Yes/NA	CV mortality (6/2)	2.4 (0.5–11.8)	
Walsh et al. 2005 [24] Busselton Health Study	1926 adults living in the rural town of Busselton, Western Australia	49.8 (17–89)	49.6	1981	20	> 4.0 (101)	NR/NR	CV mortality (170/21)	1.5 (0.9–2.5)	Age, sex, BMI, smoking, diabetes, total cholesterol, triglycerides, BP, hypertensive therapy, exercise, and thyroid disease
Rodondi et al. 2005 [13] Health, Aging, and Body Composition Study	2730 community-dwelling adults in the metropolitan areas of Pittsburgh, PA and Memphis, TN, USA	74.7 (70–79)	51	NR	4	≥ 4.5 (338)	No (only in a SA)/NA	Total mortality (283/41)	1.20 (0.83–1.74)	Age, sex, race, smoking, diabetes, prevalent CVD, poor or fair health, BP, total cholesterol, creatinine, education, income, thyroid hormone, and ACE inhibitor use
								CV mortality (94/10)	0.74 (0.34–1.61)	
						≥ 10.0 (44)		Total mortality (283/8)	2.05 (0.90–4.68)	
								CV mortality (94/3)	2.26 (0.54–9.45)	

Cont. →

Cont. **Table 15.2**

Study	Population studied	Age, years (range or age ± SD)	Percentage of women in the study	Follow-up starting, year	Follow-up duration years	TSH cut-off mU/l (no. of participants with abnormal TSH)	Exclusion of thyroid hormone/antithyroid drug users	Type of outcomes (no. of outcomes in euthyroid/subclinical hypothyroid participants)	HR (95% CI)	Adjustments
Cappola et al. 2006 [22] Cardiovascular Health Study	3233 community-dwelling adults in 4 US communities: Washington County, MD; Pittsburgh (Allegheny County), PA; Sacramento County, CA; and Forsyth County, NC	72.7 (≥65)	59.6	1989–1990	12.5	>4.5 (496)	Yes^b/Yes	Total mortality (1170/233); CV mortality (474/101)	1.14 (0.98–1.32); 1.16 (0.92–1.46)	Age, sex, prevalent CVD, thyroid medication, race, smoking, diabetes, LDL-cholesterol, lipid-lowering drugs, hypertension, BMI, and CRP
Parle et al. 2001 [23]	1171 community-dwelling adults in Birmingham, UK	70.4 (>60)	57.2	1988–1989	8.2	>5.0 (69)	Yes/Yes	Total mortality (444/25); CV mortality (118/10)	0.9 (0.6–1.4)^c; 1.4 (0.7–2.6)^c	Age and sex
Gussekloo et al. 2004 [27] Leiden 85-plus Study	558 adults living in one urban district in Leiden, The Netherlands	85 (all aged 85)	66	1997–1999	3.7	>4.8 (30)	Yes/Yes	Total mortality (180/6); CV mortality (75/2)	0.55 (0.24–1.25); 0.47 (0.11–1.90)	Sex and education

SD standard deviation, *TSH* thyroid-stimulating hormone, *HR* hazard ratio, *95% CI* 95% confidence interval, *NA* not applicable, *CHD* coronary heart disease, *CV* cardiovascular, *BP* blood pressure, *NR* not reported, *SA* sensitivity analysis, *ACE* angiotensin-converting enzyme, *CVD* cardiovascular disease, *BMI* body mass index, *CRP* C-reactive protein

[a] All studies were population-based studies. A population-based study was defined as a random sample of the general population.

[b] This study also accounted for thyroid hormone use in the follow-up, analyzing it as a time-dependent covariate.

[c] Study author provided relative risk value for subclinical hypothyroidism after exclusion of 18 participants with low T₄, and relative risk value for subclinical hyperthyroidism after exclusion of 2 participants with high T₄.

In the previously described Health, Aging, and Body Composition Study, Rodondi et al. also assessed the effect of SHypo on all-cause mortality and cardiovascular mortality. Among the 338 participants (12.4%) with SHypo, the authors found no increase in total mortality and cardiovascular mortality after the 4-year follow-up. Even after classifying the participants with SHypo according to increasing TSH levels, risks were increased for those with TSH levels above 10.0 mU/l but remained statistically not significant (Table 15.2).

Cappola et al. analyzed the data from the Cardiovascular Health Study with respect to subclinical thyroid dysfunction [22]. The Cardiovascular Health Study is a population-based, longitudinal study of cardiovascular risk factors that enrolled 5,888 adults age 65 years or older in four US communities. After the exclusion of people taking thyroid medication or medication that might have altered thyroid testing (prednisone, amiodarone) and participants with overt hyperthyroidism at baseline, 3,233 participants were included in the analysis. Euthyroidism was defined as TSH of 0.45–4.50 mU/l, SHypo as TSH of more than 4.50 mU/l but less than 20 mU/l, with a normal free T_4 concentration, and SHyper as TSH of 0.10–0.44 mU/l or less than 0.10 mU/l, with a normal free T_4. In this study, 15% had SHypo and 1.5% SHyper. After adjustment for relevant confounders, the HR for SHypo and cardiovascular mortality was 1.16 (95% CI 0.92–1.46) and that for all-cause mortality 1.14 (95% CI 0.98–1.32). Of note, 142 of 496 participants with SHypo (27%) used thyroid replacement medication during follow-up. When this covariate was included in the model, these risks remained statistically not significant, suggesting that thyroid replacement therapy for SHypo has no effect on mortality outcomes. For participants with SHyper, the HR was 0.94 (95% CI 0.49–1.83) for cardiovascular mortality and 1.08 (95% CI 0.72–1.62) for all-cause mortality (Table 15.3).

Parle et al. followed 1,191 individuals from Birmingham UK who were older than 60 years at the time of baseline measurements for 10 years to study the effect of thyroid dysfunction on mortality [23]. The mean age was 70.4 years and the normal range for TSH levels 0.5–5.0 mU/l. After the exclusion of participants who were taking thyroxine or antithyroid medication at baseline, 8% had SHypo and 6% SHyper. The authors repeated TSH and T_4 measurement at yearly intervals in those with abnormal baseline TSH values. Thirty of 76 participants with SHypo at baseline (40%) developed overt hypothyroidism and began thyroxine replacement treatment over follow-up. A TSH level over 5.0 mU/l compared to those with a TSH level within the reference range did not affect cardiovascular or all-cause mortality (HR 1.4, 95% CI 0.7–2.6, and HR 0.9, 95% CI 0.6–1.4, respectively). Observed causes of death in participants with normal or raised TSH levels did not significantly differ from age-specific mortality data from the WHO databank for England and Wales recorded in the same period. For participants with SHyper at baseline, there was an increased risk in total and cardiovascular mortality after 2, 3, 4, and 5 years. However, after 10 years of follow-up, a pattern of increased cardiovascular and total mortality was found only for participants with SHyper at baseline (HR 1.6, 95% CI 0.8–2.9, and HR 1.2, 95% CI 0.9–1.8, respectively, Table 15.3).

Risk in the very elderly was studied in the Leiden 85-Plus Study, in which adults age 85 years were followed for 4 years [27]. TSH levels of 0.3–4.8 mU/l were considered normal. Of the 558 participants with thyroid-function assessment at baseline, 5% had SHypo, 3% SHyper, and 4% were on thyroid medication. Mortality was very high, as 37% of the participants died during follow-up. Thyroid status was a strong predictor of mortality: participants with normal TSH levels had higher mortality than those with low TSH levels. Adjusting for potential confounders did not significantly change the results. The HR of mortality per standard deviation increase in TSH levels (2.71 mU/l) was 0.76 (95% CI 0.62–0.92). Moreover, subgroup analysis of participants taking thyroid medication showed that, in those with high levels of TSH and low levels of T_4, i.e., those with suboptimal thyroid replacement, survival was higher, suggesting that taking thyroxine was more harmful than beneficial in this very elderly population. If the results are presented as HR between SHypo and the normal population instead of per standard deviation increases in TSH levels, a pattern of decreased total mortality is found for participants with SHypo (HR 0.55, 95% CI 0.24–1.25, Table 15.2). Potential explanations for these age differences might be competing causes of death among older adults (e.g., due to cancer) or more competing risk factors for coronary heart disease among older adults (e.g., age, sex) [25]. Other potential explanations are related to the thyroid physiology itself in older adults (decreased

Table 15.3 Subclinical hyperthyroidism and the risk of mortality. (Adapted from [25], with permission from Annals of Internal Medicine)

Study[a]	Population studied	Age (range or age ± SD) years	Percentage of women in the study	Follow-up starting year	Follow-up duration years	TSH cut-off mU/l (no. of participants with abnormal TSH)	Exclusion thyroid hormone/antithyroid drug users	Type of outcomes (no. of outcomes in euthyroid/subclinical hypothyroid participants)	HR (95% CI)	Adjustments
Walsh et al. 2005 [24] Busselton Health Study	1926 adults living in the rural town of Busselton, Western Australia	49.8 (17–89)	49.6	1981	20	<0.4 mU/l (37)	NR/NR	CV mortality (170/3)	1.0 (0.2–4.3)	Age, sex, BMI, smoking, diabetes, total cholesterol, triglycerides, BP, hypertensive therapy, exercise, and thyroid disease
Cappola et al. 2006 [22] Cardiovascular Health Study	3233 community-dwelling adults in 4 US communities: Washington County, MD; Pittsburgh (Allegheny County), PA; Sacramento County, CA and Forsyth County, NC	72.7 (≥65)	59.6	1989–1990	12.5	<0.45 mU/l (47)	Yes[b]/Yes	Total mortality (1170/24) CV mortality (474/9)	1.08 (0.72–1.62) 0.94 (0.49–1.83)	Age, sex, prevalent CVD, thyroid medication, race, smoking, diabetes, LDL cholesterol, lipid-lowering drugs, hypertension, BMI, and CRP
Parle et al. 2001 [23]	1171 community-dwelling adults in Birmingham, UK	70.4 (>60)	57.2	1988–1989	8.2	<0.44 mU/l (76)	Yes/Yes	Total mortality (444/33) CV mortality (118/11)	1.2 (0.9–1.8)[c] 1.6 (0.8–2.9)[c]	Age and sex
Gussekloo et al. 2004 [27] Leiden 85-plus Study	558 adults living in one urban district in Leiden, The Netherlands	85 (all aged 85)	66.0	1997–1999	3.7	<0.3 mU/l (17)	Yes/Yes	Total mortality (180/7) CV mortality (75/3)	1.20 (0.59–2.69) 1.38 (0.43–4.39)	Sex and education

SD standard deviation, *TSH* thyroid-stimulating hormone, *HR* hazard ratio, *95% CI* 95% confidence interval, *NR* not reported, *CV* cardiovascular, *BMI* body mass index, *BP* blood pressure, *CVD* cardiovascular disease, *CRP* C-reactive protein

[a] All studies were population-based studies; [b] This study also accounted for thyroid hormone use in the follow-up, analyzing it as a time-dependant covariate; [c] Study author provided RR for subclinical hyperthyroidism after exclusion of 18 participants with low T4, and RR for subclinical hypothyroidism after exclusion of 2 participants with a high T4.

thyroid hormone action at the tissue level, reduced thyroid hormone metabolism) [28]. High TSH in the elderly might also be a compensatory mechanism for some perturbations, whereas in younger adults it is caused by thyroid dysfunction.

We recently pooled the results of these prospective studies in a meta-analysis [25], including data from the above-mentioned studies as well as from two longitudinal population-based studies that did not measure T_4 levels and therefore could not formally exclude participants with overt hypothyroidism, as most people with TSH elevation have subclinical and not overt hypothyroidism [29, 30]. In the absence of a consensus, we did not pre-specify a TSH cut-off to define SHypo, and performed a sensitivity analysis by limiting the analysis to studies with a TSH cut-off of at least 4.5 mU/l [2]. Using a random effects model, we found a pattern of modestly increased risk for total and cardiovascular mortality associated with SHypo [summary relative risk (RR) for total mortality 1.12, 95% CI 0.99–1.26, and for cardiovascular mortality summary RR 1.18, 95% CI 0.98–1.42) [25]. Sensitivity analysis excluding the studies that did not measure T_4 levels led to similar results. Study quality was heterogeneous and we considered formal adjudication procedures and adjudication without knowledge of thyroid status as the main quality criteria. Pooling only studies of the highest quality yielded lower point estimates. Limiting the analysis to two studies that adjusted for most cardiovascular risk factors also yielded lower point estimates [13, 22]. As suggested by the studies that included older patients, age seemed to influence the results [23, 27]. Increased total and cardiovascular mortality was only seen in participants age less than 65 years with SHypo. However, these sensitivity analyses must be considered with caution considering the small number of studies for each group. Moreover, studies of the highest quality were also those with older patients. For SHyper, we did not specify a TSH cut-off, in the absence of a consensus, but all studies had a cut-off within a small range, 0.3–0.5 mU/l. Based on a random effects model, the summary RR was 1.12 (95% CI 0.89–1.42) for total mortality and 1.19 (95% CI 0.81–1.76) for cardio-

vascular deaths. We found no differences by mean age but lower point estimates were obtained for higher-quality studies.

The study by Åsvold et al. published after our meta-analysis, seems to confirm that age might be an important effect modifier of TSH levels [31]. The Nord-Trøndelag Health Study (HUNT Study), prospectively analyzed the association between thyrotropin levels and cardiovascular mortality in 17,311 women and 8,002 men older than 40 years without known thyroid disease, cardiovascular disease, or diabetes mellitus at baseline. Mean age was 60 years. During a median follow-up of 8.3 years, the authors found a linear and positive association of thyrotropin levels within the reference range (0.5–3.5 mU/l) with coronary heart disease mortality in women, but not in men. Parle et al. found the reverse association in participants with a mean age of 70 years. Åsvold et al. also mentioned that participants with SHypo had increased mortality, but without presenting the results in numbers [32]. A positive association with coronary heart disease remains to be confirmed over the full range of TSH values in this study.

15.4 Conclusions

SHypo represents a potentially modifiable risk factor for HF and cardiovascular and total mortality. Given the high prevalence of thyroid dysfunction, even a small increase in those events among people with SHypo would have important public health implications. However, the elderly population represents a different subgroup, in which a high TSH level might be neutral or even protective at very old age in terms of total mortality. For SHyper, due to the scarcity of data, the association with mortality outcome needs further research. To date, there is no randomized controlled trial assessing HF or mortality outcome following thyroid hormone substitution. Final proof of the benefits of treating individuals with abnormally high TSH levels can only come from well-designed randomized, placebo-controlled clinical trials [33].

Key Points

- Subclinical thyroid dysfunction is the condition seen in patients who have an abnormal level of thyrotropin and a normal level of free thyroxine.

- Subclinical hypothyroidism is associated with a moderately elevated risk of heart failure events among older adults with a thyrotropin level of 7–10 mU/l. This issue has not been examined in cohorts of younger adults.

- Subclinical thyroid dysfunction represents a potentially modifiable risk factor for mortality. Adults aged less than 65 years with subclinical hypothyroidism might be at increased risk for all-cause and for cardiovascular mortality. The situation might be reversed in the very elderly. Data are more limited for subclinical hyperthyroidism.

- Before screening for thyroid dysfunction in the general population can be recommended, randomized, placebo-controlled trials of treatment of subclinical thyroid dysfunction with measurement of clinical outcomes, such as cardiovascular disease, as end points should be performed to assess the efficacy of thyroxine replacement or antithyroid medications.

References

1. Helfand M (2004) Screening for subclinical thyroid dysfunction in nonpregnant adults: a summary of the evidence for the US Preventive Services Task Force. Ann Intern Med 140:128–141
2. Surks MI, Ortiz E, Daniels GH et al (2004) Subclinical thyroid disease: scientific review and guidelines for diagnosis and management. JAMA 291:228–238
3. Haugen B (2003) When isn't the TSH normal and why? Clinical implications and causes. Paper presented at the 12th Annual Meeting of the American Association of Clinical Endocrinologists (AACE), 14–18 May 2003, San Diego, California
4. Lee S (2003) When is the TSH normal? New criteria for diagnosis and management. Paper presented at the 12th Annual Meeting of the American Association of Clinical Endocrinologists (AACE), 14–18 May 2003, San Diego, California
5. Hollowell JG, Staehling NW, Flanders WD et al (2002) Serum TSH, T4, and thyroid antibodies in the United States population (1988 to 1994): National Health and Nutrition Examination Survey (NHANES III). J Clin Endocrinol Metab 87:489–499
6. Parle JV, Franklyn JA, Cross KW et al (1991) Prevalence and follow-up of abnormal thyrotrophin (TSH) concentrations in the elderly in the United Kingdom. Clin Endocrinol (Oxf) 34:77–83
7. Sawin CT, Castelli WP, Hershman JM et al (1985) The aging thyroid. Thyroid deficiency in the Framingham Study. Arch Intern Med 145:1386–1388
8. Cooper DS (2001) Clinical practice. Subclinical hypothyroidism. N Engl J Med 345:260–265
9. Ladenson PW, Singer PA, Ain KB et al (2000) American Thyroid Association guidelines for detection of thyroid dysfunction. Arch Intern Med 160:1573–1575
10. Villar H, Saconato H, Valente O, Atallah A (2007) Thyroid hormone replacement for subclinical hypothyroidism. Cochrane Database Syst Rev (3):CD003419
11. Gottdiener JS, Arnold AM, Aurigemma GP et al (2000) Predictors of congestive heart failure in the elderly: the Cardiovascular Health Study. J Am Coll Cardiol 35:1628–1637
12. Biondi B, Palmieri EA, Lombardi G, Fazio S (2002) Effects of subclinical thyroid dysfunction on the heart. Ann Intern Med 137:904–914
13. Rodondi N, Newman AB, Vittinghoff E et al (2005) Subclinical hypothyroidism and the risk of heart failure, other cardiovascular events, and death. Arch Intern Med 165:2460–2466
14. Rodondi N, Bauer D, Cappola A et al (2008) Subclinical thyroid dysfunction, cardiac function and the risk of heart failure: The Cardiovascular Health Study. J Am Coll Cardiol 52:1152–1159
15. Manowitz NR, Mayor GH, Klepper MJ, DeGroot LJ (1996) Subclinical hypothyroidism and euthyroid sick syndrome in patients with moderate-to-severe congestive heart failure. Am J Ther 3:797–801
16. Fruhwald FM, Ramschak-Schwarzer S, Pichler B et al (1997) Subclinical thyroid disorders in patients with dilated cardiomyopathy. Cardiology 88:156–159
17. Canaris GJ, Manowitz NR, Mayor G, Ridgway EC (2000) The Colorado Thyroid Disease Prevalence Study. Arch Intern Med 160:526–534
18. Kanaya AM, Harris F, Volpato S et al (2002) Association between thyroid dysfunction and total cholesterol level in an older biracial population: The Health, Aging and Body Composition Study. Arch Intern Med 162:773–779
19. Althaus BU, Staub JJ, Ryff-De Leche A et al (1988) LDL/HDL-changes in subclinical hypothyroidism: possible risk factors for coronary heart disease. Clin Endocrinol (Oxf) 28:157–163
20. Hak AE, Pols HA, Visser TJ et al (2000) Subclinical hypothyroidism is an independent risk factor for atherosclerosis and myocardial infarction in elderly women: the Rot-

terdam Study. Ann Intern Med 132:270–278

21. Monzani F, Caraccio N, Kozakowa M et al (2004) Effect of levothyroxine replacement on lipid profile and intima-media thickness in subclinical hypothyroidism: a double-blind, placebo-controlled study. J Clin Endocrinol Metab 89:2099–2106

22. Cappola AR, Fried LP, Arnold AM et al (2006) Thyroid status, cardiovascular risk, and mortality in older adults. JA-MA 295:1033–1041

23. Parle JV, Maisonneuve P, Sheppard MC et al (2001) Prediction of all-cause and cardiovascular mortality in elderly people from one low serum thyrotropin result: a 10-year cohort study. Lancet 358:861–865

24. Walsh JP, Bremner AP, Bulsara MK et al (2005) Subclinical thyroid dysfunction as a risk factor for cardiovascular disease. Arch Intern Med 165:2467–2472

25. Ochs N, Auer R, Bauer DC et al (2008) Meta-analysis: subclinical thyroid dysfunction and the risk for coronary heart disease and mortality. Ann Intern Med 148:832–845

26. Imaizumi M, Akahoshi M, Ichimaru S et al (2004) Risk for ischemic heart disease and all-cause mortality in subclin-ical hypothyroidism. J Clin Endocrinol Metab 89:3365–3370

27. Gussekloo J, van Exel E, de Craen AJ et al (2004) Thyroid status, disability and cognitive function, and survival in old age. JAMA 292:2591–2599

28. Cooper DS (2004) Thyroid disease in the oldest old: the exception to the rule. JAMA 292:2651–2654

29. Aho K, Gordin A, Palosuo T et al (1984) Thyroid autoimmunity and cardiovascular diseases. Eur Heart J 5:43–46

30. Bauer DC, Rodondi N, Stone KL, Hillier TA (2007) Thyroid hormone use, hyperthyroidism and mortality in older women. Am J Med 120:343–349

31. Åsvold BO, Bjøro T, Nilsen TIL et al (2008) Thyrotropin levels and risk of fatal coronary heart disease: The HUNT Study. Arch Intern Med 168:855–860

32. Auer R, Rodondi N (2008) Thyrotropin levels and coronary heart disease mortality [letter]. Arch Intern Med 168:2498–2499; author reply 2499

33. Ladenson PW (2008) Cardiovascular consequences of subclinical thyroid dysfunction: more smoke but no fire. Ann Intern Med 148:880–881

Low Triiodothyronine Syndrome as a Powerful Predictor of Death in Heart Failure

16

Giorgio Iervasi, Laura Sabatino and Giuseppina Nicolini

Abstract Thyroid hormone (TH) has a critical role in cardiovascular homeostasis under both physiological and pathological conditions. THs, in particular the biologically active triiodothyronine (T_3), modulate cardiac contractility, heart rate, diastolic function, and systemic vascular resistance through genomic, and nongenomic-mediated effects. In heart failure (HF), the main alteration of thyroid function is referred to as "low-T_3 syndrome," characterized by a reduction in serum T_3 with normal levels of thyroxine (T_4) and thyrotropin (thyroid-stimulating hormone, TSH). This syndrome, which affects approximately one-third of patients with more severe HF, is commonly interpreted as an adaptive factor minimizing the catabolic phenomena of illness. However, this interpretative hypothesis is now questioned: experimental data have shown potential negative effects of the low-T_3 state in the progressive deterioration of cardiac function and myocardial remodeling in HF. In addition, prognostic studies have shown that T_3 levels are a strong predictor of mortality in HF patients, also adding prognostic power to conventional cardiac parameters. All these data, together with the evidence of some benefit of administration of synthetic THs administration to HF patients in pilot studies, indicate that placebo-controlled prospective studies are now needed in order to better define the safety and prognostic effects of long-term treatment with synthetic THs in HF.

Keywords Thyroid hormones • Low-T_3 syndrome • Mild hypothyroidism • Cardiovascular effects • Heart failure • Prognosis and survival

16.1 Introduction

Nearly 10 million people in the United States and Europe suffer from chronic heart failure (HF), and 1 million patients are diagnosed with HF each year. HF represents a major public healthcare and economic problem in Western countries, being one of the principal causes of morbidity, mortality, and hospitalization. Also, chronic HF is one of the most common reasons for general practitioner consultations by people 65–70 years old. The population-based cohort Rotterdam Study of 7,983 participants showed that survival after diagnosis was 63% at 1 year, 51% at 2 years, and 35% at 5 years [1].

Neuroendocrine activation is important in the progression of HF, and inhibition of neurohormones has long-term benefit in terms of mortality and morbidity. Experimental and clinical findings strongly support the concept that thyroid hormone (TH) also

G. Iervasi (✉)
C.N.R. Clinical Physiology Institute, S. Cataldo Research Campus, Pisa, Italy

G. Iervasi, A. Pingitore (eds.), *Thyroid and Heart Failure*.
© Springer-Verlag Italia 2009

plays a fundamental role in cardiovascular homeostasis. In HF, the main and earliest alteration of thyroid function is what is referred to as "low-T$_3$ syndrome," which is characterized by a reduction in serum total triiodothyronine (T$_3$) and free T$_3$ with normal levels of thyroxine (T$_4$) and thyrotropin (thyroid-stimulating hormone, TSH). This syndrome, which may affect one-third of patients with advanced HF (corresponding to 1 million people living in the United States and Europe), is conventionally regarded as an adaptive mechanism reducing the catabolic processes of illness. However, in recent years this interpretative model has been widely debated. The principal goal of the present chapter is to review the main pathophysiological and clinical links between altered thyroid metabolism and HF during the progression from organ-specific (i.e., cardiovascular) disease to systemic disorder.

16.2 Cardiovascular Actions of Thyroid Hormone: Cellular, Neurohumoral, and Hemodynamic Effects

Whatever its initial cause, HF represents progressive structural and functional derangement of the cardiovascular system, mainly mediated by persistent, toxic activation of sodium-retaining, vasoconstrictive neuroendocrine systems and of proinflammatory cytokines. The natural consequence is that the evolution and prognosis of HF is closely dependent on the derangement of neurohumoral systems. TH significantly and directly affects both cardiovascular- and neuroendocrine-related systems. A convincing argument in favor of a pathophysiological relationship between the progression of HF and the appearance of a hypothyroid-like state secondary to a reduction in the biologically active hormone T$_3$ should be founded on evidence of molecular, cellular, and neurohumoral actions resulting from a TH defect able to induce an HF-like state.

16.2.1 Physiology of the Thyroid System: General Aspects

The thyroid gland secretes just a small amount (4–6 μg/day) of T$_3$ [2]. In humans, most T$_3$ (nearly 20–25 μg/day) derives from conversion in peripheral tissues from the prohormone T$_4$, which is uniquely

secreted by the thyroid [2]. For the conversion of T$_4$ into T$_3$, two iodothyronine 5′-monodeiodinases have been identified: type 1, also termed D1, and type 2, also termed D2. A third monodeiodinase, type 3 (D3), catalyzes the inactivation pathway of T$_4$ by generating the biologically inactive hormone reverse T$_3$ (rT$_3$) [3]. The deiodinative pattern, taken as a whole, constitutes the principal homeostatic system that controls circulating and intracellular concentrations of the active form T$_3$ in the body's various peripheral districts. By an extreme simplification we can say that type 1 deiodinase is the major source of circulating T$_3$ and type 2 deiodinase is responsible for the local production of T$_3$ in the tissues [4]. However, more recent data seem to support the hypothesis that D2 is responsible for the production of significant amounts of circulating T$_3$, at least in humans [5].

The major actions of TH are the result of the interaction of T$_3$ with its specific nuclear receptor (TR). In humans, two TR isoforms, TRα and TRβ, have been described, both of which bind T$_3$ and mediate TH-regulated gene expression.

Although most of the effects of TH are nuclear-mediated, there is clear evidence of additional, nongenomic, rapid (seconds or minutes) actions of T$_3$ and T$_4$ [6]. The signal transduction pathways modulated by TH include cell-surface G-protein-coupled receptors and activation of the mitogen-activated protein kinase (MAPK) cascade or P13 kinase. Nongenomic and genomic actions of TH may interface, as documented by TH-induced activation of the MAPK pathway that promotes translocation to the nucleus of serine phosphorylated TRβ1. Effects of TH on the mitochondria may also be included as extranuclear actions of the hormone, although THs also have been documented to regulate some gene expression in the mitochondria, including those involved in ATP turnover.

16.2.2 Cardiac Effects of Thyroid Hormone

Thyroid hormone regulates various cardiac structural and functional proteins, as extensively discussed in other chapters. T$_3$ signaling is critical for proper heart function, regulating the expression of the myosin heavy chain isoforms α-MHC and β-MHC by increasing the expression of the former and decreasing that of the latter [7]. Moreover, T$_3$ stimulates nearly all of the enzyme systems involved in Ca^{2+} and ion flux. In adults, SERCA2 is responsible for cytosolic Ca^{2+} homeostasis by regulating the amount of Ca^{2+} released during each cardiac cycle. Phospholamban inhibits SERCA2 through a decrease in its affinity for Ca^{2+} [8]. Thyroid hormone stimulates SERCA2 [9] and inhibits phospholamban, so that the ratio of phospholamban to Ca^{2+}-ATPase is higher in hypothyroid hearts. TH also exerts important effects on the electrophysiological properties of cardiac myocytes [10–12]; in particular, TH shares the regulation of voltage-gated potassium channels at the molecular level.

Ventricular remodeling is a critical process in the development and progression of HF. An interesting potential link between the cardiac phenotype observed in HF and the cardiac hypothyroid state is the so-called fetal gene recapitulation, a pattern characterized by an increase in β-MHC and phospholamban and a decrease in α-MHC and SERCA2 [13]. A fetal gene program is activated in failing human hearts; a hypothyroid state induces in the heart a fetal gene program that is similar in pattern to the one seen in HF, and that is reversible with TH treatment. In a rat model of starvation-induced low-T_3 syndrome, cardiac α-MHC mRNA content was significantly reduced compared with controls, the decline being linearly related to the decrease in serum T_3 [14]. Systolic and diastolic left ventricular function was impaired, as demonstrated by the reduction of both $+dP/dt$ and the mean left ventricular relaxation time. Importantly, supplementation with synthetic L-T_3 normalized the α-MHC isoform and SERCA2 contents, despite persistent food restriction, improved systolic and diastolic heart performance. These results are in line with those described by Ladenson et al. in a case report of a young man with dilated cardiomyopathy and hypothyroidism; in this patient, the restoration of euthyroidism resulted in a gradual and substantial improvement in the ventricular ejection fraction and functional capacity, accompanied by an 11-fold increase in ventricular α-MHC mRNA levels [15].

In addition, the importance for ventricular geometry and mechanical function of the extracellular matrix in maintaining myocyte alignment has been increasingly recognized [16, 17]. Metalloproteinases regulate the turnover of myocardial extracellular matrix proteins. Accumulating experimental evidence indicates an important role for the reduced activity of matrix metalloproteinases in the patho-

genesis and progression of left ventricular dysfunction. TH seems to play a key role in the regulation of metalloproteinases; the administration of L-T_3 in rats is accompanied by an increase in serum and left ventricular metalloproteinase action and, consequently, by a reduction of extracellular matrix [18].

16.2.3 Vascular Effects of Thyroid Hormone: General Aspects

TH markedly affects the peripheral vascular tone [19]. Administration of synthetic TH is followed by a rapid reduction in peripheral vascular resistance [20, 21]; this effect is secondary either to local release of vasodilators, which follows the increased metabolic activity and oxygen consumption induced by the hormone, or to a direct effect of TH on vascular smooth muscle (VSM) cells [22].

Both T_3 and T_4 have vasodilatory effects, those of the former being more prominent than those of the latter. At present, however, the multiple mechanisms by which TH per se influences the peripheral vasculature have not been fully explained. The endothelium is likely a pressure sensor, secreting factors with vasodilatory action and modulating responsiveness to counteracting vasoconstrictors. THs may modulate VSM tone through the synthesis and release of endothelium-derived relaxing molecules such as nitric oxide (NO) and of unidentified diffusible endothelium-derived hyperpolarizing factors (EDHF) that act via the opening of potassium channels. THs interact directly with VSM cells of isolated rabbit mesenteric artery, causing dilation [23]; in particular, T_4 was found to be more potent than T_3 in inducing vascular relaxation in rat mesenteric resistance vessels [24]. Moreover, in vitro studies demonstrated that exposure to T_3 of VSM cells isolated from rat aorta caused these cells to relax rapidly. This effect was independent of cyclic adenosine monophosphate (cAMP) and NO formation [21]. Indeed, primary cultures of vascular endothelial cells exposed to T_3 do not show NO production, indicating that T_3 interacts directly with VSM cells to cause relaxation. In rat skeletal muscle resistance arteries, T_3 is more effective than T_4 in inducing vasodilation [25]. This dilation appears to have both endothelium-dependent and endothelium-independent components because T_3 dilation was attenuated by N^G- nitro-L-arginine, indomethacin, and glibenclamide. Analysis of all the cited studies highlights a wide variety of somewhat contrasting data that prevents the drawing of definitive conclusions; however, the different methods and experimental approaches adopted may partially explain the disparate results reported on the vascular effects of THs.

An additional remark is that, in hypothyroid rats, renal sensitivity to endothelium-dependent and NO-mediated vasodilators is also diminished; the decreased responsiveness to vasodilation in renal vessels may partially explain the observed increase in total vascular resistance in the presence of a hypothyroid state [26]. The impaired water excretion occurring in hypothyroidism may thus reflect the alteration in renal plasma flow and glomerular filtration rate secondary to increased systemic resistance and generalized vascular contraction together with a reduced cardiac output, all of which are corrected by substitution treatment with synthetic TH.

16.2.4 Effects of Thyroid Hormone on Myocardial Flow

A reduction of vasomotor tone induced by THs has also been documented in the coronary arteries. A direct, dose-dependent effect of THs within a few seconds of administration has been described in rat coronary arteries, suggesting a nongenomic mechanism of vasodilating action of the hormone that is independent of cAMP, guanosine monophosphate (GMP), or NO generation [27]. A coronary vasodilator effect of TH has been observed in various animal models, e.g., after hypothermic global ischemia in an ex vivo canine heart, in in vivo anesthetized rabbit and rat models, and in an ischemia–reperfusion isolated rat heart model [27–30]. Notably, the vasodilatory effects of T_3 in the heart occur only in the ventricles, not in the atria [30].

An important additional finding is that type 2 deiodinase is expressed in cultured human coronary artery cells and human aortic cells [31]. The presence of D2, which represents the main enzyme involved in the local supply of biologically active T_3 from the conversion of T_4, suggests that VSM cells are indeed potential physiological targets for the action of THs [21, 31]. Moreover, the identification of different TR mRNA isoforms in vascular cells points to a classic genomic action of T_3 [31]. Based on the above finding, it is plausible to postulate that, besides the nongenomic effects of T_3 on vascular tone, the hormone may modulate VSM cell contractility by regulating the cellular phenotype through classic nuclear transcription mechanisms.

16.2.5 Microcirculatory Effects of Thyroid Hormones

Until now, very few studies have been carried out to investigate the in vivo role of THs on the microcirculation. Recent data from our laboratory have shown that T_3 causes a dose-dependent dilation of hamster cheek pouch arterioles within a few minutes of its administration [32]. Arteriolar relaxation is abolished by NO synthase (NOS) inhibition, indicating a correlation between T_3-induced dilation and NOS activation. NO is known to activate a soluble guanylate cyclase in neighboring cells that leads to an increase in cGMP, inducing the relaxation of VSM [21, 33]. These results support the hypothesis that NO is the main factor in T_3-induced arteriolar dilation in vivo, at least in experimental animal models. Interestingly, the same studies demonstrated that T_4 causes arteriolar dilation, but the time to dilation was significantly different for T_4 and T_3. Moreover, the effect of T_4 was abolished by iopanoic acid, which inhibits both type 1 and type 2 deiodinase, indicating that local conversion of T_4 to T_3 is crucial for the dilation induced by THs. Conversely, local application of propylthiouracil (PTU), an elective inhibitor of type 1 deiodinase, does not change the vascular response to T_4. Taken together, these results suggest that local T_4-to-T_3 conversion plays an important physiological role in the dilation induced by THs in the microcirculation in vivo and in the regulation of T_3-mediated vascular tone.

16.2.6 Thyroid Hormone and Neuroendocrine Systems: How Do the Two Systems Cross-Talk?

TH produces marked neuroendocrine responses. Low thyroid function can influence many of the neurohumoral systems involved in vascular tone and plasma volume regulation. In particular, TH modulates the sympathetic and plasma renin-angiotensin-aldosterone systems, and activates natriuretic peptide transcription and synthesis. Plasma levels of TH appear to be directly correlated with renin activity and plasma levels of angiotensin II and aldosterone [34, 35]. Patients with chronic hypothyroidism show enhanced sympathetic activity that may contribute significantly to peripheral vasoconstriction; the increased sympathetic efflux may overcome a down-regulation of postsynaptic vasoconstrictor α-adrenoceptors, which is described in hypothyroid states. This is at variance with what is observed in normal physiology, in which a positive relationship exists between TH and the number and activity of noradrenergic receptors.

The number and function of vasodilatory β-adrenoceptors are also reduced in hypothyroidism and represents a major cause of the decrease in renin secretion together with a reduction in liver angiotensinogen production. Hypothyroidism may reduce plasma angiotensinogen by 71%, plasma renin activity by 73%, and plasma angiotensin II by 81%, at least in rats [34]. Inhibition of the renin–angiotensin system could lead to significant vasodilation, volume depletion, and hypotension if not sufficiently compensated by the activation of opposite pressor and salt-retentive systems. As a matter of fact, T_3 deprivation, besides increasing sympathetic efflux, may release the normal inhibition of vasopressin induced by TH, thus favoring vasoconstriction and maintaining intravascular volume. Interestingly, despite the reduction in angiotensin II levels, plasma aldosterone is frequently found to be normal or even increased in hypothyroidism [36]; this fact could be in keeping with either an adrenal supersensitivity to angiotensin II, as in some forms of low-renin, salt-sensitive hypertension, or reduced renal clearance. TH also causes significant changes in angiotensin receptor density, especially in the angiotensin II subtype: angiotensin II subtype density increased by 168% in hypothyroid rats [34]. Angiotensin II plays an important role in the control of cardiomyocyte growth, hypertrophy, and fibrosis. The increase in angiotensin II receptor gene expression, as documented in hypothyroid rats, may thus represent an additional mechanism favoring regression to the fetal gene program, which is induced by low circulating levels of THs [37, 38].

Finally, hypothyroidism down-regulates the activity of cardiac natriuretic peptides at the level of vascular, glomerular, and tubular receptors by decreasing receptor effects on vasodilation and natriuresis. The net effect of all these neuroendocrine actions, coupled with the lack of direct

T_3-dependent vasodilation, produces an increase in vascular resistance. At the kidney level, this may lead to a decrease in glomerular filtration and medullary flow rate with impairment of glomerular–tubular balance and increase in sodium reabsorption, both corrected by hormonal replacement therapy [39]. Interesting pathophysiological data on the relationships between thyroid function and neuroendocrine aspects in the absence of cardiovascular disease have been derived from a human model of acute severe hypothyroidism secondary to total thyroidectomy [40]. The main finding of the study was that hypothyroidism induced an increase in blood pressure levels, particularly diastolic, reversible with TH replacement therapy. Importantly, in the hypothyroid state, mean values for plasma catecholamines were in the upper normal range. Norepinephrine decreased significantly as well as epinephrine, although to a lesser degree of significance, during L-T_4 treatment. In addition, mean aldosterone and cortisol levels were significantly higher then the corresponding values measured under L-T_4 therapy. Overall, the data indicate that sympathoadrenal stimulation is observed during acute hypothyroidism, as a possible mechanism counteracting the concomitant, hypothyroid-induced decrease in myocardial inotropism and cardiac output. An important proof in favor of a direct action of THs on the neuroendocrine system in HF is derived from a recent placebo-controlled study from our group that will be extensively discussed in Chapter 20. Ten patients with cardiopathy who had low T_3 levels underwent 3-day synthetic L-T_3 infusion. After administration of T_3, plasma norepinephrine, N-terminal pro B-type natriuretic peptide (NT-proBNP), and aldosterone significantly decreased. This preliminary result clearly indicates that, in cardiomyopathic conditions, short-term L-T_3 replacement therapy also significantly improves the neuroendocrine profile.

16.2.7 Hemodynamic Effects of Thyroid Hormone

When overall genomic and nongenomic cellular effects of TH on the heart and vascular system are considered, it is not surprising that these hormones play a pivotal role in ardiovascular homeostasis and whole, body performance. To use a forced simplification, the cardiovascular system is comparable to a mechanical, central pump (heart) and a system of ducts (vessels) that generate and maintain pressure gradients among various circulatory districts in order to guarantee a capillary flow that is proportional to tissue needs. Cardiac output is the volume of blood ejected by the heart per unit time and is defined as the product of the stroke volume and the heart rate. Cardiac output may increase dependent on an increase in diastolic filling volume (the so-called Sterling mechanism) and/or a reduction in end-systolic volume secondary to increased inotropism. Peripheral resistance can be defined as the ratio between the pressure fall and the flow throughout a vascular segment.

Both diastolic and systolic functions, which depend closely on the relaxation and contractile properties of the heart, respectively, are clearly influenced by TH [19, 41, 42]. Furthermore ventricular contractile function is significantly influenced by changes in hemodynamic conditions secondary to the TH-induced reduction in peripheral vascular tone. The observed rapid changes in systolic pump efficiency after TH administration strongly depend on central and peripheral hormonal effects that act synergetically to improve systolic performance. The final hemodynamic result is that TH homeostasis preserves a positive ventricle-arterial coupling, thus leading to a more favorable balance for heart work [19]. Replacement doses of TH in patients with HF and low T_3 syndrome appear to induce a decrease in afterload without changing either systolic pressure or heart rate, with a consequent increase in left ventricular performance in the absence of a parallel increase in external cardiac work and myocardial oxygen consumption [43].

The importance of TH in maintaining cardiovascular homeostasis is also deducible from data showing that mild forms of TH abnormalities, e.g., subclinical hypothyroidism, alter cardiovascular function significantly [44]. In 30 female patients with a first diagnosis of subclinical hypothyroidism and without other concomitant diseases, a reduced end-diastolic left ventricular volume (decreased preload) and increased systemic vascular resistance (increased afterload), leading to impairment of cardiac pump performance, were observed [44]. The resulting worsening in cardiac pump efficiency was due to the reduction of stroke volume, and cardiac output, because heart rate was unaffected. Importantly, all these altered parameters normalized after TH replacement therapy. Even more interest-

ing is the good relationship found between TSH, as the best biochemical marker of whole-body thyroid hypofunction, and the parameters of systolic left ventricular performance [44]. All the data, taken together, indicate that changes in preload and afterload are a reasonable explanation for the documented decrease in systolic pump performance observed in subclinical hypothyroidism, without the need to invoke simultaneous impairment in myocardial inotropic function.

In the intact organism, the cardiovascular system is responsible for all O_2 exchanges and total renewal of the body's metabolic products. Energy expenditure may be another parameter under TH control, potentially affecting hemodynamics. TH is known to modulate tissue metabolic demands, oxygen consumption, and heat production. On the basis of these considerations, it is conceivable that some hemodynamic adjustments (e.g., cardiac output and vascular changes) also follow primary modifications in metabolic demand. In this context, the decrease in cardiac output and increase in peripheral arterial resistance and diastolic blood pressure of the hypothyroid state may be interpreted as the final result of an adaptive response to the reduction in tissue metabolic activities.

16.3 Mild Thyroid Hypofunction and Heart Failure Evolution: A "Total Body" Pathophysiological Interpretative Model

The negative effects on the cardiovascular system observed during the evolution of HF and potentially ascribed to a low T_3 state cannot be explained solely by the adverse effects of mild thyroid hypofunction on cardiac inotropism and peripheral vascular resistance. The loss of euthyroid status affects virtually all physiological systems, including the central nervous system and musculoskeletal apparatus. In particular, psychological depression and worsening of exercise capacity, both contributing to a deterioration in quality of life that parallels the reduction in cardiovascular performance, may be in part the direct negative consequence of a reduction in biologically active T_3 [45, 46]. A low T_3 state may thus significantly participate via a variety of multiorgan mechanisms to the progression of HF towards a systemic disorder with a poor prognosis (Fig. 16.1).

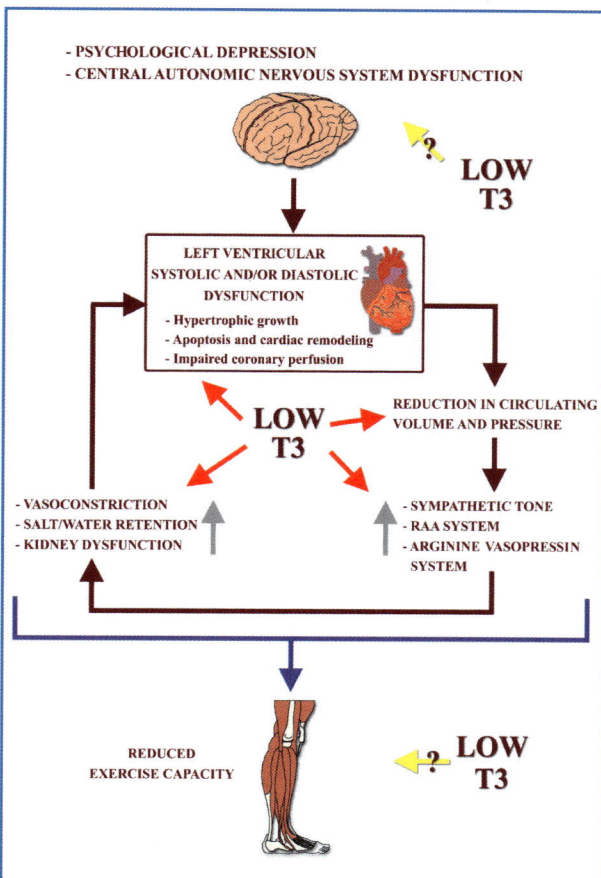

Fig. 16.1 Possible multiorgan negative effects of a low-T₃ state, favoring progression of heart failure and worsening of patient quality of life. *Yellow arrows* indicate a not yet well-documented but probable negative effect. *Red arrows* indicate an already documented or very likely negative effect

16.4 Thyroid Hormones in Heart Failure: Clinical Evidence

A low T_3 state is not a rare finding in patients with HF [42] and has been noted in 20–30% of patients with dilated cardiomyopathy [47–49]. The incidence of low T_3 syndrome correlates with clinical status, with a significantly higher incidence in patients in NYHA functional classes III–IV than in those in NYHA I–II [48, 50]. A strong association between the reduction in biologically active T_3 and mortality was clearly documented in a large unselected population of hospitalized cardiac patients [51]. At present, the concept that altered thyroid metabolism contributes to progression of HF is mainly supported by five clinical observational studies [47–49, 52, 53] all showing the important

role of a low T_3 state in the prognostic stratification of patients with HF (Table 16.1).

In the above-cited studies, the altered thyroid metabolism was assessed by means of various parameters indicating disturbed T_4 peripheral conversion, such as a reduction in circulating levels of T_3 [49, 48, 53], a low free T_3 index/reverse T_3 ratio [47], and a low free T_3/free T_4 ratio in serum [52]. Irrespective of the parameter used, all these studies showed that an altered peripheral TH pathway was in every case associated with a high incidence of fatal events (cardiac or cumulative death). The study of Hamilton et al. [47] is particularly important because it was the first clinical study that tried to correlate the progression of HF with thyroid status; in that study it was shown that a low free T_3 index/reverse T_3 ratio was associated with a poor outcome in 84 inpatients with advanced congestive HF. Similar results were documented in the study of Opasich et al. [48], in which 199 cardiomyopathic patients with moderate to severe HF hospitalized for assessment of cardiac transplantation were enrolled. The incidence of cardiac death was significantly higher in patients with low T_3 syndrome than in those without (48% vs. 21%, respectively). The results of more recent study by Kozdag et al. [52], which enrolled 111 in patients with ischemic and nonischemic dilated cardiomyopathy, confirmed the relatively higher probability of cardiac death in patients with a low free T_3/free T_4 ratio (cut-off value ≤ 1.7). This altered thyroid pattern also correlated with a worse diastolic function, identified as a restrictive type of diastolic filling. In a study from our group that enrolled 281 inpatients with nonischemic and ischemic HF, total T_3 and left ventricular ejection fraction were found to be the only independent predictive variables of both cardiac and cumulative death (Tables 16.2 and 16.3) [53]. Moreover, mortality rate was significantly affected by the presence of a low T_3 state as documented by the time course of the Kaplan–Meier curves (Fig. 16.2). Using the best cut-off value of 0.20 for left ventricular ejection fraction, as assessed by ROC curve (sensitivity = 31%, specificity = 84%), in combination with the lower limit of the normal range of total T_3 (80 ng/dl), four subgroups of patients were identified. The survival of patients with reduced left ventricular ejection fraction and total T_3 was lower than that of patients with a similar ejection fraction but normal total T_3, thus showing the power of total T_3 concentration in discrimi-

Table 16.1 Main results from observational studies on the relationship between thyroid state and prognosis in patients with heart failure

Authors, year	Patients	Parameter	Follow-up	Main reported results	Survival
Hamilton et al. 1990 [47]	ACHF $n = 84$	FT$_3$ index/rT$_3$ ratio	7.3±6.6[a] months	FT$_3$I/rT$_3$ ratio (>4)	100%
				FT$_3$I/rT$_3$ ratio (≤ 4)	37%
Opasich et al. 1996 [48]	DCMP $n = 199$	TT$_3$	417 ± 259 days	Normal T$_3$, low T$_3$	79%
					52%
Kozdag et al. 2005 [52]	DCMP $n = 111$	FT$_3$/FT$_4$ ratio	12 ± 8 months	FT$_3$/FT$_4$ (> 1.7) specificity	71%
				FT$_3$/FT$_4$ (≤ 1.7) sensitivity	100%
Pingitore et al. 2005 [49]	DCMP $n = 281$	TT$_3$/FT$_3$ LVEF	12 ± 7 months	Normal T$_3$ and LVEF(> 20%)	90%
				Normal T$_3$ and LVEF(< 20%)	83%
				Low TT$_3$ and LVEF(> 20%)	73%
				Low T$_3$ and LVEF(< 20%)	61%
Passino et al. 2008 [53]	HF $n = 442$	FT$_3$/BNP	36 months (median)	Low BNP, normal FT$_3$	84%
				Low T$_3$, low BNP	69%
				High BNP, normal FT$_3$	60%
				High BNP, low FT$_3$	28%

[a] Mean ± SD

ACHF advanced congestive heart failure, *FT$_3$* free T$_3$, *rT$_3$* reverse T$_3$, *DCMP* dilated cardiomyopathy, *TT$_3$* total T$_3$, *LVEF* left ventricular ejection fraction, *HF* heart failure, *BNP* brain natriuretic peptide

Table 16.2 Univariate and multivariate logistic regression analysis for cardiac death in patients with heart failure. (Experimental data from [49])

Variables[a]	Odds ratio	95% CI	p value
Univariate regression			
sex	3.3	1.2–8.7	0.02
ejection fraction	0.6	0.4–0.8	0.002
end-diastolic diameter	1.5	1.1–2.0	0.02
total T$_3$	0.7	0.5–0.9	0.004
Multivariate regression			
sex	3.0	1.0–8.4	0.04
total T$_3$	0.6	0.5–0.8	0.003
ejection fraction	0.6	0.4–0.9	0.03

[a] Only variables found to be significant are listed

Table 16.3 Univariate and multivariate logistic regression analysis for cumulative death in patients with heart failure. (Experimental data from [49])

Variables[a]	Odds ratio	95% CI	p value
Univariate regression			
age	1.4	1.0–1.9	0.04
ejection fraction	0.6	0.4–0.8	< 0.001
end-diastolic diameter	1.5	1.1–1.9	0.01
total T$_3$	0.5	0.4–0.67	< 0.001
free T$_3$	0.7	0.5–0.9	0.005
β-Blockers	0.5	0.2–0.9	0.04
Obesity	0.4	0.2–0.8	0.01
NYHA	1.3	1.1–1.6	0.006
Multivariate regression			
total T$_3$	0.5	0.4–0.7	< 0.001
ejection fraction	0.5	0.4–0.8	< 0.001

[a] Only variables found to be significant are listed

nating patients at very high risk of death. These findings well fit the common clinical observation of different outcomes in patients with similar but severely impaired left ventricular ejection fraction.

All the above mentioned results, taken as whole, clearly indicate that a low T$_3$ state is not a mere surrogate of other, more powerful indicators of poor outcome, such as left ventricular ejection fraction. In addition, in this era of cost-effectiveness and of highly technological and expensive clinical proce-dures, it is well worth also looking for accessible, low-cost instruments that can facilitate diagnostic and/or prognostic decision-making. Total (or free) T$_3$ measurement is an easily interpretable, simple, and reliable blood test, technically undemanding, very inexpensive, and accessible to all medical centers [54], unlike most of the known biohumoral

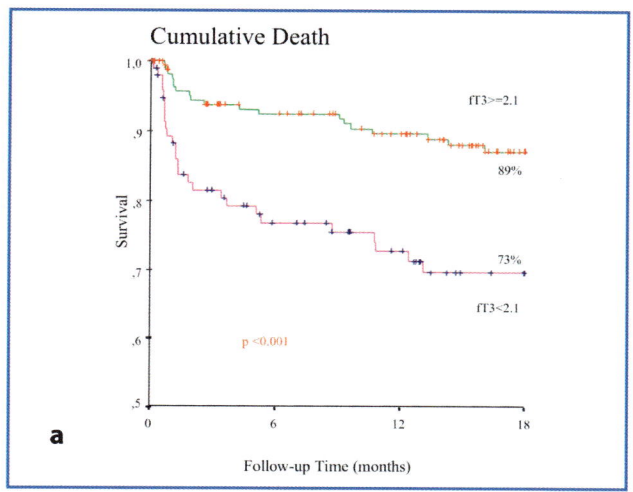
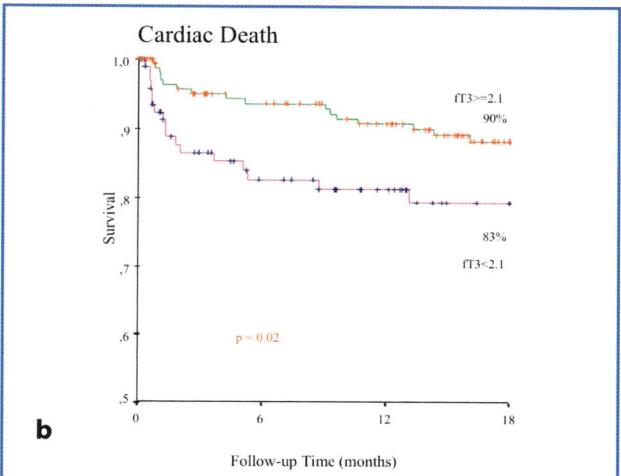

Fig. 16.2 Kaplan-Meier survival curves of patients with a low-T_3 state ($n = 103$) versus those with normal T_3 levels ($n = 178$): cumulative death (**a**) and cardiac death (**b**). (Experimental data from [49])

markers of HF. Results from the previous study by our group [49] have been significantly reinforced by very recent additional findings [53] on 442 patients. A low free T_3 concentration independently predicts a worse outcome, especially in those patients with higher brain natriuretic peptide (BNP) concentration. Both free T_3 and BNP, together with NYHA classification, were shown to be independent predictors of cardiac mortality among a wide range of clinical variables. The additive prognostic power of free T_3 measurement was highlighted by the analysis of the survival curve of those patients with combined high BNP and low free T_3, who showed the highest mortality (28%), and the survival curve of those with combined low BNP and normal free T_3, who showed the lowest mortality (84%), and by the observation that a low free T_3 value was able to identify higher risk of death in patients with relatively low BNP.

From an interpretative point of view, the occurrence of low T_3 syndrome may be considered the final result of a progressive impairment of TH peripheral metabolism, which begins in the early stages of cardiac dysfunction. In a human model of disease, as represented by asymptomatic or mildly symptomatic patients with idiopathic dilated cardiomyopathy, signals of altered TH metabolism were particularly found in patients with more depressed left ventricular function and early symptoms of HF [55]. In that study, circulating T_3 was broadly but significantly correlated with left ventricular ejection fraction; also, it was the only inde-

pendent biohumoral predictor of clinical symptoms, whereas BNP was the most important predictor of left ventricular dysfunction. By considering the values for left ventricular ejection fraction and NYHA functional class, natriuretic peptides (i.e., BNP and artrial natriuretic peptide) were found to be more related to worsened left ventricular dysfunction only, whereas T_3/T_4 ratio – as a rough but valid clinical index of T_4 peripheral conversion – was found to be more related to the combination of left ventricular dysfunction and early appearance of clinical symptoms of HF. These results, when analyzed together with the previous findings of other authors showing a higher incidence of low T_3 syndrome in patients with overt HF [47–49], would suggest a continuous relationship between progression of left ventricular impairment, presence of symptoms of HF of whatever origin, and progression of an altered peripheral TH metabolism. Progressive T_3 reduction and the occurrence of a "true" low T_3 syndrome may represent two consecutive steps of the same process. In an early phase, when left ventricular dysfunction is still not associated with overt symptoms and full activation of the neuroendocrine vasoactive sodium-retaining systems, T_3 is predominantly related to cardiac function and can thus be considered a marker of cardiac impairment. Conversely, when cardiac disease progresses toward overt HF, and the occurrence of true low T_3 syndrome increases over time, T_3 concentrations are not yet related to cardiac dysfunction [49] but instead represent a marker of multisystem involvement and thus an important prognostic predictor of death [47–49, 52, 53]. Subclinical mild primary hypothyroidism, characterized by increased thyrotropin levels in the presence of normal values of free TH₃, has also been linked to increased mortality in patients with diagnosed ischemic or nonischemic cardiac disease. Unlike low T₃ syndrome, which can be considered a disorder of peripheral thyroid metabolism developing progressively during the evolution of several systemic diseases, subclinical primary hypothyroidism is a disorder of the thyroid gland. In the large prospective observational study cited above [56], survival time was significantly lower in subclinical hypothyroidism than in euthyroid patients when cardiac and cumulative deaths were considered. The observed negative prognostic impact of any form of mild thyroid hypofunction in cardiac patients suggests that a normal thyroid status is essential for maintaining systemic and cardiovascular homeostasis [19, 41]; when a normal thyroid status is persistently lost, increased whole-body and cardiovascular vulnerability is observed.

However, demonstrating causality is much more difficult than demonstrating an association, and additional findings are necessary to investigate this important issue and to yield more conclusive information.

Pathophysiological studies in animals and humans are needed to better define the potential role of altered thyroid metabolism, as observed throughout the evolution of HF. Large, multicenter, placebo-controlled prospective studies could provide information on the safety and prognostic effects of long-term treatment with synthetic TH or TH analogues. Important issues should be a clear definition of primary and secondary end points (mortality, hospitalization, quality of life, side effects, etc.) as well as type, dosage, and schedule of treatment.

Moreover, the finding of D2 (and D3) gene expression in the cardiovascular system implies a sophisticated mechanism of local bioavailability of TH and opens the way to potentially interesting therapeutic perspectives involving novel molecular and pharmacological strategies in the treatment of HF.

16.5 Conclusions

Emerging experimental and clinical observations seem to indicate the close link between a low T₃ state and the evolution and prognosis of HF.

Acknowledgments The authors wish to thank Maria Scarlattini for her technical support in the experimental work cited here and to Laura Mazza and Giuliano Kraft for their professional contribution to the revision of the manuscript.

Key Points

- Signaling of biologically active thyroid hormone T₃ is critical for proper heart and vascular function.

- In heart failure, the main and earliest alteration of thyroid function is referred to as "low T₃ syndrome" and is characterized by a reduction in serum T₃ but with normal levels of T₄ and TSH.

- Low T₃ syndrome is found in 20–30% of patients with dilated cardiomyopathy. The incidence of correlates with clinical status.

- A low T₃ state may play a significant role, through a variety of multiorgan mechanisms, in the progression of heart failure towards a systemic and prognostically unfavorable disorder.

- The concept that altered thyroid metabolism contributes to progression of heart failure in humans is supported by observational studies showing the association of a low T₃ state with a high incidence of fatal events.

References

1. Bleumink GS, Knetsch AM, Sturkenboom MC et al (2004) Quantifying the heart failure epidemic: prevalence, incidence rate, lifetime risk and prognosis of heart failure The Rotterdam Study. Eur Heart J 25:1614–1619

2. Pilo A, Iervasi G, Vitek F et al (1990) Thyroidal and peripheral production of 3,5,3¢-triiodothyronine in humans by mental analysis. Am J Physiol 258:E715–726

3. Bianco AC, Salvatore D, Gereben B et al (2002) Biochemistry cellular and molecular biology, and physiological roles of the iodothyronine selenodeiodinases. Endocr Rev 23:38–89

4. Croteau W, Davey JC, Galton VA et al (1996) Cloning of the mammalian type II iodothyronine deiodinase. A selenoprotein differentially expressed and regulated in human and rat brain and other tissues. J Clin Invest 98:405–417

5. Maia AL, Kim BW, Huang SA et al (2005) Type 2 iodothyronine deiodinase is the major source of plasma T3 in euthyroid humans. J Clin Invest 115:2524–2533

6. Davis PJ, Davis FB (2002) Nongenomic actions of thyroid hormone on the heart [review]. Thyroid 12:459–466

7. Dillmann WH, Barrieux A, Shanker R (1989) Influence of thyroid hormone on myosin heavy chain mRNA and other messenger RNAs in the rat heart. Endocr Res 15:565–577

8. Koss KL, Kranias EG (1996) Phospholamban: a prominent regulator of myocardial contractility. Circ Res 79:1059–1063

9. Kiss, E, Jakab G, Kranias EG et al (1994) Thyroid hormone-induced alterations in phospholamban protein expression. Regulatory effects on sarcoplasmic reticulum Ca2+ transport and myocardial relaxation. Circ Res 75:245–251

10. Shimoni, Y, Severson D, Giles W (1995) Thyroid status and potassium currents in rat ventricular myocytes. Am J Physiol 268:H576–H583

11. Guo, W, Kamiya K, Hojo M et al (1998) Regulation of Kv4.2 and Kv1.4 K+ channel expression by myocardial hypertrophic factors in cultured newborn rat ventricular cells. J Mol Cell Cardiol 30:1449–1455

12. Bosch RF, Wang Z, Li GR et al (1999) Electrophysiological mechanisms by which hypothyroidism delays repolarization in guinea pig hearts. Am J Physiol 277:H211–H220

13. Kinugawa K, Wayne A, Minobe BS et al (2001) Signaling pathways responsible for fetal gene induction in the failing human heart. Evidence for altered thyroid hormone receptor gene expression. Circulation 103:1089–1094

14. Katzeff, HL, Powell SR, Ojamaa K (1997) Alterations in cardiac contractility and gene expression during low-T3 syndrome: prevention with T3. Am J Physiol Endocrinol Metab 273:951–956

15. Ladenson PW, Sherman SI, Baughman KL et al (1992) Reversible alterations in myocardial gene expression in a young man with dilated cardiomyopathy and hypothyroidism. Proc Natl Acad Sci U S A 89:5251–5255

16. Spinale FG (2002) Matrix metalloproteinases. Regulation and dysregulation in the failing heart. Circ Res 90:520–530

17. Peterson JT, Hallak H, Johnson L et al (2001) Matrix metalloproteinase inhibition attenuates left ventricular remodeling and dysfunction in a rat model of progressive heart failure. Circulation 103:2303–2309

18. Ghose RS, Mishra S, Ghosh G et al (2007) Thyroid hormone induces myocardial matrix degradation by activating matrix metalloproteinase-1. Matrix Biol 26:269–279

19. Klein, I, Ojamaa K (2001) Thyroid hormone and the cardiovascular system. N Engl J Med 344:501–509

20. Klein I (1990) Thyroid hormone and the cardiovascular system. Am J Med 88:631–637

21. Ojamaa K, Klemperer JD, Klein I (1996) Acute effects of thyroid hormone on vascular smooth muscle. Thyroid 6:505–512

22. Ojamaa K, Petrie JF, Balkman C (1994) Posttranscriptional modification of myosin heavy-chain gene expression in the hypertrophied rat myocardium. Proc Natl Acad Sci U S A 91:3468–3472

23. Ishikawa T, Chijiwa T, Hagiwara M et al (1989) Thyroid hormones directly interact with vascular smooth muscle strips. Mol Pharmacol 35:760–765

24. Zwaveling J, Pfaffendorf M, Van Zwieten PA (1997) The direct effects of thyroid hormones on rat mesenteric resistance arteries. Fundam Clin Pharmacol 11:41–46

25. Rosler B (1967) Thyroxine and triiodothyronine protein complexes in serum Mesocricetus auratus and Gerbillus pyramidum [in German]. Acta Biol Med Ger 18:597–606

26. Vargas F, Moreno JM, Rodriguez-Gomez I et al (2006) Vascular and renal function in experimental thyroid disorders. Eur J Endocrinol 154:197–212

27. Yoneda K, Takasu N, Higa S et al (1998) Direct effects of thyroid hormones on rat coronary artery: nongenomic effects of triiodothyronine and thyroxine.Thyroid 8:609–613

28. Liu Q, Cianachan AS, Lopaschuk GD (1998) Acute effects of triiodothyronine on glucose and fatty acid metabolism during reperfusion on ischemic rat hearts. Am J Physiol 275: E392–E399

29. Klemperer JD, Zelano J, Helm RE et al (1995) Triiodothyronine improves left ventricular function without oxygen wasting effects after global hypothermic ischemia. J Thorac Cardiovasc Surg 109:457–465

30. Kimura K, Shinozaki Y, Jujo S et al (2006) Triiodothyronine acutely increases blood flow in the ventricles and kidneys of anesthetized rabbits. Thyroid 16:357–360

31. Mizuma H, Marukami M, Mori M (2001) Thyroid hormone activation in human vascular smooth muscle cells: expression of type II iodothyronine deiodinase. Circ Res 88:313–318

32. Colantuoni A, Marchiafava PL, Lapi D et al (2005) The effects of tetraiodothyronine and triiodothyronine on hamster cheek pouch microcirculation. Am J Physiol Heart Circ Physiol 288:H1931–1936

33. Feng Q, Hedner T (1980) Endothelium-derived relaxing factor (EDRF) and nitric oxide (NO). II. Physiology, pharmacology and pathophysiological implications. Clin Physiol 10:503–526

34. Marchant C, Brown L, Sernia C (1993) Renin-angiotensin system in thyroid dysfunction in rats. J Cardiovasc Pharmacol 22:449–455

35. Ganong WF (1982) Thyroid hormones and renin secretion. Life Sci 30:577–584

36. Fletcher AK, Weetman AP (1998) Hypertension and hypothyroidism. J Hum Hypertens 12:79–82

37. Vergaro G, Emdin M (2008) Cardiac angiotensin receptor expression in hypothyroidism: back to fetal gene programme? J Physiol 1:7–8

38. Carneiro-Ramos MS, Diniz GP, Almeida JR et al (2007)

Cardiac angiotensin II type I and type II receptors are increased in rats submitted to experimental hypothyroidism. J Physiol 583:213–223

39. Villabona C, Sahun M, Roca M et al (1999) Blood volumes and renal function in overt and subclinical primary hypothyroidism. Am J Med Sci 318:277–280

40. Formei E, Iervasi G (2002) The role of thyroid hormone in blood pression homeostasis: evidence from short-term hypothyroidism in humans. J Clin Endocrinol Metab 87:1996–2000

41. Kahaly GJ, Dillmann WH (2005) Thyroid hormone action in the heart. Endocr Rev 26:704–728

42. Klein I, Danzi S (2007) Thyroid disease and the heart. Circulation 116:1725–1735

43. Pingitore A, Galli E, Barison A et al (2008) Acute effects of triiodothyronine replacement therapy in patients with chronic heart failure and low-T3 syndrome: a randomized, placebo-controlled study. J Clin Endocrin Metab 93:1351–1358

44. Ripoli A, Pingitore A, Favilli B et al (2005) Does subclinical hypothyroidism affect cardiac pump performance? Evidence from a magnetic resonance imaging study. J Am Coll Cardiol 45:439–445

45. Davis JD, Stern RA, Flashman LA (2003) Cognitive and neuropsychiatric aspects of subclinical hypothyroidism: significance in the elderly. Curr Psychiatry Rep 5:384–390

46. Caraccio N, Natali A, Sironi A et al (2005) Muscle metabolism and exercise tolerance in subclinical hypothyroidism: a controlled trial of levothyroxine. J Clin Endocrin Metab 90:4057–4062

47. Hamilton MA, Stevenson LW, Lu M et al (1990) Altered thyroid hormone metabolism in advanced heart failure. J Am Coll Cardiol 16:91–95

48. Opasich C, Pacini F, Ambrosino N et al (1996) Sick euthyroid syndrome in patients with moderate-to-severe chronic heart failure. Eur Heart J 17:1860–1866

49. Pingitore A, Landi P, Taddei MC et al (2005) Triiodothyronine levels for risk stratification of patients with chronic heart failure. Am J Med 118:132–136

50. Ascheim DD, Hryniewicz K (2002) Thyroid hormone metabolism in patients with congestive heart failure: the low triiodothyronine state. Thyroid 12:511–515

51. Iervasi G, Pingitore A, Landi P et al (2003) Low-T3 syndrome: a strong prognostic predictor of death in patients with heart disease. Circulation 107:708–713

52. Kozdag G, Ural D, Vural A et al (1995) Relation between free triiodothyronine/free thyroxine ratio, echocardiographic parameters and mortality in dilated cardiomyopathy. Eur J Heart Fail 7:113–118

53. Passino C, Pingitore A, Landi P et al (2009) Prognostic value of combined measurement of brain natriuretic peptide and triiodothyronine in heart failure. J Card Fail 15:35–40

54. De Groot LJ (ed) (1989) Thyroid function tests and effects of drugs on thyroid function. Saunders, Philadelphia, USA

55. Pingitore A, Iervasi G, Barison A et al (2006) Early activation of an altered thyroid hormone profile in asymptomatic or mildly symptomatic idiopathic left ventricular dysfunction. J Card Fail 12: 520–526

56. Iervasi G, Molinaro S, Landi P et al (2007) Association between increased mortality and mild thyroid dysfunction in cardiac patients. Arch Intern Med 167:1–7

Carmine Zoccali and Francesca Mallamaci

Abstract The kidney is a major physiological player in the metabolism of thyroid hormones. Chronic renal insufficiency alters the synthesis, distribution, and elimination of thyroid hormones and disturbs central (hypothalamo-pituitary) control of thyroid function. Studies have shown that inflammation is a relevant component in the low triiodothyronine (T_3) levels commonly observed in patients with chronic renal insufficiency associated with chronic kidney disease. Recent surveys and prospective cohort studies have coherently pointed out the important contribution of low-T_3 to cardiomyopathy and to the high risk of death in patients with end-stage renal disease (ESRD). However, even though a role for low T_3 in the high risk of adverse clinical outcomes associated with this condition seems likely, direct proof is lacking. Mechanistic studies and exploratory intervention trials in ESRD patients with low-T_3 are needed to further investigate the nature of the association between T_3 and clinical outcome, as concluded from observational studies in this very high risk population.

Keywords T_3 • TSH • CKD • ESRD • Inflammation • LVH • LV dysfunction • Cardiomyopathy • Cardiovascular risk • Death • CRP, IL-6 • Dialysis

17.1 Introduction

In general terms the control of thyroid hormone synthesis is ensured by two major mechanisms. The first is centered on the thyroid-stimulating hormone (TSH) versus thyroxine (T_4) and triiodothyronine (T_3) feedback loop, whereby TSH stimulates T_4 and T_3 synthesis in the thyroid gland and is in turn inhibited by these hormones; thyrotropin-releasing hormone (TRH) is an integral part of this mechanism. This feedback loop provides a very sensitive defense against alterations in thyroid secretion. The second mechanism consists of the extrathyroidal conversion of T_4 to T_3 by various hormonal, nutritional, and disease-dependent factors, a mechanism aimed at guaranteeing rapid changes in tissue thyroid hormone availability in response to nonthyroidal illness. Extrathyroidal conversion of T_4 is a mechanism of major relevance because about 80% of the T_3 produced results from 5'-deiodination of T_4 in peripheral tissues by two T_4-5'-deiodinases (type I and type II) localized in cell membranes and in endoplasmic reticulum microsomes [1]. As discussed below, the kidney has an important role in the metabolism of thyroid hormones. For this reason, impaired renal function and the resulting accumulation of uremic waste products ("uremic toxins") may disturb thyroid physiology at various lev-

C. Zoccali (✉)
Renal and Transplantation Unit, United Hospitals,
and CNR-IBIM Clinical Epidemiology and Pathophysiology
of Renal Diseases and Hypertension Unit,
Reggio Calabria, Italy

G. Iervasi, A. Pingitore (eds.), *Thyroid and Heart Failure*.
© Springer-Verlag Italia 2009

els that include thyroid hormone production, distribution and elimination and the hypothalamo-pituitary control of the thyroid gland. Inflammation is a new aspect of the thyroid–kidney connection and a most likely trigger of low-T_3 in patients with chronic kidney disease (CKD) [2, 3]. Even though there is no study to date documenting a causal role of thyroid dysfunction in the high cardiovascular risk associated with renal insufficiency, in the last few years circumstantial evidence has been gathered that low-T_3 is strongly associated with inflammation in CKD and that it may be a relevant player in cardiomyopathy and the high risk of death of these patients.

17.2 Thyroid Hormone Metabolism and the Kidney

The kidney is the organ that, together with the liver, expresses the most abundant deiodinase activity and ensures iodide clearance by glomerular filtration of this halogen. Iodide excretion is reduced in severe CKD, which leads to iodide accumulation and increased thyroidal iodide uptake, a phenomenon that expands intrathyroidal iodide pooling and blocks thyroid hormone synthesis. Iodide accumulation probably explains the higher prevalence of goiter and hypothyroidism in patients with CKD [4, 5].

Conversion of T_4 to T_3 in the periphery is impaired in end-stage renal disease (ESRD) [4], but this disturbance apparently does not divert thyroid hormone metabolism toward the reverse T_3 (rT_3) pathway, because plasma rT_3 levels are unaltered in CKD. This finding differentiates patients with CKD from those with other chronic illnesses which instead are characterized by enhanced generation of rT_3 from T_4 [4]. Importantly, low-T_3 levels may be triggered by metabolic acidosis in ESRD [6]. Disturbances in synthesis and/or affinity to the ligand of thyroid hormone protein carriers [thyroid-hormone-binding globulin (TBG), prealbumin, and albumin] may contribute to hypothyroidism in renal insufficiency. Low serum albumin is very frequent in uremia and uremic toxins may inhibit binding to TBG and other carriers. Urea, creatinine, indoles, and phenols inhibit protein binding of T_4 [7] as well as binding of the same hormone to solid phase matrices used in clinical assays developed for measuring plasma T_4 [8]. Studies performed in the 1980s and 1990s showed that plasma TSH is unaltered in patients with CKD [4, 9]. However, the pituitary response (defined in terms of changes in plasma TSH concentration) to TRH in patients with renal insufficiency, particularly in ESRD, occurs at a later stage, has a shallower course, and lasts longer than that seen in healthy subjects [10, 11]. This alteration is currently attributed to a hypothalamic–pituitary disturbance due to accumulation of uremic toxins. The circadian TSH profile in CKD patients is characterized by an attenuated rise in TSH in the evening hours [12] and by reduced amplitude in the pulsatile component of this pituitary hormone [13]. Notwithstanding these central alterations of the TSH control system, the TSH response to T_3 and T_4 is well-maintained in these patients [9, 10]. Importantly, plasma TSH undergoes the expected rise after thyroidectomy in patients with renal insufficiency [14], which indicates that measurements of this hormone are a valid indicator of hypothyroidism in these patients [4, 15].

From a clinical point of view, a number of similarities exist between hypothyroidism and advanced renal failure: hypothermia, bowel motility disturbances and infrequent evacuation, dehydration of the skin, tiredness, and drowsiness are symptoms considered typical of both conditions. Furthermore, as previously mentioned, perhaps due to the accumulation of unknown toxin(s), goiter is more prevalent in patients in ESRD than in the general population [4, 16, 17]. Notwithstanding these similarities, the majority of patients with CKD and ESRD maintain adequate thyroid gland function, as documented by normal TSH, T_4, T_3 and rT_4 plasma profiles [4, 15].

17.3 Inflammation and Low-T_3 in End-Stage Renal Disease

CKD – ESRD in particular – is now considered as a prototypical chronic inflammatory state [18], while C-reactive protein (CRP) [18–21], a nonspecific marker of inflammation, and interleukin 6 (IL-6) [22, 23] are regarded as fundamental biomarkers for cardiovascular risk stratification in these patients. Cardiomyopathy is perhaps the most pervasive complication of ESRD [24, 25]. About one-third of patients starting renal replacement treatment display clinical evidence of heart failure [26, 27]. Chronic dialysis [28, 29] does not halt the evolution of cardiomyopathy. In the asymptomatic ESRD population, the proportion of patients with systolic dysfunction is at least seven times higher than in coeval cohorts in the community [27]. Capillary rarefaction and cardiomyocyte–capillary mismatch is the anatomical hallmark of this condition [30], and pressure and volume overload, severe anemia [31], sympathetic overactivity [32, 33], and hyperparathyroidism [34] are well-established risk factors of cardiac disease in ESRD. In recent years attention has been focused on the inflammatory pathway and a large series of biomarkers including CRP [35, 36], IL-6 [37], TNF-α [38], hypoalbuminemia [31], and fibrinogen [39] have been shown to be associated with left ventricular hypertrophy (LVH) and LV dysfunction in ESRD patients. Low albumin, in particular, appears to be a strong marker of the severity of cardiomyopathy in these patients [40, 41].

Uremia is an established cause of nonthyroidal illness [42]. About 20% of patients with ESRD have low free T_3 (fT_3) levels, while TSH is frankly subnormal in approximately 8% [3]. Thus, low-T_3 is the most common functional alteration of thyroid hormones in advanced renal failure. Low-T_3 is classically interpreted as an adaptation aimed at maintaining energy balance and at minimizing protein wasting in this condition [9]. More recently, it was hypothesized that nonthyroidal illness in ESRD patients is in part explained by chronic systemic inflammation [2]. Cytokines are of paramount importance in nonthyroidal illness. IL-6 is increased [43] and inversely related to T_3 levels in this condition [44]. Observations in patients with cancer documented that both IL-6 and TNF-α lower serum T_3 [45, 46]. Low-T_3 in ESRD is mainly attributed to impaired extrathyroidal T_4-to-T_3 conversion (21) [4]. As previously emphasized, inflammation in ESRD is strongly implicated in both the high mortality and the cardiovascular complications of this population. Nonthyroidal illness commonly occurs in various stressful conditions such as sepsis, myocardial infarction, and virtually all severe diseases [47]. Plasma T_3 is the earliest alteration of the thyroid hormone profile in nonthyroidal illness. This phenomenon represents an acute-phase response generated by activation of cytokines, IL-6 in particular [44, 48]. IL-6 administered on a long-term basis suppresses T_3 [45]. A causal role of IL-6 in thyroid dysfunction is suggested by experiments in the IL-6 knockout mouse. Bacterial endotoxin administration in this transgenic model triggers a much less pronounced reduction in plasma T_3 than

in wild-type mice [48]. Several studies have shown an association between thyroid dysfunction and inflammation in humans. CRP levels are increased in both subclinical and clinical hypothyroidism [49], and free T_4 is inversely related to plasma fibrinogen [50]. As many as 30% of patients hospitalized because of heart failure display subnormal T_3 [51], and it is well-known that this disease is associated with high IL-6 plasma levels [52]. Interestingly, CRP and IL-6 are inversely associated with T_3 in patients with ESRD [2]. This phenomenon is of clinical relevance because a parallel association exists between this thyroid hormone and ICAM and VCAM-1 (two biomarkers of endothelial activation/dysfunction) (Fig. 17.1). Circulating T_3 in ESRD patients is inversely associated with the number of cardiovascular complications including stroke, myocardial infarction, and peripheral vascular disease indicating structural damage of the cardiovascular system (Fig. 17.2). Furthermore, it was documented that in patients with CKD T_3, is very sensitive to intercurrent inflammatory–infectious processes (Fig. 17.3), confirming that inflammation acutely interferes with thyroid function in this condition also. The links between inflammation and thyroid function may be complex and perhaps bidirectional. Indeed, lipoprotein (a), a pro-atherogenic protein and an acute-phase reactant strongly associ-

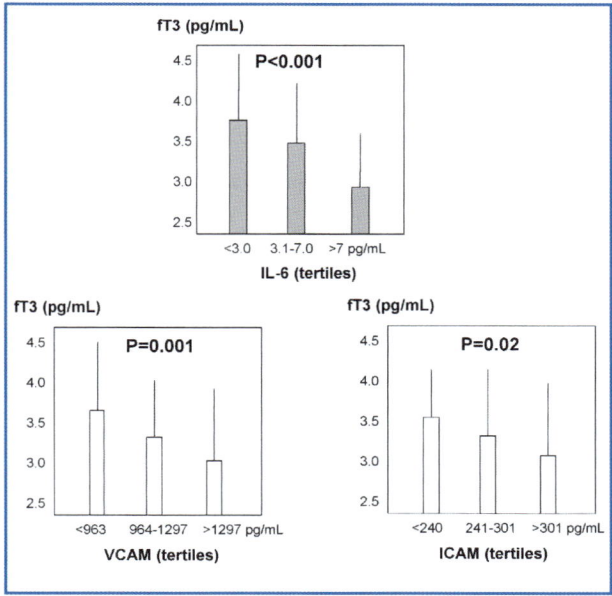

Fig. 17.1 Relationship between plasma levels of free triiodothyronine (fT_3) and IL-6 and ICAM and VCAM-1 in patients with end-stage renal disease. (Drawn from numerical data derived from [2])

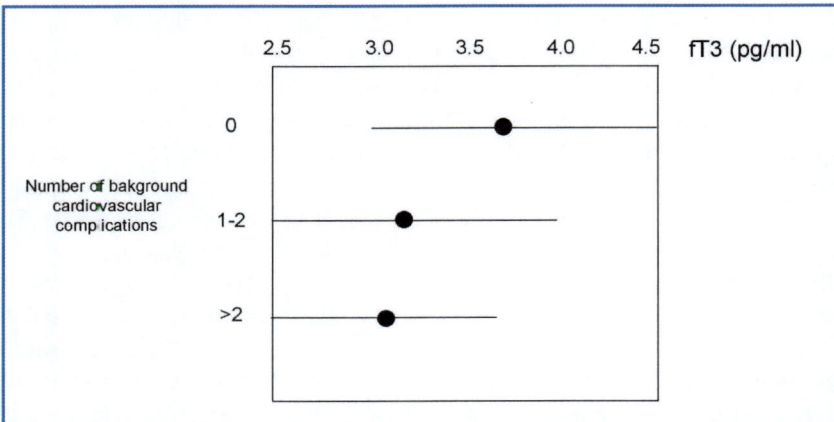

Fig. 17.2 Relationship between plasma levels of free T$_3$ and background cardiovascular complications in end-stage renal disease patients. (Drawn from numerical data derived from [2])

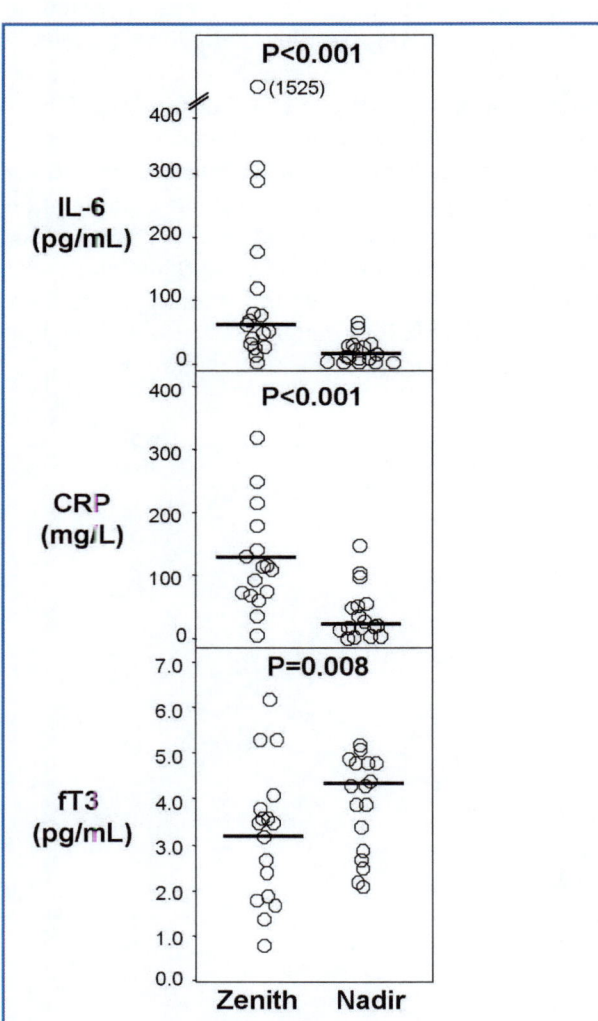

Fig. 17.3 Plasma levels of IL-6 and CRP and fT$_3$ at the zenith and the nadir of an intercurrent inflammatory–infectious process in a series of patients with CKD. (Drawn from numerical data derived from [2])

ated with CRP in ESRD [53], is significantly reduced by D-thyroxine treatment in clinically euthyroid ESRD patients [54].

Given the high risk portended by low-T$_3$ in patients with cardiac diseases (see below), the inverse association between this thyroid hormone and biomarkers of inflammation and structural cardiovascular damage may be of major importance to explain the exceedingly high overall and cardiovascular mortality of patients with advanced renal failure.

17.4 Epidemiology of Clinical and Subclinical Hypothyroidism in CKD

The notion that hypothyroidism is more frequent in patients with ESRD on dialysis has a firm basis [4]. However, until recently the influence of mild and moderate degrees of renal insufficiency on thyroid gland function was unknown. In an analysis of about 15,000 Americans participating into the NHANES III survey [55], hypothyroidism, defined on the basis of serum T$_4$ and TSH, was very frequent (23%) in patients with an estimated glomerular filtration rate (GFR) below 30 ml/min per 1.73 m^2 body surface (Fig. 17.4). In the majority of patients (56%), the disease was subclinical. This high frequency could not be attributed to confounding factors such as age, gender, or ethnicity, and the coherently inverse link between prevalence of hypothyroidism and GFR clearly indicated that renal function loss was the most relevant factor

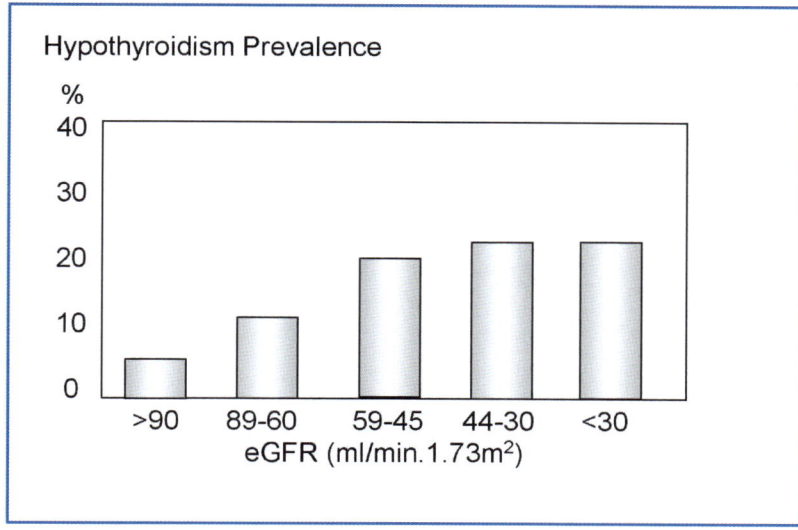

Hypothyroidism Prevalence

Fig. 17.4 Prevalence of hypothyroidism in relation to estimated glomerular filtration rate (eGFR) levels in the NHANES III cohort (see text). (Drawn from numerical data derived from [55])

explaining this association. Recent cross-sectional data from 3089 adult outpatients referred by general practitioners for routine biochemistry testing to a hospital laboratory in Italy [56] showed a prevalence of subclinical primary hypothyroidism of 7% at an estimated GFR above 90 ml/min per 1.73 m^2 and of 17.9% at an estimated GFR below 60 ml/min per 1.73 m^2. Again this association was independent of age, gender, fasting plasma glucose, cholesterol, and triglyceride concentrations. Thus, subclinical hypothyroidism is a relatively common condition in patients with moderate to severe CKD. In another recent survey in patients with advanced renal failure before dialysis the prevalence of subclinical hypothyroidism was 8% [3].

17.5 Cardiovascular Disease and Low-T$_3$ in ESRD

Low-T$_3$ in nonthyroidal illnesses is considered as a response aimed at preventing protein and energy wastage [47]. However, persistently low-T$_3$ levels may eventually become a maladaptive response [42]. In fact, low-T$_3$ entails a negative prognosis in a variety of severe diseases (see below).

T$_3$ regulates fundamental genes in myocardial cells. It up-regulates voltage-gated K channels and Na/K-ATPase and down-regulates the Na/Ca exchanger [57]. High circulating T$_3$ levels increase systolic function and cardiac output, and vice versa. Probably due to the increase in afterload and to the atherogenic effect of low levels of T$_3$ on the arterial

system [58], LV mass is either unchanged [59] or increased [60] in subclinical hypothyroidism. A causal role of T$_3$ deficiency in cardiomyopathy is supported by a recent trial in patients with nondilated cardiomyopathy, in whom synthetic L-T$_3$ replacement therapy elicited a clear-cut improvement in the neurohumoral profile (norepinephrine and N-terminal pro-B-natriuretic peptide) and in LV performance [61].

As emphasized before, LV dysfunction and LVH are pervasive complications in ESRD and are considered as a maladaptive response to various risk factors [62]. As discussed, inflammation plays a central role in the high risk of dialysis patients and inflammation markers have been consistently associated with atherosclerosis [63, 64] LV dysfunction [39] and LVH [35, 39]. Given the role of inflammation in cardiovascular diseases in these patients, the coherent association between low-T$_3$ and reduced LV function and increased LV mass appears to be of paramount importance [65] (Fig. 17.5). Intriguingly, detailed multivariate analyses revealed that these associations were highly influenced by biomarkers of inflammation. The regression coefficients of the relationships between T$_3$ and LV mass and midwall fractional shortening were indeed critically affected by the inclusion of inflammation markers in the multivariate models, particularly serum albumin (Fig. 17.6), a phenomenon in keeping with the hypothesis that low-T$_3$ is an intermediate mechanism implicated in the adverse effect of inflammation on the heart. Thus, T$_3$ and inflammation appear to be in the same causal pathway leading to car-

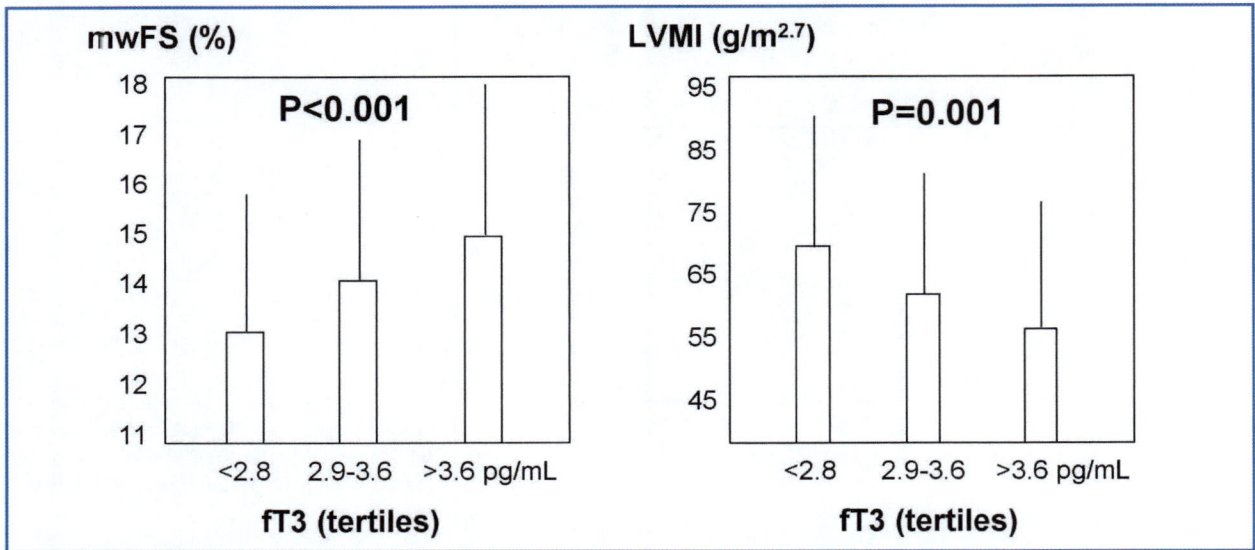

Fig. 17.5 Relationship between plasma levels of fT₃ and midwall fractional shorteninng (MWFS) and left ventricular mass index (LVMI) in end-stage renal disease patients. (Drawn from numerical data derived from [65])

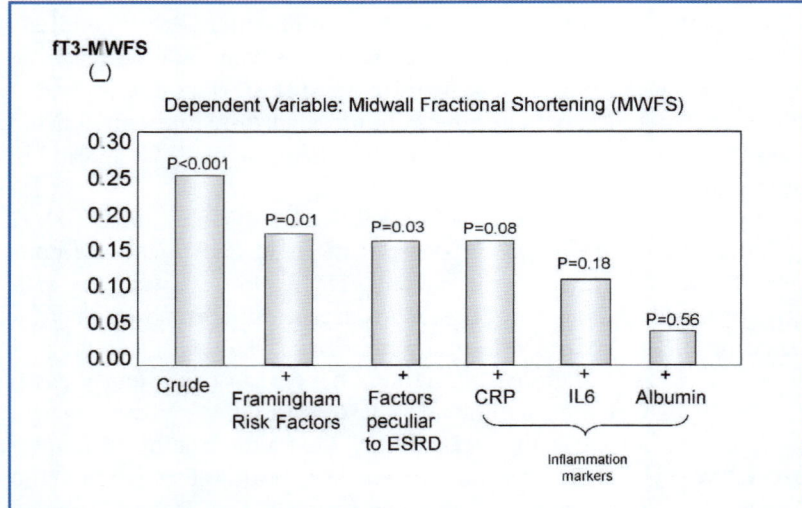

Fig. 17.6 Sequential adjustments of the fT₃–midwall fractional shortening (MWFS) relationship by multiple regression analysis. Risk factors peculiar to end-stage renal disease are hemoglobin and calcium per phosphate product. (Drawn from data reported in [65]). Multivariate analysis with LMVI as a dependent variable produced similar results [65]

diomycpathy. Of note in this study, a strong T₃–serum albumin link (Fig. 17.7) was in part independent of IL-6 and CRP. This phenomenon suggests that low-T₃ also contributes to reducing serum albumin by a mechanism or mechanisms independent of inflammation – a possibility in line with studies showing that thyroid hormone deficiency reduces protein synthesis [66] and favors transcapillary escape of albumin [67]. Thus, it can be surmised that inflammation engenders a low-T₃ state in ESRD (20) and that this condition in turn amplifies the effect of inflammation on serum albumin

(Fig. 17.8). In addition to the established direct effects of low-T₃ on cardiac performance [57], low albumin per se may be a mediator of the effects of T₃ on LV function, and videodensitometric studies have shown that myocardial texture is markedly reduced in subclinical hypothyroidism. Reduced videodensitometric characteristics of myocardial texture fully reversible after long-term L-thyroxine treatment) is indeed interpreted as an effect of enhanced transcapillary escape of albumin into the extracellular space in the myocardium [60]. Importantly regression of videodensitometric alterations after thyroid

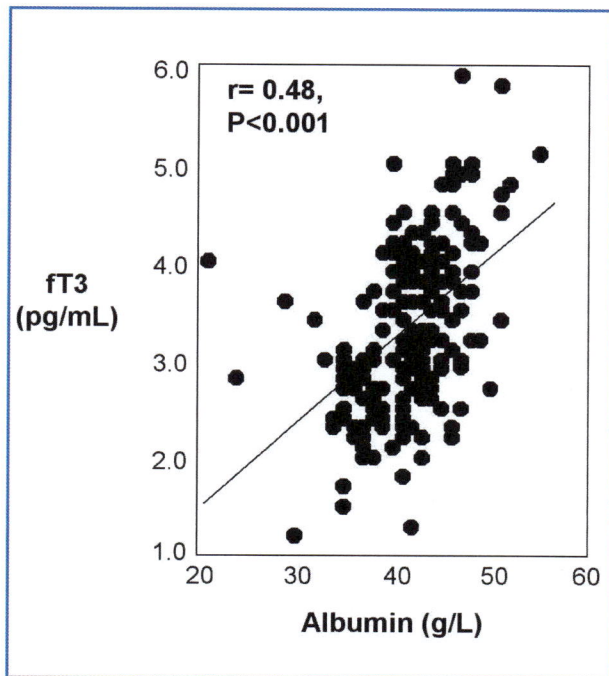

Fig. 17.7 Relationship between plasma levels of fT$_3$ and serum albumin in end-stage renal disease patients. (Drawn from numerical data derived from [2])

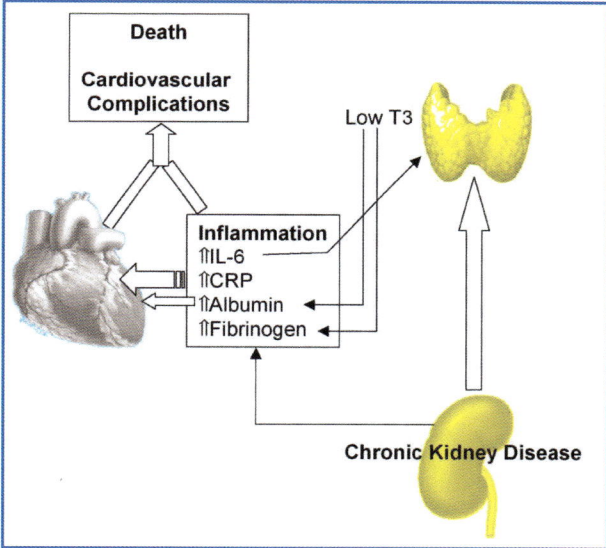

Fig. 17.8 Hypothesized relationship between inflammation, hypoalbuminemia, and left ventricular dysfunction in patients with renal insufficiency. Chronic kidney disease (CKD) engenders a low-T$_3$ syndrome by metabolic mechanisms (see text) and by inflammation. In turn, low-T$_3$ potentiates transcapillary escape of albumin and coagulation disturbances, and in directly and indirectly (particularly via hypoalbuminemia, see text) contributes to cardiomyopathy. Cardiomyopathy, inflammation, and hyperfibrinogenemia act in concert in engendering cardiovascular complications and death in patients with CKD

hormone replacement is also associated with improved myocardial performance in these patients [60]. Hypoalbuminemia is one of the strongest risk factors for progressive cardiomyopathy and heart failure in dialysis patients [40]. Therefore, low-T$_3$ may also contribute to LV dysfunction by amplifying the hypoalbuminemic effect of inflammation, a hypothesis that could be specifically tested in experimental studies and in studies employing videodensitometry.

17.6 Low-T$_3$ and Mortality in ESRD

Low-T$_3$ as well as high IL-6 predict survival in various diseases, and these two biomarkers are inversely associated with each other in ESRD. This inverse association and the relationship between LV mass and function in these patients (discussed above) suggest that depressed T$_3$ may be a risk factor for adverse outcomes in ESRD.

T$_3$ is fundamental for the regulation of cell physiology. It impinges upon cell replication and controls ion channels, oxidative phosphorylation, mitochondrial gene transcription, and the generation of numerous intracellular secondary messengers. T$_3$ is central in the adaptive response to starvation and severe illness. As briefly alluded to before, this adaptation is protective in the short term, but in the long term it may turn out to be noxious [42]. Low-T$_3$ in intensive care patients predicts 5-day mortality [68], and it is an indicator of poor prognosis in patients with liver cirrhosis [69], severe pulmonary disease [70], and cardiac disease [71].

Nonthyroidal illness in patients with CKD and ESRD has long been considered a harmless condition [72]. Since low-T$_3$ is associated with depressed myocardial performance in ESRD patients [65], this alteration should not be necessarily viewed as a favorable, compensatory adaptation to illness. Fibrinogen is elevated and inversely related with T$_3$ and portends a high risk of death in these patients [73], suggesting that the atherothrombotic potential of subclinical thyroid dysfunction in ESRD should not be overlooked. Against this background it is of major clinical relevance that T$_3$ is a very consistent predictor of death in ESRD, and that the strength of this association is not modified much by statistical adjustment for traditional and nontraditional risk factors (Fig. 17.9). In keeping with parallel cross-sectional observations on cardiomyopathy in the

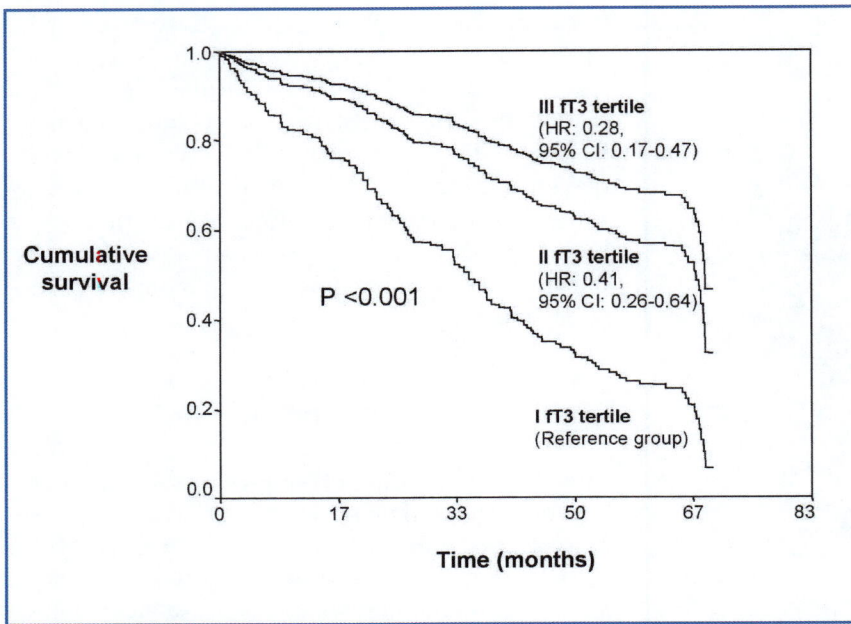

Fig. 17.9 Independent relationship between plasma levels of fT$_3$ and all-cause death in ESRD patients (multivariate Cox's regression analysis). (Drawn from data reported in [74])

same patients, inflammation and low-T$_3$ appear to be in the same causal pathway conducive to death. Indeed, T$_3$ emerged as a highly significant predictor of death in an extensive Cox's multivariate analysis including IL-6, while IL-6 was largely unassociated with death in the same model [74]. Yet IL-6 became a significant death predictor, and a quite strong one, when T$_3$ was excluded from the Cox model. This analysis confirms that T$_3$ is a relevant mediator of the adverse effects of inflammation in ESRD patients. Thyroid hormone is a major determinant of thermogenesis and energy expenditure, and resting energy expenditure (REE) is very sensitive to small doses of T$_4$. In this regard it is worth noting that REE predicted mortality in a cohort of patients on peritoneal dialysis but that the predictive value of this measurement faded after adjustment for inflammation markers and residual renal function [75].

17.7 Can T$_3$ Supplementation Provide a New Therapeutic Approach in Patients with Renal Insufficiency?

Extensive biological knowledge about the role of T$_3$ in the control of cell and organ physiology, the coherent series of observations in ESRD patients, and pilot trials of T$_3$ supplementation in other chronic conditions associated with nonthyroidal illness suggest that supplementing T$_3$ may have a favorable influence on clinical outcomes in CKD and dialysis patients with low-T$_3$. A prospective randomized trial reported beneficial effects of small doses of T$_3$ in children undergoing heart surgery [76]. Likewise, favorable hemodynamic effects of T$_3$ administration were noted in an experimental model of myocardial infarction [77] and in a very recent trial in patients with dilated cardiomyopathy [61]. However, we still lack long-term studies testing the effect of T$_3$ on mortality in patients with heart disease and, more generally, in those with nonthyroidal illness associated with chronic diseases. Near-physiologic doses of T$_3$ (50 μg/day) produce a negative nitrogen balance in patients with chronic renal failure [9], a finding considered as a warning against thyroid hormone supplementation in these patients. Yet this may only reflect correction of hypothyroidism, and any increase in protein catabolism can be prevented by adequately augmenting protein intake. The important observation that the low-T$_3$ state of ESRD can be almost fully corrected by treatment of metabolic acidosis [6] opens an interesting perspective for intervention. On the other hand, the safety of T$_3$ administration in patients with heart failure indicates that it is unlikely that T$_3$ will cause harm to CKD and ESRD patients with T$_3$ depletion.

In summary, low-T_3 is a marker of LVH and cardiomyopathy and an independent predictor of death in hemodialysis patients. These observations lend support to the hypothesis that this alteration is implicated in the high risk of this population. Mechanistic studies and exploratory intervention trials in ESRD patients with low-T_3 are needed to further investigate the nature of the association between T_3 and clinical outcomes unraveled by observational studies in this very high-risk population.

Key Points

- Impairment of renal function and the resulting accumulation of uremic waste products ("uremic toxins") may disturb thyroid physiology at various levels, including thyroid hormone production, distribution, and elimination and involve the hypothalamo-pituitary control of the thyroid gland.

- In patients with chronic kidney disease (CKD) T_3 is very sensitive to intercurrent inflammatory–infectious processes and appears to be inversely related to biomarkers of inflammation such as interleukin-6 and C-reactive protein.

- Subclinical hypothyroidism is a relatively common condition in patients with moderate to severe CKD.

- Low-T_3 is associated with left ventricular (LV) hypertrophy and LV systolic dysfunction in patients with end-stage renal disease (ESRD).

- Low-T_3 predicts death and cardiovascular outcomes in ESRD. T_3 supplementation may be useful to curb the exceedingly high rate of cardiovascular complications of CKD. Clinical trials in this area are a research priority.

References

1. Bianco AC, Kim BW (2006) Deiodinases: implications of the local control of thyroid hormone action. J Clin Invest 116:2571–2579
2. Zoccali C, Tripepi G, Cutrupi S et al (2005) Low triiodothyronine: a new facet of inflammation in end-stage renal disease. J Am Soc Nephrol 16:2789–2795
3. Carrero JJ, Qureshi AR, Axelsson J et al. (2007) Clinical and biochemical implications of low thyroid hormone levels (total and free forms) in euthyroid patients with chronic kidney disease. J Intern Med 262:690–701
4. Kaptein EM, Quion-Verde H, Chooljian CJ et al. (1988) The thyroid in end-stage renal disease. Medicine (Baltimore) 67:187–197
5. Ramirez G, Jubiz W, Gutch CF et al. (1973) Thyroid abnormalities in renal failure. A study of 53 patients on chronic hemodialysis. Ann Intern Med 79:500–504
6. Wiederkehr MR, Kalogiros J, Krapf R (2004) Correction of metabolic acidosis improves thyroid and growth hormone axes in haemodialysis patients. Nephrol Dial Transplant 19:1190–1197
7. Spaulding SW, Gregerman RI (1972) Free thyroxine in serum by equilibrium dialysis: effects of dilution specific ions and inhibitors of binding. J Clin Endocrinol Metab 34:974–982
8. Hochstetler LA, Flanigan MJ, Lim VS (1994) Abnormal endocrine tests in a hemodialysis patient. J Am Soc Nephrol 4:1754–1759
9. Lim VS, Flanigan MJ, Zavala DC et al (1985) Protective adaptation of low serum triiodothyronine in patients with chronic renal failure. Kidney Int 28:541–549
10. Czernichow P, Dauzet MC, Broyer M et al (1976) Abnormal TSH, PRL and GH response to TSH releasing factor in chronic renal failure. J Clin Endocrinol Metab 43:630–637
11. Duntas L, Wolf CF, Keck FS et al (1992) Thyrotropin-releasing hormone: pharmacokinetic and pharmacodynamic properties in chronic renal failure. Clin Nephrol 38:214–218
12. Pasqualini T, Zantleifer D, Balzaretti M et al (1991) Evidence of hypothalamic-pituitary thyroid abnormalities in children with end-stage renal disease. J Pediatr 118:873–878
13. Wheatley T, Clark PM, Clark JD et al (1989) Abnormalities of thyrotrophin (TSH) evening rise and pulsatile release in haemodialysis patients: evidence for hypothalamic-pituitary changes in chronic renal failure. Clin Endocrinol (Oxf) 31:39–50
14. Spector DA, Davis PJ, Helderman et al (1976) Thyroid function and metabolic state in chronic renal failure. Ann Intern Med 85:724–730

15. Kaptein EM (1996) Thyroid hormone metabolism and thyroid diseases in chronic renal failure. Endocr Rev. 17:45–63

16. Ramirez G, O'Neill W Jr, Jubiz W, Bloomer HA (1976) Thyroid dysfunction in uremia: evidence for thyroid and hypophyseal abnormalities. Ann Intern Med 84:672–676

17. Castellano M, Turconi A, Chaler E et al (1996) Thyroid function and serum thyroid binding proteins in prepubertal and pubertal children with chronic renal insufficiency receiving conservative treatment undergoing hemodialysis or receiving care after renal transplantation. J Pediatr 128:784–790

18. Zoccali C, Mallamaci F, Tripepi G (2003) Inflammation and atherosclerosis in end-stage renal disease. Blood Purif 21:29–36

19. Zimmermann J, Herrlinger S, Pruy A et al (1999) Inflammation enhances cardiovascular risk and mortality in hemodialysis patients. Kidney Int 55:648–658

20. Stenvinkel P, Wanner C, Metzger T et al (2002) Inflammation and outcome in end-stage renal failure: does female gender constitute a survival advantage? Kidney Int 62:1791–1798

21. Yeun JY, Levine RA, Mantadilok V et al (2000) C-Reactive protein predicts all-cause and cardiovascular mortality in hemodialysis patients. Am J Kidney Dis 35:469–476

22. Pecoits-Filho R, Barany P, Lindholm B et al (2002) Interleukin-6 is an independent predictor of mortality in patients starting dialysis treatment. Nephrol Dial Transplant 17:1684–1688

23. Zoccali C, Tripepi G, Mallamaci F (2006) Dissecting inflammation in ESRD: do cytokines and C-reactive protein have a complementary prognostic value for mortality in dialysis patients? J Am Soc Nephrol 17:S169–S173

24. Parfrey PS, Griffiths SM, Harnett JD et al (1990) Outcome of congestive heart failure, dilated cardiomyopathy, hypertrophic hyperkinetic disease and ischemic heart disease in dialysis patients. Am J Nephrol 10:213–221

25. Zoccali C (2007) How important is echocardiography for risk stratification in follow-up of patients with chronic kidney disease? Nat Clin Pract Nephrol 3:178–179

26. Foley RN, Parfrey PS, Harnett JD et al (1995) Clinical and echocardiographic disease in patients starting end-stage renal disease therapy. Kidney Int 47:186–192

27. Zoccali C, Benedetto FA, Mallamaci F et al (2004) Prognostic value of echocardiographic indicators of left ventricular systolic function in asymptomatic dialysis patients. J Am Soc Nephrol 15:1029–1037

28. Foley RN, Parfrey PS, Kent GM et al (2000) Serial change in echocardiographic parameters and cardiac failure in end-stage renal disease. J Am Soc Nephrol 11:912–916

29. Zoccali C, Benedetto FA, Tripepi G et al (2006) Left ventricular systolic function monitoring in asymptomatic dialysis patients: a prospective cohort study. J Am Soc Nephrol 17:1460–1465

30. Amann K, Breitbach M, Ritz E et al (1998) Myocyte/capillary mismatch in the heart of uremic patients. J Am Soc Nephrol 9:1018–1022

31. Harnett JD, Foley RN, Kent GM et al (1995) Congestive heart failure in dialysis patients: prevalence, incidence, prognosis, and risk factors. Kidney Int 47:884–890

32. Zoccali C, Mallamaci F, Tripepi G et al. (2002) Norepinephrine and concentric hypertrophy in patients with end-stage renal disease. Hypertension 40:41–46

33. Cice G, Ferrara L, Di BA et al (2001) Dilated cardiomyopathy in dialysis patients – beneficial effects of carvedilol: a double-blind placebo-controlled trial. J Am Coll Cardiol 37:407–411

34. Drueke T, Fauchet M, Fleury J et al (1980) Effect of parathyroidectomy on left-ventricular function in haemodialysis patients. Lancet 1:112–114

35. Wang AY, Wang M, Woo J et al (2004) Inflammation, residual kidney function, and cardiac hypertrophy are interrelated and combine adversely to enhance mortality and cardiovascular death risk of peritoneal dialysis patients. J Am Soc Nephrol 15:2186–2194

36. Ayus JC, Mizani MR, Achinger SG et al (2005) Effects of short daily versus conventional hemodialysis on left ventricular hypertrophy and inflammatory markers: a prospective controlled study. J Am Soc Nephrol 16:2778–2788

37. Losito A, Kalidas K, Santoni S et al (2003) Association of interleukin-6 -174G/C promoter polymorphism with hypertension and left ventricular hypertrophy in dialysis patients. Kidney Int 64:616–622

38. Erten Y, Tulmac M, Derici U et al (2005) An association between inflammatory state and left ventricular hypertrophy in hemodialysis patients. Ren Fail 27:581–589

39. Zoccali C, Benedetto FA, Mallamaci F et al (2003) Fibrinogen inflammation and concentric left ventricular hypertrophy in chronic renal failure. Eur J Clin Invest 33:561–566

40. Foley RN, Parfrey PS, Harnett JD et al (1996) Hypoalbuminemia, cardiac morbidity, and mortality in end-stage renal disease. J Am Soc Nephrol 7:728–736

41. Zoccali C, Benedetto FA, Mallamaci F et al (2001) Prognostic impact of the indexation of left ventricular mass in patients undergoing dialysis. J Am Soc Nephrol 12:2768–2774

42. De Groot LJ (1999) Dangerous dogmas in medicine: the nonthyroidal illness syndrome. J Clin Endocrinol Metab 84:151–164

43. Bartalena L, Brogioni S, Grasso L et al (1994) Relationship of the increased serum interleukin-6 concentration to changes of thyroid function in nonthyroidal illness. J Endocrinol Invest 17:269–274

44. Boelen A, Platvoet-ter Schiphorst MC, Wiersinga WM (1993) Association between serum interleukin-6 and serum 3,5,3?-triiodothyronine in nonthyroidal illness. J Clin Endocrinol Metab 77:1695–1699

45. van der PollT, Romijn JA, Wiersinga WM et al (1990) Tumor necrosis factor: a putative mediator of the sick euthyroid syndrome in man. J Clin Endocrinol Metab 71:1567–1572

46. Stouthard JM, van der Poll T, Endert E et al (1994) Effects of acute and chronic interleukin-6 administration on thyroid hormone metabolism in humans. J Clin Endocrinol Metab 79:1342–1346

47. Chopra IJ (1996) Nonthyroidal illness syndrome or euthyroid sick syndrome? Endocr Pract 2:45–52

48. Boelen A, Maas MA, Lowik CW et al (1996) Induced illness in interleukin-6 (IL-6) knock-out mice: a causal role of IL-6 in the development of the low 3,5,3'-triiodothyronine syndrome. Endocrinology 137:5250–5254

49. Christ-Crain M, Meier C, Guglielmetti M et al (2003) Elevated C-reactive protein and homocysteine values: cardiovascular risk factors in hypothyroidism? A cross-sectional and a double-blind placebo-controlled trial. Atheroscle-

rosis 166:379–386

50. Chadarevian R, Bruckert E, Giral P et al (1999) Relationship between thyroid hormones and fibrinogen levels. Blood Coagul Fibrinolysis 10:481–486

51. Iervasi G, Pingitore A, Landi P et al (2003) Low-T3 syndrome: a strong prognostic predictor of death in patients with heart disease. Circulation 107:708–713

52. Deng MC, Erren M, Lutgen A et al (1996) Interleukin-6 correlates with hemodynamic impairment during dobutamine administration in chronic heart failure. Int J Cardiol 57:129–134

53. Kaysen GA, Kumar V (2003) Inflammation in ESRD: causes and potential consequences. J Ren Nutr 13:158–160

54. Bommer C, Werle E, Walter-Sack I et al (1998) D-thyroxine reduces lipoprotein(a) serum concentration in dialysis patients. J Am Soc Nephrol 9:90–96

55. Lo JC, Chertow GM, Go AS et al (2005) Increased prevalence of subclinical and clinical hypothyroidism in persons with chronic kidney disease. Kidney Int 67:1047–1052

56. Chonchol M, Lippi G, Salvagno G et al (2008) Prevalence of subclinical hypothyroidism in patients with chronic kidney disease. Clin J Am Soc Nephrol 3:1296–1300

57. Klein I, Ojamaa K (2001) Thyroid hormone and the cardiovascular system. N Engl J Med 344:501–509

58. Hak AE, Pols HA, Visser TJ et al (2000) Subclinical hypothyroidism is an independent risk factor for atherosclerosis and myocardial infarction in elderly women: the Rotterdam Study. Ann Intern Med 132:270–278

59. Biondi B, Palmieri EA, Lombardi G et al (2002) Effects of subclinical thyroid dysfunction on the heart. Ann Intern Med 137:904–914

60. Monzani F, Di B, V Caraccio N et al (2001) Effect of levothyroxine on cardiac function and structure in subclinical hypothyroidism: a double blind placebo-controlled study. J Clin Endocrinol Metab 86:1110–1115

61. Pingitore A, Galli E, Barison A et al (2008) Acute effects of triiodothyronine (T3) replacement therapy in patients with chronic heart failure and low-T3 syndrome: a randomized placebo-controlled study. J Clin Endocrinol Metab 93:1351–1358

62. Zoccali C, Mallamaci F, Tripepi G (2003) Traditional and emerging cardiovascular risk factors in end-stage renal disease. Kidney Int Suppl S105–S110

63. Zoccali C, Benedetto FA, Mallamaci F et al (2000) Inflammation is associated with carotid atherosclerosis in dialysis patients. Creed Investigators. Cardiovascular Risk Extended Evaluation in Dialysis Patients. J Hypertens 18:1207–1213

64. Stenvinkel P, Heimburger O, Jogestrand T (2002) Elevated interleukin-6 predicts progressive carotid artery atherosclerosis in dialysis patients: association with Chlamydia pneumoniae seropositivity. Am J Kidney Dis 39:274–282

65. Zoccali C, Benedetto F, Mallamaci F et al (2006) Low triiodothyronine and cardiomyopathy in patients with end-stage renal disease. J Hypertens 24:2039–2046

66. Hansen JM, Lassen NA, Munck O et al (1979) Metabolic turnover rate and transcapillary escape rate of albumin before and during treatment of myxoedema: on the pathogenesis of the oedema formation [proceedings]. J Physiol 293:81P–82P

67. Wheatley T, Edwards OM (1983) Mild hypothyroidism and oedema: evidence for increased capillary permeability to protein. Clin Endocrinol (Oxf) 18:627–635

68. Peeters RP, Wouters PJ, van Toor H et al (2005) Serum 3,3?,5?-Triiodothyronine (rT3) and 3,5,3?-triiodothyronine/rT3 are prognostic markers in critically ill patients and are associated with postmortem tissue deiodinase activities. J Clin Endocrinol Metab 90:4559–4565

69. Rink C, Siersleben U, Haerting J et al (1991) Development of the low-T3-syndrome and prognosis assessment in patients with liver cirrhosis. Gastroenterol J 51:138–141

70. Scoscia E, Baglioni S, Eslami A et al (2004) Low triiodothyronine (T3) state: a predictor of outcome in respiratory failure? Results of a clinical pilot study. Eur J Endocrinol 151:557–560

71. Iervasi G, Molinaro S, Landi P et al (2007) Association between increased mortality and mild thyroid dysfunction in cardiac patients. Arch Intern Med 167:1526–1532

72. Lim VS (2001) Thyroid function in patients with chronic renal failure. Am J Kidney Dis 38:S80–S84

73. Zoccali C, Mallamaci F, Tripepi G et al (2003) Fibrinogen mortality and incident cardiovascular complications in end-stage renal failure. J Intern Med 254:132–139

74. Zoccali C, Mallamaci F, Tripepi G et al (2006) Low triiodothyronine and survival in end-stage renal disease. Kidney Int 70:523–528

75. Wang AY, Sea MM, Tang N et al (2004) Resting energy expenditure and subsequent mortality risk in peritoneal dialysis patients. J Am Soc Nephrol 15:3134–3143

76. Chowdhury D, Parnell VA, Ojamaa K et al (1999) Usefulness of triiodothyronine (T3) treatment after surgery for complex congenital heart disease in infants and children. Am J Cardiol. 84:1107–9 A10

77. Dyke CM, Yeh T, Jr, Lehman JDet al. (1991) Triiodothyronine-enhanced left ventricular function after ischemic injury. Ann Thorac Surg 52:14–19

Abstract Existing data clearly demonstrate that depression is an independent risk factor for poor prognosis in patients with cardiovascular diseases, including chronic congestive heart failure (CHF). However, the mechanisms underlying this relationship are not fully understood. Low-triiodothyronine (T_3) syndrome is reported in CHF as well as in depression and may be associated with both these disorders. Both heart and brain are sensitive to thyroid hormone fluctuations even within normal limits. In cardiovascular patients, growing evidence indicates a strong association between a drop in T_3 concentration and the incidence and progression of CHF. While the evidence suggests a strong link between depression, low-T_3 syndrome, and the severity of CHF, to date no systematic investigations have documented this relationship. One preliminary study found that depressed patients with coronary artery disease had a higher prevalence of CHF and lower T_3 concentration than nondepressed patients, suggesting that an association between depression and low-T_3 syndrome may be clinically important in patients with CHF. Compensation of low-T_3 syndrome in these patients improves ventricular performance. Treatment of depressed patients with T_3 accelerates the effects of antidepressants, including treatment-resistant cases of depression. Compensation of low-T_3 syndrome in patients with CHF and depression may lead to improvement in both cardiovascular function and mental function.

Keywords Chronic heart failure • Coronary artery disease • Triiodothyronine • Depression • Low-T_3 syndrome • Reverse T_3 • Hypothalamus–pituitary–thyroid (HPT) axis • Deiodinase • Pathogenesis • Hypothyroidism • B-type natriuretic peptides • Treatment-resistant depression

18.1 Chronic Heart Failure

Chronic congestive heart failure (CHF) is a syndrome in which the heart is unable to pump enough blood to meet the needs of the body's tissues. CHF is associated with important clinical and social consequences. The risk of mortality is six to nine times higher in patients with CHF than in the general population. The lifetime risk for CHF approaches 20%, and mortality approaches 25% after 1 year and 50% after 5 years [1]. For people over 65, it is the leading cause of death. Rehospitalization rates are about 50% within 12 months after discharge. Despite therapeutic advances, CHF-associated morbidity and mortality continue to increase [2].

The most frequent cause of CHF is coronary artery disease (CAD), followed by hypertension,

R. Bunevičius (✉)
Institute of Psychophysiology and Rehabilitation,
Kaunas University of Medicine, Palanga, Lithuania

G. Iervasi, A. Pingitore (eds.), *Thyroid and Heart Failure*.

valvular heart disease, and cardiomyopathy. An impaired pumping action of the heart triggers a number of hormonal and neuroendocrine mechanisms that tend to correct the diminished blood flow. These corrective responses are helpful only in the short term as they increase the work of the failing heart and thus in the long term damage the heart. Specific mechanisms include activation of the sympathetic nervous system, the renin–angiotensin–aldosterone system, and the immune system, and myocyte remodeling [3, 4]. Certain molecules, such as nitric oxide and hormones of the heart, so-called natriuretic peptides, may play a positive role in CHF. Other factors, such as gender, race, arrhythmias, hypercoagulability, and inflammation factors, are associated with severity and outcomes of CHF [5].

Existing data clearly demonstrate that mental depression is an independent risk factor for poor prognosis in patients with cardiovascular diseases, including CHF [6]. However, the mechanisms underlying this relationship are not fully understood. Low-triiodothyronine (T_3) syndrome is reported in CHF [7] as well as in depression [8], providing a possible link between the two disorders.

18.2 Depression

Depression is a major public health problem and research priority. It is a chronic, disabling mental disorder with a high rate of recurrence and the fourth leading cause of disease burden, accounting for 4.4% of total disability. Depression causes the largest amount of nonfatal disease burden, accounting for almost 12% of total years lived with disability worldwide [9]. Every year it affects about 8% of the population [10], making it the leading cause of impairment in adults in North America and Western Europe [9]. Impairment in daily functioning caused by depression or anxiety exceeds that caused by other chronic diseases, such as hypertension, diabetes, and back or neck problems [11]. Epidemiological studies have shown that when a person is diagnosed with major depression, he or she has a significantly greater risk of dying within 1 year than does someone who is not depressed. The negative effect of depression on mortality is especially evident in patients with a serious somatic disease, such as cancer, stroke, or heart disease, including CHF [12].

The prevailing biological hypothesis of depression suggests that mood disorders are associated with dysregulation of amines in the brain. Norepinephrine and serotonin are the neurotransmitters most often implicated in the pathophysiology of depression [13]. Dysfunction of these neurotransmitters may cause dysregulation of various neuroendocrine axes, such as the adrenal axis, the growth hormone axis, and the thyroid axis. Among the dysfunctions of the thyroid axis, low-T_3 syndrome is frequently reported in depressed patients [8].

18.3 Low-T_3 Syndrome

A decrease in serum T_3 concentration and a parallel increase in reverse T_3 concentration are common findings in many illnesses, e.g., trauma, starvation, and after surgical operations. These changes in hypothalamus–pituitary–thyroid (HPT) axis function, taken together, are referred to as low-T_3 syndrome. In the fasting state, this shift from production of the metabolically potent thyroid hormone T_3 toward production of the metabolically inactive thyroid hormone reverse T_3 suggests a compensatory role. However, in chronic illnesses, such as CHF and depression, a low-T_3 concentration can produce its own negative consequences. These HPT axis changes have also been called "euthyroid sick syndrome" (ESS), a term tending to minimize their clinical significance. An alternative designation, which does not presume metabolic significance, is "nonthyroidal illness syndrome" [14]. A marked decrease in serum thyroid hormone concentration in patients with severe nonthyroidal illness is associated with a high probability of death, while recovery from an underlying illness is usually accompanied by the reversal of thyroid abnormalities [14].

Secretion of thyroid hormones is controlled by the pituitary thyroid-stimulating hormone (TSH), which in turn is stimulated by hypothalamic thyrotropin-releasing hormone (TRH) and suppressed by negative feedback from serum thyroid hormones. The thyroid gland secretes several hormones, including T_4, T_3, and reverse T_3. The main secretion of the thyroid gland is T_4, and the thyroid gland is the only source of this hormone. In contrast, no more than 20% of the biologically more active hormone T_3 is secreted by the thyroid gland. The remainder of T_3 production is in other tissues, by the enzymatic removal of iodine from the T_4 molecule by deiodinases, which exist in several forms. Type I deiodinase (D1) is located primarily in liver and kidney and is responsible for producing as much as 80% of T_3. Type II deiodinase (D2) is located primarily in the brain and in muscles, including the heart in humans, and contributes to tissue T_3 concentration. Type III deiodinase (D3) converts T_4 into reverse T_3, which is inactive, and degrades T_3 [15]. T_3 penetrates cell membranes and is responsible for the majority of the genomic and nongenomic effects of thyroid hormones.

A principal mechanism underlying low serum concentration of T_3 in patients with nonthyroidal illness is the reduced activity of D1 in the liver. Increased concentrations of cytokines, such as interleukin-6 and tumor necrosis factor α, are responsible for impaired expression of hepatic D1. Other mechanisms involved in the pathogenesis of low-T_3 syndrome include a decrease in the concentration of thyroid-hormone-binding proteins and the decreased secretion of TRH and TSH. Dopamine secretion and prolonged hypercortisolemia may each play a role [14]. However, the role of neurohormones in the pathogenesis of the low-T_3 syndrome remains largely unknown.

18.4 Heart Failure and Depression

As mentioned above, depression is common in patients with cardiovascular diseases. Increased rates of depression are reported in CAD, after myocardial infarction (MI), and in CHF [12, 16]. Depression is a risk factor for the development of CAD [17], and the risk of being affected with CAD is 60% higher in depressed patients. Depression worsens the prognosis of heart disease, increasing disability, reducing quality of life, and increasing mortality in patients with CAD and following MI [18]. In patients with CAD, depression doubles mortality. In post-MI patients, depression more than doubles mortality. Some studies have reported a dose–response relationship between severity of depression and the prognosis of the CAD [19]. The impact of depression on treatment outcome, including survival after coronary artery bypass surgery, is also unfavorable. CAD is the most common cause of CHF, and, among patients with CHF, rates of depression are reportedly from 11% to 48% in outpatients and exceed 70% in inpatients [20]. The high variance in the reported prevalence of depres-

sion may be related to many factors. However, it is clear that in patients with heart disease clinical depression is much more prevalent than in the general population, in which the rate is about 8% [10].

Depression is a clinically important co-morbid condition in CHF. It increases the risk of CHF development in the elderly, especially in women, and in patients with other risk factors for CHF, such as hypertension [21]. Depression in patients with CHF is associated with a poor prognosis and is an independent risk factor for death, re-hospitalization, and functional decline [22]. Co-morbid depression significantly increases health care costs in patients with CHF, and its negative impact on the quality of life is greater than that of heart malfunction, as evidenced by increased N-terminal-pro-B-type natriuretic peptide (NT-pro-BNP) concentrations or decreased left ventricular ejection fraction [23].

It is important to understand the mechanisms by which depression increases the morbidity, mortality, and costs associated with CHF. Current knowledge implicates psychosocial factors, such as noncompliance with treatment, and poor social and emotional support. Psychobiological mechanisms point to inflammation factors, which are found to be increased in depressed CHF patients compared to nondepressed CHF patients. Depression and CHF share some mechanisms that may worsen outcomes of heart disease, including increased adrenergic activation and dysregulation of autonomic function and heart rhythm. In a seeming paradox, hypocholesterolemia is also related to a marked increase in mortality in advanced heart failure [24]. Despite increasing information about links between depression and CHF, there is no accepted model that accommodates potential mechanisms. Moreover, some perhaps important mechanisms have not yet been studied. Dysfunction in thyroid hormone metabolism, frequently found in depression and CHF, is such a mechanism.

18.5 Heart Failure and Low-T_3 Syndrome

Effects of thyroid hormones on the functioning of the cardiovascular system have been known for many years and are observed in both hyperthyroidism and hypothyroidism. T_3 increases cardiac inotropy and chronotropy. It influences contractile function by regulating the transcription of myocyte-specific genes [4]. T_3 also directly affects vascular smooth muscle cells, promoting relaxation of resistant arterioles and decreasing peripheral vascular resistance. Normal thyroid hormone concentrations are required for normal cardiovascular functioning; an excess or a deficiency of thyroid hormones disorganizes it.

There are several heart diseases that are accompanied by low-T_3 syndrome. After myocardial infarction, cardiac surgery in adults and children, and cardiac arrest, as well as in CHF, serum T_3 concentrations decline. This decline is related to worsened cardiovascular functioning and worsened outcomes of the heart disease or of surgery [25–27].

Low-T_3 syndrome represents the most prevalent alteration in thyroid hormone metabolism in CHF, affecting about one-third of these patients [26]. As T_3 concentration decreases, functional impairment increases, as assessed by the New York Heart Association functional classification. However, even patients with mild and compensated CHF display some early manifestations of low-T_3 syndrome [28]. In CHF patients, the low-T_3 syndrome is associated with poor left ventricular function, tachyarrhythmia, and increased mortality [4]. The low-T_3 concentration in CHF is a stronger predictor of poor outcome than is dyslipidemia, age, or left ventricular ejection fraction.

As the heart fails, a change occurs in the dynamics of an important regulatory system. The heart normally secretes cardiac B-type natriuretic peptides (BNP), including NT-pro-BNP, and thyroid hormones stimulate its secretion [29]. With heart failure, BNP and NT-pro-BNP concentrations markedly increase [30], despite the usual decline in T_3 concentration.

The low-T_3 syndrome shares several biochemical and clinical characteristics with hypothyroidism, and both syndromes are found in CHF. Functionally and phenotypically, the failing heart resembles the hypothyroid heart. Shared characteristics include somatic symptoms such as weakness, dyspnea, edema, cold intolerance, and psychological symptoms such as sleep apnea and depression. Decreased cardiac output and contractility together with increased peripheral vascular resistance are found in both hypothyroidism and CHF. These conditions share autonomic features: increased norepinephrine concentration, overexpression of sympathetic tone, and underexpression of parasympathetic (vagal) tone. Changes in cardiac

gene expression are also similar in CHF and hypothyroidism. Positively regulated T_3 genes such as SERCA-2 and α-MHC are down-regulated, and negatively regulated genes such as β-MHC are up-regulated [31].

The above data suggest that treatment with thyroid hormones improves cardiac function in patients with CHF as it does in patients with hypothyroidism. Experimental data indicated that T_3 supplementation normalizes cardiac function in the low-T_3 syndrome caused by starvation. In heart transplantation, T_3 has been used to resuscitate donor hearts with poor function, in recipients to improve myocardial aerobic metabolism, and to increase heart function in potential donors after cerebral death. It was reported that after heart surgery in both children and adults administration of T_3 improved cardiovascular functioning [27]. T_3 supplementation was shown to alter gene transcription in the myocardium of infants undergoing cardiopulmonary bypass surgery [32]. Evidence is accumulating that normalization of T_3 concentration is beneficial to CHF patients as well. Preliminary data indicate that treatment of the low-T_3 syndrome with T_3 or with the thyroid hormone analogue diiodothyropropionic acid improves cardiovascular functioning in CHF patients [33]. Recent data showed that short-term treatment with T_3 in low-T_3 syndrome patients with CHF due to dilated cardiomyopathy significantly improved both neuroendocrine profile and ventricular performance [34]. These data strengthen the need for further controlled trials with more patients and longer periods of T_3 administration.

It has been suggested that T_3, but not T_4, should be used for interventions in low-T_3 syndrome because of impaired peripheral T_4 conversion to T_3 by D1 in liver. Intravenous administration of TRH was shown to restore serum T_3 concentrations in patients with low-T_3 syndrome [35]. Moreover, treatment with antidepressant drugs stimulates T_3 production in the brain and increases its concentration in serum [36]. However, there are no data on the effects of treatment with TRH or with antidepressant drugs on cardiovascular function and HPT axis function in patients with CHF.

18.6 Depression and Low-T_3 Syndrome

Functional impairment of the thyroid gland may cause significant alterations in the functioning of the adult brain, leading to serious mental deficits such as dementia or depression. Although most overtly hypothyroid or hyperthyroid patients show mental deficits, predominantly depression, most depressed patients are euthyroid. A small proportion of patients with recognized major depression demonstrate subclinical hypothyroidism, of which an exaggerated TSH response to TRH injection is a characteristic. At the same time, between one quarter and one third of depressed patients demonstrate a blunted TSH response to TRH [37], which is believed to be a biological marker of depression. Involvement of the HPT axis, as evidenced by the TSH response to TRH stimulation in female patients with major depression, is illustrated in Figure 18.1 [37]. Basal TSH levels in major depression are usually normal or low normal. The most common thyroid axis finding in depression is transient hyperthyroxinemia [38], which may be accompanied by increased concentrations of reverse T_3 and decreased concentrations of T_3 [8]. Such changes in the peripheral thyroid hormone economy together with a blunted TSH response to TRH stimulation are typical features of the low-T_3 syndrome, which is reported in a significant proportion of depressed patients [8]. Recovery from depression, like recovery from other nonthyroid illnesses, results in normalization of TSH secretion as well as normalization of thyroid hormone concentrations in serum and in cerebrospinal fluid [39]. Thyroid hormone

metabolism in the brain undergoes a specific change in depressed patients during recovery. Increasing T_3 concentrations could be a precondition for the recovery of depressed patients [36].

The evidence of a relationship between thyroid dysfunction and mental state has evoked interest in using thyroid hormones in the treatment of mental disorders. Several clinical trials have confirmed the clinical value of thyroid hormones in the treatment of depression. Specifically, there is good evidence that a small dose of T_3 can accelerate the effects of tricyclic antidepressants, including treatment-resistant cases of depression. The role of T_3 in augmenting the antidepressive effects of selective serotonin reuptake inhibitors (SSRIs) in the majority of studies also showed positive results [40]. In one large study, augmentation with T_3 was a useful treatment in depressed patients who experienced unsatisfactory results with two previous antidepressant medications [41]. Another strategy using thyroid hormones in some mood disorders, such as rapid-cycling bipolar disorder or treatment-resistant depression, employs supraphysiological doses of T_4 [36]. It was reported recently that the antidepressant effect of T_3 augmentation of SSRIs was correlated with significant changes in the brain's bioenergetic metabolism [42]. This suggests that T_3 is an important factor regulating bioenergetic processes in the brain and that these processes are related to the manifestation and treatment of depressive disorders.

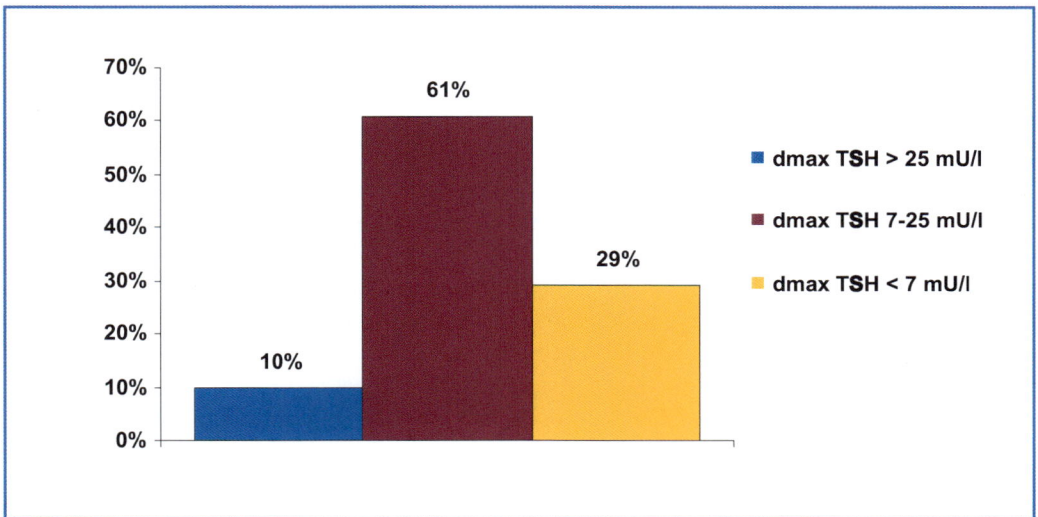

Fig. 18.1 *TSH* response to TRH stimulation (d_{max} TSH) in 41 female patients with major depression [37]. d_{max} TSH > 25 mU/l demonstrates subclinical hypothyroidism; d_{max} TSH 7–25 mU/l demonstrates euthyroidism; d_{max} TSH < 7 mU/l demonstrates a blunted TSH response, which is believed to be a biological marker of depression

Even mild fluctuations in thyroid hormone concentration within the normal range may affect mental functioning. It was reported that subclinical hypothyroidism is related to depression, and euthyroid patients with treated Graves' disease exhibit a high prevalence of affective disorders [43]. Subtle relationships between thyroid function, even within the normal range, and response to antidepressant treatment were demonstrated in patients with major depression. Serum T_3 concentrations in the low normal range and serum T_4 concentrations in the high normal range are found in replacement therapy of hypothyroidism with T_4. This pattern of thyroid hormones corresponds to the low-T_3 syndrome and is related to increased psychiatric morbidity [44]. Thyroid hormone replacement with a combination of T_4 and T_3 restores a normal T_3/T_4 ratio and improves mental functioning in some but not all patients [45]. It was summarized that the majority of patients subjectively prefer combined treatment with T_4 and T_3 [46].

Evidence that thyroid hormones interact with neural tissues affecting mood and cognition in adults may have several explanations. Thyroid hormones in the adult brain regulate the expression of several genes that may affect mood and cognition, including the gene for corticotropin-releasing hormone, and the genes for neurotrophins, such as nerve growth factor and brain-derived neurotrophic factor. In addition, by genomic and possibly nongenomic mechanisms, T_3 interacts with several important neurotransmitters, such as serotonin and norepinephrine, which are crucial for mood regulation, and with acetylcholine, which is crucial for cognition [40]. Decreased T_3 concentration in the low-T_3 syndrome may affect these mechanisms, causing depression, as happens in hypothyroidism. Treatment with T_3, which restores T_3 concentrations to normal, may improve mental status as well as cardiac function.

18.7 Depression and Low-T_3 syndrome in CHF

As mentioned above, depression is a common finding in CHF. However, this co-morbidity has not been investigated with regard to the low-T_3 syndrome, which is frequently reported in both conditions. A schematic hypothetical model of thyroid–heart–brain interactions is presented in

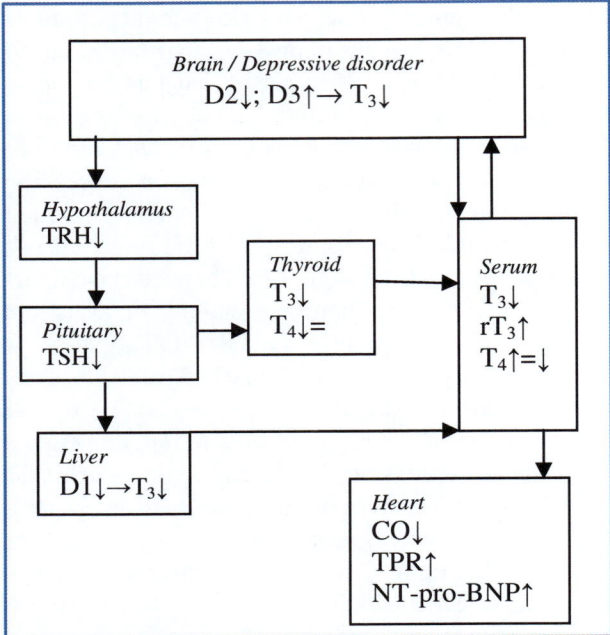

Fig. 18.2 Model of the brain–thyroid–heart interaction in patients with congestive heart failure with depressive disorder and low-T3 syndrome. *D1* type I deiodinase, *D2* type II deiodinase, *D3* type III deiodinase, *CO* cardiac output, *TPR* total peripheral resistance, *NT-pro-BNP* pro-B-type natriuretic peptide

Figure 18.2. In this model, depression, through its effects on the HPT axis and on T_3 production in the brain, may contribute to additional decreases in serum T_3 concentration in patients with CHF, which in turn, may worsen hemodynamics (e.g., reduced cardiac output and peripheral resistance), cardiac function, and outcomes of CHF. However, other models of interaction between the thyroid axis and depression in CHF should be considered.

For example, in an alternative model, low-T_3 syndrome caused by CHF may affect thyroid hormone homeostasis in the brain and result in depression in patients vulnerable to mood disorders. In this model, depression is a function of low-T_3 syndrome, and an association between the two does not result in a decline in cardiac function. Vulnerability to depression is associated with the short allele of a functional polymorphism in the promoter region of the serotonin transporter gene (5-HTTLPR) in conjunction with stressful life events [47]. Chronic heart disease such as CHF may be considered as a stressful life event. It was demonstrated recently in patients with chronic CAD that carriers of the short allele of 5-HTTLPR were more vulnerable to depression, perceived stress, and high norepinephrine secretion, suggesting that these factors may contribute to worse cardiovascular outcomes [48]. These findings may be extrapolated to CHF with low-T_3 syndrome. In this model, low-T_3 syndrome may interact with the short allele of 5-HTTLPR and predispose to depression in patients with CHF. On the other hand, low-T_3 syndrome may have more specific effects on the brain. D2 polymorphism, which is responsible for T_3 production in the brain, and D1 polymorphism, which is responsible for circulating T_3 concentrations, interacting with low-T_3 syndrome may result in brain hypothyroidism, at least in those parts of the brain responsible for cognition [49] and for mood.

Other factors, such as thyroid disease, treatment with thyroid medication or amiodarone, inflammation, age, and sex, as well as personality traits may also affect thyroid function or mood, contributing to an association between depressive disorder and low-T_3 syndrome in patients with CHF. For example, activation of inflammatory processes may be a primary mechanism responsible for worsened outcomes in CHF; this activation, as discussed earlier, may contribute to depressive disorder as well as to low-T_3 syndrome. In this model, however, depression and/or low-T_3 syndrome are markers of a primary mechanism and are without significant pathophysiological impact on cardiac function. Finally, a model that considers low-T_3 syndrome and depression as adaptations to chronic illnesses that minimize catabolism and physical activity of patients with chronic disease must be acknowledged. However, in this model, low-T_3 syndrome and depression have positive effects on cardiac function and outcome in patients with CHF, and such benefits have not been found in the majority of the studies.

While the evidence summarized above suggests a strong link between depression, low-T_3 syndrome, and CHF, to date no direct systematic investigations exist documenting the relationship between depression and low-T_3 syndrome in patients with CHF. One preliminary study [50] found that depressed patients with CAD participating in a rehabilitation program had lower T_3 concentrations and higher NT-pro-BNP concentrations than nondepressed patients. Significant correlations between NT-pro-BNP concentrations and thyroid hormone concentrations in the total sample of patients were found in that study. Higher NT-pro-BNP concentrations were related to lower total T_3 concentrations, with higher reverse T_3 concentrations and higher free T_4 concentrations. There were no significant correlations between depression and hormonal variables in the total sample of patients. However, in men, higher scores of depression were related to lower total T_3 concentrations and to higher NT-pro-BNP concentrations. Correlations between scores of depression, NT-pro-BNP concentrations, and total T_3 concentrations remained significant in the subgroup of male patients with CHF (Fig. 18.3), suggesting that an association between depression and low-T_3 syndrome is of clinical importance in patients with CHF, especially in men.

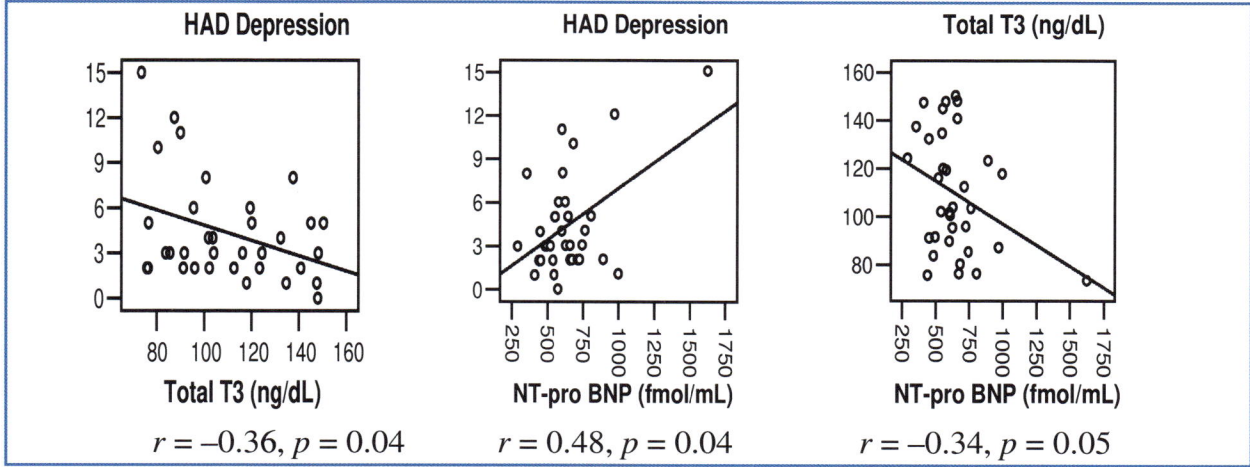

Fig. 18.3 Correlations between concentrations of the cardiac B-type natriuretic peptide NT-pro-BNP, and total T3, and depression scores on the Hospital Anxiety and Depression (HAD) scale in male patients with heart failure. (Bunevicius et al., unpublished data)

Further research is needed to assess the association between depression and low-T_3 syndrome as well as to reveal an impact of such an association on mechanisms affecting cardiac morbidity and mortality in patients with CHF. It should include interventions designed to compensate for the T_3 deficiency in CHF patients with low-T_3 syndrome. What effects do such compensations have on heart function and on mental function? These interventions may include treatment with T_3 or with its analogues, treatment with human recombinant TSH, treatment with TRH or with its analogues, and treatment with antidepressant drugs. CHF patients with depression and low-T_3 syndrome may be a target population for such studies.

Acknowledgments The author wishes to thank Dr. Arthur J. Prange Jr, Boshamer Professor of Psychiatry at the University of North Carolina at Chapel Hill, for his contributions to the content and structure of this chapter.

Key Points

- Depression is an independent risk factor for a poor prognosis in patients with chronic congestive heart failure (CHF).

- Low-triiodothyronine (T_3) syndrome is another independent risk factor for a poor prognosis in patients with CHF.

- Low-T_3 syndrome is reported in patients with depression.

- Preliminary data suggest that low-T_3 syndrome mediates the link between depression and poor cardiac functioning in patients with coronary artery disease and in CHF.

- Treatment with T_3 in depressed patients augments the effects of antidepressants.

- Compensation of low-T_3 syndrome in CHF patients improves cardiovascular function.

- Compensation of low-T_3 syndrome in patients with CHF and depression may lead to improvement in cardiovascular function and improvement in mood.

References

1. Levy D, Kenchaiah S, Larson M et al (2002) Long-term trends in the incidence of and survival with heart failure. N Engl J Med 347:1397–1402

2. Heywood JT, Saltzberg MT (2005) Strategies to reduce length of stay and costs associated with decompensated heart failure. Curr Heart Fail Rep 2:140–147

3. Parish RC, Evans JD (2008) Inflammation in chronic heart failure. Ann Pharmacother 42:1002–1016

4. Portman MA (2008) Thyroid hormone regulation of heart metabolism. Thyroid 18:217–225

5. Jessup M, Brozena S (2003) Heart failure. N Engl J Med 348:2007–2018

6. Rutledge T, Reis VA, Linke SE et al (2006) Depression in heart failure: a meta-analytic review of prevalence, intervention effects, and associations with clinical outcomes. J Am Coll Cardiol 48:1527–1537

7. Pingitore A, Landi P, Taddei MC et al (2005) Triiodothyronine levels for risk stratification of patients with chronic heart failure. Am J Med 118:132–136

8. Premachandra BN, Kabir MA, Williams IK (2006) Low T3 syndrome in psychiatric depression. J Endocrinol Invest 29:568–572

9. Ustun TB, Ayuso-Mateos JL, Chatterji S et al (2004) Global burden of depressive disorders in the year 2000. Br J Psychiatry 184:386–392

10. Kessler RC, Chiu WT, Demler O et al (2005) Prevalence, severity, and comorbidity of 12-month DSM-IV disorders in the National Comorbidity Survey Replication. Arch Gen Psychiatry 62:617–627

11. Cook EL, Harman JS (2008) A comparison of health-related quality of life for individuals with mental health disorders and common chronic medical conditions. Public Health Rep 123:45–51

12. Burg MM, Abrams D (2004) Depression in chronic medical illness: the case of coronary heart disease. J Clin Psychol 57:1323–1337

13. Malhi GS, Parker GB, Greenwood J (2005) Structural and functional models of depression: from sub-types to substrates. Acta Psychiatr Scand 111:94–105

14. De Groot LJ (2006) Non-thyroidal illness syndrome is a manifestation of hypothalamic-pituitary dysfunction, and in view of current evidence, should be treated with appropriate replacement therapies. Crit Care Clin 22:57–86

15. Bianco AC, Larsen PR (2005) Intracellular pathways of iodothyronine metabolism. In: Braverman LE, Utiger RD (eds) Werner and Ingbar's The Thyroid: a fundamental and clinical text, 9th edn. Lippincott Williams and Wilkins, Philadelphia, pp 109–134

16. Gottlieb SS, Khatta M, Friedmann E et al (2004) The influence of age, gender, and race on the prevalence of depression in heart failure patients. Am Coll Cardiol 43:1542–1549

17. Lett HS, Blumenthal JA, Babyak MA et al (2004) Depression as a risk factor for coronary artery disease: evidence, mechanisms, and treatment. Psychosom Med 66:305–315

18. van Melle JP, de Jonge P, Spijkerman TA et al (2004) Prognostic association of depression following myocardial infarction with mortality and cardiovascular events: a meta-analysis. Psychosom Med 66:814–822

19. Lespérance F, Frasure-Smith N, Talajic M, Bourassa MG (2002) Five-year risk of cardiac mortality in relation to initial severity and one-year changes in depression symptoms after myocardial infarction. Circulation 105:1049–1053

20. Vaccarino V, Kasl SV, Abramson J, Krumholz HM (2001) Depressive symptoms and risk of functional decline and death in patients with heart failure. J Am Coll Cardiol 38:199–205

21. Abramson J, Berger A, Krumholz HM, Vaccarino V (2001) Depression and risk of heart failure among older persons with isolated systolic hypertension. Arch Intern Med 161:1725–1730

22. Murberg TA, Furze G (2004) Depressive symptoms and mortality in patients with congestive heart failure: a six-year follow-up study. Med Sci Monit 10: CR643–648

23. Müller-Tasch T, Peters-Klimm F, Schellberg D et al (2007) Depression is a major determinant of quality of life in patients with chronic systolic heart failure in general practice. J Card Fail 13:818–824

24. Horwich TB, Hamilton MA, MacLellan WR, Fonarow GC (2002) Low serum total cholesterol is associated with marked increase in mortality in advanced heart failure. J Card Fail 8:216–224

25. Friberg L, Drvota V, Bjelak AH et al (2001) Association between increased levels of reverse triiodothyronine and mortality after acute myocardial infarction. Am J Med 111:699–703

26. Ascheim DD, Hryniewicz K (2002) Thyroid hormone metabolism in patients with congestive heart failure: the low triiodothyronine state. Thyroid 12:511–515

27. Klemperer JD (2002) Thyroid hormone and cardiac surgery. Thyroid 12:517–521

28. Shanoudy H, Soliman A, Moe S et al (2001) Early manifestations of "sick euthyroid" syndrome in patients with compensated chronic heart failure. J Card Fail 7:146–152

29. Schultz M, Faber J, Kistorp C et al (2004) N-terminal-pro-B-type natriuretic peptide (NT-pro-BNP) in different thyroid function states. Clin Endocrinol (Oxf) 60:54–59

30. Doust JA, Glasziou PP, Pietrzak E, Dobson AJ (2004) A systematic review of the diagnostic accuracy of natriuretic peptides for heart failure. Arch Intern Med 164:1978–1984

31. Danzi S, Klein I (2004) Thyroid hormone and the cardiovascular system. Minerva Endocrinol 29:139–150

32. Danzi S, Klein I, Portman MA (2005) Effect of triiodothyronine on gene transcription during cardiopulmonary by-pass in infants with ventricular septal defect. Am J Cardiol 95:787–789

33. Morkin E, Pennock GD, Spooner PH et al (2002) Clinical and experimental studies on the use of 3,5-diiodothyropropionic acid, a thyroid hormone analogue, in heart failure. Thyroid 12:527–533

34. Pingitore A, Galli E, Barison A et al (2008) Acute effects of triiodothyronine (T3) replacement therapy in patients with chronic heart failure and low-T3 syndrome: a randomized, placebo-controlled study. J Clin Endocrinol Metab 93:1351–1358

35. Van den Berghe G, de Zegher F, Baxter RC et al (1998) Neuroendocrinology of prolonged critical illness: effects of exogenous thyrotropin-releasing hormone and its combination with growth hormone secretagogues. J Clin Endocrinol Metab 83:309–319

36. Baumgartner A (2000) Thyroxine and the treatment of affective disorders: an overview of the results of basic and clinical research. Int J Neuropsychopharmacol 3:149–165

37. Bunevicius R, Lasas L, Kazanavicius G, Prange AJ Jr (1996) Pituitary responses to thyrotropin releasing hormone in depressed women with thyroid gland disorders. Psychoneuroendocrinology 21:631–639

38. Williams M, Harris R, Dayan C et al (2008) Thyroid function and the natural history of depression: findings from the Caerphilly Prospective Study (CaPS) and a meta-analysis. Clin Endocrinol (Oxf) Aug 4 [Epub ahead of print]

39. Kirkegaard C, Faber J (1991) Free thyroxine and 3,3?,5?-triiodothyronine levels in cerebrospinal fluid in patients with endogenous depression. Acta Endocrinol (Copenh) 124:166–172

40. Lifschytz T, Segman R, Shalom G et al (2006) Basic mechanisms of augmentation of antidepressant effects with thyroid hormone. Curr Drug Targets 7:203–210

41. Nierenberg AA, Fava M, Trivedi MH et al (2006) A comparison of lithium and T(3) augmentation following two failed medication treatments for depression: a STAR*D report. Am J Psychiatry 163:1519–1530

42. Iosifescu DV, Bolo NR, Nierenberg AA et al (2008) Brain bioenergetics and response to triiodothyronine augmentation in major depressive disorder. Biol Psychiatry 63:1127–1134

43. Bunevicius R, Velickiene D, Prange AJ Jr (2005) Mood and anxiety disorders in women with treated hyperthyroidism and ophthalmopathy caused by Graves' disease. Gen Hosp Psychiatry 27:133–139

44. Saravanan P, Simmons DJ, Greenwood R et al (2005) Partial substitution of thyroxine with tri-iodothyronine in patients on thyroxine replacement therapy: results of a large community-based randomised controlled trial. Clin Endocrinol Metab 90: 805–812

45. Bunevicius R, Kazanavicius G, Zalinkevicius R, Prange AJ Jr (1999) Effects of thyroxine as compared with thyroxine plus triiodothyronine in patients with hypothyroidism. N Engl J Med 340: 424–429

46. Escobar-Morreale HF, Botella-Carretero JI, Escobar del Rey F, Morreale de Escobar G (2005) Treatment of hypothyroidism with combinations of levothyroxine plus liothyronine [review]. J Clin Endocrinol Metab 90:4946–4954

47. Caspi A, Sugden K, Moffitt TE et al (2003) Influence of life stress on depression: moderation by a polymorphism in the 5-HTT gene. Science 301:386–389

48. Otte C, McCaffery J, Ali S, Whooley MA (2007) Association of a serotonin transporter polymorphism (5-HTTL-PR) with depression, perceived stress, and norepinephrine in patients with coronary disease: the Heart and Soul Study. Am J Psychiatry 164:1379–1384

49. de Jong FJ, Peeters RP, den Heijer T et al (2007) The association of polymorphisms in the type 1 and 2 deiodinase genes with circulating thyroid hormone parameters and atrophy of the medial temporal lobe. J Clin Endocrinol Metab 92:636–640

50. Bunevicius R, Varoneckas G, Prange AJ Jr et al (2006) Depression and thyroid axis function in coronary artery disease: impact of cardiac impairment and gender. Clin Cardiol 29:170–174

Section **IV**

Treatment:
Present and Future Options

Treatment Options for Primary Thyroid Disease in Patients with Heart Failure

19

Anthony Toft and Kate Gaskell

Abstract The management of thyroid disease is usually straightforward. However, the presence of heart failure, whether due to primary thyroid disease or not, presents challenges to both diagnosis and management. Effective care requires an understanding of non-thyroidal illness and the effect of drugs on thyroid hormone metabolism, and a willingness to adapt treatment to the individual patient rather than adhering slavishly to guidelines.

Keywords Amiodarone • Atrial fibrillation • Carbimazole • Cardiomyopathy • Cardioversion • Iodine-131 • Non-thyroidal illness • Propranolol • Subclinical hyperthyroidism • Subclinical hypothyroidism • Thromboembolism • Thyrotropin • Thyrotropin-receptor antibody • Thyroxine

19.1 Hyperthyroidism

"The pulse was 156 in a minute, very full and hard, alike in both wrists, irregular as to strength, and intermitting at least once in six beats... (she) had twice or thrice been seized in the night with a sense of constriction and difficulty of breathing, which was attended with a spitting of a small quantity of blood... (the thyroid) occupied both sides of her neck, so as to have reached an enormous size, ... the eyes were protruded from their sockets, and the countenance exhibited an appearance of agitation and distress, especially on any muscular exertion... (she) had oedematous swelling of her legs and thighs...".

This description by Parry [1] of a patient he attended in 1786 was the first to associate atrial fibrillation and heart failure with hyperthyroidism due to what is now known as Graves' disease. The changes to the cardiovascular system in hyperthyroidism include increased resting heart rate, con-

tractility, ejection fraction, and blood volume and decreased systemic vascular resistance. As a result, cardiac output may increase as much as threefold [2]. It is surprising how well most patients tolerate these changes, complaining only of palpitations and breathlessness on exertion. There is evidence for a reversible cardiomyopathy with left ventricular ejection fraction decreasing on exercise [3], but overt cardiac failure is rare in patients under the age of 60 unless there has been long-standing severe thyrotoxicosis. Even in older patients there are often other contributing factors, such as hypertension and ischaemic or valvular heart disease. Although bilateral ankle edema is an early feature of cardiac failure, in patients with hyperthyroidism it is more likely to result from vasodilatation, reversal of the day:night ratio of urinary sodium and water excretion [4], and pulmonary hypertension [5].

19.1.1 Establishing the Diagnosis in Patients with Cardiac Failure

In Parry's patient, the clinical diagnosis of Graves' disease would now be obvious. There

A. Toft (✉)
Endocrine Clinic, Royal Infirmary, Edinburgh, Scotland, UK

G. Iervasi, A. Pingitore (eds.), *Thyroid and Heart Failure.*
© Springer-Verlag Italia 2009

would almost certainly have been a bruit audible over the enlarged vascular goitre and, for cardiac failure to have been present in such a relatively young patient, concentrations of serum free thyroxine (fT$_4$) and free triiodothyronine (fT$_3$) would have been markedly elevated and probably greater than 60 pmol/l (normal 9–21) and 20 pmol/l (normal 3–7), respectively. Isotope imaging would have shown a diffuse and increased uptake by the goitre and the concentration of the thyroid-stimulating hormone (TSH) receptor antibody (TRAb) in excess of 40 IU/l (normal less than 1.5). It is in the elderly with hyperthyroidism, however, that cardiac failure and atrial fibrillation are most likely to occur. The clinical diagnosis of hyperthyroidism in this group may not be so obvious. Weight loss may be obscured by fluid retention and oedema, reduced appetite and weakness due to proximal myopathy attributed to the debility of cardiac failure. There may be neither goitre nor ophthalmopathy. Even nodular thyroid disease, increasingly common with age, may not be palpable and only evident on isotope imaging. The hyperthyroidism of nodular thyroid disease is milder than in patients with Graves' disease and its duration longer. In up to 50% of patients, fT$_4$ is in the upper part of the reference range and fT$_3$ is elevated – so-called T$_3$ hyperthyroidism. Although less than 1% of patients with new-onset atrial fibrillation have evidence of overt hyperthyroidism [6], a diagnosis of hyperthyroidism should be considered in patients with atrial fibrillation or cardiac failure for which there is no obvious cause or in whom the complications are unexpected in the context of established heart disease. That such a policy is by no means universal is highlighted by the finding that 13% of patients with idiopathic atrial fibrillation attending a large teaching hospital cardiology clinic were found to have biochemical evidence of hyperthyroidism [7].

19.1.2 Subclinical Hyperthyroidism

The increasing availability of accurate tests of thyroid function has led to earlier diagnosis and treatment of hyperthyroidism than was possible even 25 years ago, when assays for TSH were less sensitive. It has been established that even the mildest form of overproduction of thyroid hormones, subclinical hyperthyroidism, in which a suppressed serum TSH concentration is associated with serum T$_3$ and T$_4$ concentrations within their respective reference ranges, is a risk factor for atrial fibrillation [8, 9]. The risk of developing atrial fibrillation is five times that of the control population and is no less than is the case for overt thyrotoxicosis [10]. One explanation for this unexpected finding is that subclinical hyperthyroidism is most commonly associated with nodular thyroid disease, which is typically found in those over 70 years of age. Such patients are likely to have other established heart diseases, themselves independent risk factors for atrial fibrillation. Even increases in thyroid hormone concentrations within their reference ranges are sufficient to trigger the dysrhythmia and precipitate or worsen cardiac failure in susceptible patients.

19.1.3 Hyperthyroidism or Non-thyroidal Illness?

Thyroid function tests may be altered in non-thyroidal illness and mimic biochemical hyperthyroidism. Several mechanisms are involved; these include suppression of TSH release due to increased concentrations of dopamine, cytokines, cortisol, and somatostatin; reduction in the extrathyroidal conversion of T$_4$ to T$_3$, also a feature of treatment with amiodarone; displacement of thyroid hormones from plasma proteins by drugs, such as furosemide in the management of cardiac failure; changes in the affinity characteristics and in the serum concentrations of thyroid hormone binding proteins; and methodological problems associated with free T$_3$ and T$_4$ measurements [11]. The finding of a suppressed serum TSH concentration with a raised free T$_4$ concentration of 25–40 pmol/l is not an uncommon finding in patients with significant non-thyroidal illness, such as atrial fibrillation and cardiac failure. Indeed, in a large series of hospitalised patients, a low serum TSH concentration was three times as likely to be due to non-thyroidal illness than to hyperthyroidism [12]. In most patients with significant non-thyroidal illness serum total T$_3$ will be low-normal, but if it is in the upper part of the reference range this may be due to a fall from a previously elevated concentration in a patient with hyperthyroidism due to impaired T_4 to T_3 conversion. In the absence of ophthalmopathy or goitre, measurement of the TSH receptor antibody and isotope imaging may be helpful in detecting Graves' disease or impalpable nodular thyroid disease. If there still remains doubt, a trial of antithyroid drugs for a period of 3–6 months may be indicated.

19.1.4 Treatment of Cardiac Failure and Atrial Fibrillation

19.1.4.1 Reducing the Tachycardia

As in any patient with cardiac failure, treatment with diuretics such as furosemide is essential. In the presence of atrial fibrillation, digoxin is unlikely to be effective. There is not only a reduced sensitivity of the heart to digoxin in hyperthyroidism, but also increased renal clearance [13]. Indeed, failure to slow the ventricular rate in patients with atrial fibrillation, despite normally adequate doses of digoxin, should raise the clinical suspicion of hyperthyroidism, particularly if there is a response to the addition of a small dose of a β-adrenoceptor antagonist such as propranolol. There have been isolated reports of cardiovascular collapse in Chinese people with thyrotoxic cardiomyopathy within hours of the administration of propranolol [14, 15]. However, the consensus is that this class of drugs is an essential primary treatment of hyperthyroid heart failure, whether atrial fibrillation is present or not, by improving the tachycardia-mediated aspect of ventricular dysfunction without altering systolic or diastolic performance [2]. Propranolol in an oral dose of 160 mg daily, preferably as a slow-release preparation, will reduce heart rate significantly to less than 100 beats per minute within 24 h in the majority of patients [16]. Although a $β_1$-selective agent such as atenolol will be equally effective in reducing heart rate, it is less useful in ameliorating the tremor and anxiety. It should be emphasised that β-adrenoceptor blockade does not abolish the tachycardia of hyperthyroidism but is a useful interim adjunct therapy until antithyroid drugs restore thyroid hormone concentrations to normal.

19.1.4.2 Reducing Thyroid Hormone Concentrations

Antithyroid Drugs

Although propranolol, but not other β-adrenoceptor antagonists, inhibits the peripheral conversion of T_4 to T_3, with a rise in the serum concentration of the metabolically inactive reverse T_3, the changes are minor and confer no clinical benefit [17].

Carbimazole, its active metabolite, methimazole, and propylthiouracil act by inhibiting thyroid hormone synthesis. Patients begin to notice an improvement in their symptoms after some 2–3 weeks of treatment with carbimazole in a dose of 40 mg daily. The equivalent dose for methimazole is 30 mg and for propylthiouracil 400 mg, taken as 200 mg twice daily. In most patients, serum T_3 and T_4 concentrations will have returned to their reference ranges by 6–8 weeks [18]. The normal maintenance dose for carbimazole is 5–15 mg daily. Adjustment to the dose in the early weeks of treatment is guided by clinical response and concentrations of thyroid hormones, as there is a delay in pituitary thyrotrophs recovering from suppression by previously elevated serum T_3 and T_4 concentrations. At this stage, it is possible to record a misleadingly low serum TSH of < 0.01 mU/l in the presence of normal or low serum T_3 and T_4 concentrations [19]. After 6–8 weeks of antithyroid drug therapy, the best guide to the appropriate dose of carbimazole is the serum TSH concentration. Once thyroid function is stable, ablative treatment with iodine-131 is an option. The alternative is to continue with carbimazole long-term rather than run the risk of recurrent hyperthyroidism and its cardiovascular consequences if antithyroid drugs are stopped after a conventional period of 12–18 months. In this respect, it has been shown that antithyroid drugs are safe and cost-effective if given continuously for 10 years or more [20].

Iodine-131

Within a few days of treatment with iodine-131 there may be a radiation-induced leak of stored thyroid hormones into the circulation and a significant increase in the serum concentrations of both T_3 and

T$_4$ [21]. In most patients with hyperthyroidism due to Graves' disease or nodular thyroid disease, this transient increase in serum thyroid hormone concentrations is of no significance, but in those with thyrocardiac disease the worsening of thyrotoxicosis may have serious clinical consequences and may even precipitate thyroid crisis.

Pre-treatment with antithyroid drugs does not prevent an increase in serum T$_3$ and T$_4$ concentrations after iodine-131 therapy, but any increase is from a lower baseline [22] and not harmful. This pattern is consistent with the observation that antithyroid drug therapy can reduce the content of both T$_3$ and T$_4$ in the thyroid gland of patients with Graves' disease by over 95% [23]. Almost 20 years ago, a survey of members of the American Thyroid Association found that 31% of correspondents prescribed antithyroid drugs before and 40% after iodine-131 treatment [24]. It would be surprising, however, if patients with thyrocardiac disease or hyperthyroid patients with unrelated cardiac conditions, such as ischaemic or valvular heart disease, were not rendered euthyroid prior to iodine-131 therapy and during the 6–8 weeks before radioiodine is effective.

Treatment with antithyroid drugs before, and probably after, iodine-131 therapy renders the thyroid relatively radioresistant and increases the risk of treatment failure [25, 26]. The effectiveness of carbimazole is not diminished if it is withdrawn for as little as 24–48 h before and after iodine-131 administration [27]. There is some evidence that propylthiouracil confers even greater radioresistance [28], but suggestions that this antithyroid drug should be withdrawn for at least 2 weeks either side of iodine-131 treatment are impractical, exposing a vulnerable patient to uncontrolled hyperthyroidism. It is likely that any radioresistance resulting from antithyroid drug therapy will be overcome by the use of the high doses of iodine-131 of 400–600 MBq (11–16 mCi) administered by most endocrinologists to patients with thyrocardiac disease in order to achieve euthyroidism as quickly as possible and in the knowledge that hypothyroidism within 2–4 months is likely. In the authors' clinic, patients with severe hyperthyroidism or with thyrocardiac disease are first rendered euthyroid with carbimazole. The antithyroid drug is stopped 72 h before treatment with 400 MBq iodine-131 and re-started in the same dose 72 h after therapy and continued for a period of 6 weeks. Review of the patient at 8 weeks allows a meaningful assessment of thyroid status.

The presence of significant active thyroid eye disease would be an indication for long-term treatment with carbimazole rather than with iodine-131. The high doses of glucocorticoids recommended to ameliorate any radiation-induced deterioration in orbitopathy would be unwise in patients with cardiac failure [29].

19.1.4.3 Reducing the Risk of Thromboembolism

The risk of thromboembolism in patients with thyrotoxic atrial fibrillation has not been quantified adequately. Opinions range from advocating warfarin for most patients [30] to the view that in younger patients with no evidence of structural heart disease or hypertension the risk of anticoagulation may outweigh the benefits [2]. There is some evidence that the risk of systemic embolisation is significantly less in atrial fibrillation due to hyperthyroidism than in mitral stenosis or ischaemic heart disease [31]. However, it is likely that the presence of cardiac failure enhances any risk of thromboembolism in patients with thyrotoxic atrial fibrillation, and anticoagulants would seem sensible in this context, particularly if elective cardioversion is anticipated. Clearly, any decision about anticoagulants should be tailored to individual patients, and the elderly in whom compliance may be in doubt or with a history of falls would be candidates for treatment with aspirin rather than warfarin. Anti-coagulant control may be difficult because hyperthyroidism is associated with an increased sensitivity to warfarin [32].

19.1.4.4 Timing of Cardioversion

It is unlikely that a patient with thyrotoxic atrial fibrillation complicated by cardiac failure and, therefore, likely to be associated with other forms of heart disease will revert to stable sinus rhythm spontaneously. The chances of successful elective electrical cardioversion are probably under 20% but are less dependent on the duration of atrial fibrillation than on the absence or presence of structural heart disease [33]. Despite the low success rate, one attempt at cardioversion is worthwhile, but it should be delayed until serum TSH concentrations have been detectable for at least 6 weeks, given that the effects of hyperthyroidism on cardiac function persist for that length of time after restoration of thyroid hormone concentrations to normal [3].

19.1.5 Problems Posed by Amiodarone

"A 70 year old man presented with weight loss of 7 kg over a period of two months, associated with a reduced appetite, worsening breathlessness and bilateral leg oedema, despite treatment with furosemide, spironolactone, and ramipril, prescribed after he had sustained an anterior myocardial infarction complicated by the development of atrial fibrillation and congestive cardiac failure nine months earlier. He had also been taking amiodarone 200 mg daily but, because of the development of exfoliative dermatitis, this had been replaced by digoxin some two months before. Examination revealed him to be in atrial fibrillation with a ventricular rate of 160 beats per minute and in biventricular failure. He was noted for the first time to have a small nodular goitre. Serum fT_4 was markedly elevated at 80 pmol/l (normal 9–21) and total T_3 marginally raised at 2.8 nmol/l (normal 1.1–2.6). Serum TSH concentration was less than 0.05 mU/l. Uptake of iodine-131 by the thyroid at 4 h was negligible and ultrasound examination confirmed the presence of a multinodular goitre."

This case illustrates many of the features of amiodarone-induced thyrotoxicosis, which carries a high mortality in the presence of left ventricular dysfunction [34]. Amiodarone in a dose of 200 mg daily provides more than fifty times the recommended intake of iodine. As iodine is one of the building blocks for thyroid hormone synthesis, excess iodine will precipitate hyperthyroidism in patients in whom there is underlying autonomous thyroid dysfunction, as in Graves' disease or nodular goitre. This is known as type I amiodarone-induced thyrotoxicosis and it tends to be more severe in areas of iodine deficiency. The disproportionately high ratio of T_4 to T_3 in this form of hyperthyroidism is a reflection of decreased peripheral monodeiodination of thyroxine to triiodothyronine. Amiodarone has a half-life of some

50 days as it is stored in fat, which becomes a slow-release depot of iodine. As a result, amiodarone-induced thyrotoxicosis may present many months after the anti-dysrhythmic drug has been withdrawn.

As iodine uptake is negligible in patients with amiodarone-induced thyrotoxicosis, the initial treatment is with carbimazole, which may have to continue indefinitely if amiodarone is deemed the best treatment for chronic atrial fibrillation. If amiodarone can be withdrawn, it may be possible to administer an ablative dose of iodine-131 once there has been recovery of iodine uptake. This therapy would allow the future use of amiodarone without fear of precipitating hyperthyroidism. In patients with severe amiodarone-induced thyrotoxicosis, treatment with carbimazole alone may not reduce serum thyroid hormone concentrations adequately within weeks as would normally be expected. In that situation the addition of potassium perchlorate, which inhibits the uptake of iodine by the thyroid, is indicated.

In type II amiodarone-induced thyrotoxicosis, there is a chemical thyroiditis in patients with an inherently normal thyroid gland, with release of preformed thyroid hormones. Hyperthyroidism is transient, lasting for several weeks, and often followed by an equally short-lived phase of hypothyroidism. There are no investigations that reliably distinguish between the type I and type II forms, but the presence of goitre, ophthalmopathy, pretibial myxedema, and TSH-receptor antibodies in the serum favours a diagnosis of type I amiodarone-induced thyrotoxicosis.

A "wait and see" policy may be appropriate in patients thought to have type II amiodarone-induced thyrotoxicosis and was favoured by both European and American thyroidologists in a recent survey [35]. However, given the frequent uncertainty in distinguishing between the two forms, a pragmatic approach is to treat all patients with carbimazole [36], and to withdraw the antithyroid drug if the serum TSH concentration becomes elevated – an indication of the hypothyroid phase of amiodarone-induced thyroiditis.

It is obviously important that thyroid function is assessed prior to starting treatment with amiodarone, but such a sensible policy is honoured more in the breach than in the observance, perhaps understandably in the charged atmosphere of dealing with an ill patient in the emergency room.

19.2 Hypothyroidism

Overt hypothyroidism, in which the serum fT_4 concentration is low and serum TSH concentration elevated, usually in excess of 20 mU/l (normal < 4.5), is characterised by decreased heart rate, myocardial contractility, and cardiac output and by increased systemic vascular resistance and mild diastolic hypertension. In addition, there may be raised total and low-density lipoprotein (LDL) cholesterol, endothelial dysfunction, and increased arterial stiffness. These changes predispose patients to cardiovascular disease and, ultimately, cardiac failure.

However, in both primary care and hospital practice, there is now a low threshold for measuring thyroid function, and most patients identified with thyroid failure have the mildest form, or subclinical hypothyroidism, in which serum fT_4 is in the lower part of the reference range and serum TSH elevated, but usually less than 10 mU/l. The patient with long-standing profound hypothyroidism with cardiac failure, pleural and pericardial effusions, and ascites is vanishingly rare in clinical practice. The usual challenges are the initiation of thyroid hormone replacement in patients with overt hypothyroidism, symptomatic ischaemic heart disease, and cardiac failure, when subclinical hypothyroidism should be treated, and determining the appropriate dose of thyroxine.

19.2.1 Initiation of Thyroxine Therapy

Although it is reasonable to prescribe a full replacement dose of thyroxine of 100–150 μg daily to a patient immediately following total thyroidectomy for differentiated thyroid carcinoma, the received medical wisdom, no doubt based on accumulated anecdotal evidence, is that in the elderly and in those with symptomatic ischaemic heart disease or cardiac failure, thyroxine should be prescribed in a low dose of 25 μg daily and increased incrementally by 25 μg every 6–8 weeks until serum TSH is normal. The only significant study of the effects of thyroxine therapy in patients with co-existent hypothyroidism and angina pectoris was conducted almost 50 years ago [37]. Angina improved in 38% of patients, was unchanged in 46%, and deteriorated in 16%. There can be no hard or fast rule about how to treat patients with cardiovascular disease

and overt hypothyroidism, which is now more likely to be an associated condition rather than causative. Each patient should be considered on his or her merits.

"A 65-year-old woman with a history of myocardial infarction complicated by the development of cardiac failure two years previously presented with several episodes of central chest pain radiating to the jaw and left arm, each lasting up to 30 min during the preceding 24 h. Thyroid function tests performed two weeks earlier because of a strong family history of thyroid disease revealed a serum fT_4 concentration of 7 pmol/l (normal 9–21) and TSH of 23.0 mU/l (normal less than 4.5). She had been started on treatment with thyroxine in a dose of 25 μg daily and had taken this medication for three days. ECG revealed a sinus bradycardia of 50 beats per min and 1.5 mm horizontal ST-segment depression in leads II, III, and aVF. Serum troponin was less than 0.2 μg/l."

It is unlikely that thyroxine prescribed in the low dose of 25 μg daily for a period of 3 days was related to the development of the acute coronary syndrome, and it is equally unlikely that delaying cardiovascular intervention for several weeks until thyroid function tests were restored to normal with thyroxine would have been in the patient's best interest. The advice should be to proceed to angiography and, probable, re-vascularisation of the affected right coronary artery as soon as possible. However, in a patient with established ischaemic heart disease who experiences angina every 2–3 weeks after strenuous exercise, which is quickly relieved by glyceryl trinitrate, it would be appropriate to start thyroxine treatment in the anticipation that there would be no change in the severity of symptoms.

As there are no slow-release forms of triiodothyronine available, it is inappropriate to use combinations of synthetic triiodothyronine and thyroxine or thyroid extract in the treatment of patients with significant cardiac disease, as there is a peak serum T_3 concentration 1–2 h after ingestion that may be sufficient to induce symptomatic tachycardia.

19.2.2 Bioavailability of Thyroxine

An increasing number of drugs have been shown to reduce the absorption of thyroxine. Those relevant to patients with cardiovascular disease include: ferrous sulphate prescribed, to reverse the iron deficiency anaemia induced by long-term use of aspirin; calcium salts, given prophylactically to an ageing population to prevent reduction in bone mineral density; and proton-pump inhibitors, such as omeprazole, widely used in the treatment of gastro-oesophageal reflux disease. A rise in serum TSH concentration in a patient previously well-controlled on a stable dose of thyroxine should prompt a review of other medication rather than an immediate assumption of poor compliance. There are several generic preparations of thyroxine and there are issues about their bioequivalence [38]. It is wise to insist that the same preparation of thyroxine is dispensed after each prescription refill.

19.2.3 Subclinical Hypothyroidism – To Treat or Not?

Rather surprisingly, a large cross-sectional population study concluded that subclinical hypothyroidism was an independent risk factor for atherosclerosis and myocardial infarction in elderly women, comparable to smoking, diabetes mellitus, and hypercholesterolaemia [39]. However, this finding was neither confirmed in the longitudinal component of the study nor in a 10-year cohort study [40]. Randomised controlled trials of the effect of thyroxine replacement in patients with subclinical hypothyroidism failed to show a reduction in either total or LDL-cholesterol [41], or an improvement in well-being in patients with a serum TSH concentration of less than 10 mU/l who were considered to be symptomatic [42].

Minor decreases in myocardial contractility can be detected by echocardiography in patients with subclinical hypothyroidism [43], but the clinical significance of such observations is far from clear for most patients. However, any subtle decrease in myocardial contractility may be important in the context of cardiac failure and it would be reasonable to treat with thyroxine in such circumstances.

There is a consensus that patients with subclinical hypothyroidism and a serum TSH concentration greater than 10 mU/l should be treated, as some 5% of such patients per year develop overt thyroid failure. It makes sense to "nip things in the bud" rather than wait for symptoms to develop or run the risk of lost follow-up.

A raised serum TSH concentration but a normal serum free T$_4$ in the presence of cardiac failure may be temporary and a manifestation of the changes in thyroid function with time in relation to recovery from non-thyroidal illness [12] or the transient hypothyroid phase of an amiodarone-induced thyroiditis.

19.2.4 How Much Thyroxine?

The majority of patients with primary hypothyroidism feel well while taking thyroxine in a dose that restores both serum TSH and fT$_4$ to their respective reference ranges, as recommended by the American Thyroid Association [44]. For most clinicians, this means an fT$_4$ in the upper part of the reference range and a TSH in the lower part of its reference range, e.g., serum fT$_4$ 19 pmol/l, serum TSH 0.5 mU/l. Some patients only achieve a sense of well-being if serum TSH is suppressed and fT$_4$ is high normal or even elevated, albeit less than 30 pmol/l. Although a suppressed serum TSH is not recommended in patients taking thyroxine replacement therapy [45], this guidance is based on misinterpretation of important studies [8, 40, 46]. There is no evidence that a suppressed serum TSH is harmful if the serum T$_3$ concentration is unequivocally normal. However, in view of the lack of agreement about what constitutes the correct dose of thyroxine, and adhering to the practice of wishing to do no harm, it would be judicious to adjust the dose of thyroxine replacement in patients with cardiac disease so that serum TSH is normal.

Key Points

- β-Adrenoceptor antagonists are an integral part of the treatment of thyrotoxic atrial fibrillation and cardiac failure.

- Subclinical hyperthyroidism is a risk factor for atrial fibrillation.

- Pre-treatment with antithyroid drugs before and after iodine-131 therapy should be standard practice in patients with hyperthyroid atrial fibrillation and/or cardiac failure.

- Thyroid function should be assessed prior to treatment with amiodarone.

- There is no evidence that treatment of subclinical hypothyroidism in patients with a serum TSH concentration of < 10 mU/l is of benefit.

References

1. Parry CH (1825) Collections from the unpublished medical writings. Underwood, London, vol 2, pp 111–120
2. Klein I, Danzi S (2007) Thyroid disease and the heart. Circulation 116:1725–1735
3. Forfar JC, Muir AL, Sawers SA et al (1982) Abnormal left ventricular function in hyperthyroidism: evidence for a possible reversible cardiomyopathy. N Engl J Med 307:1165–1170
4. Bell GM, Sawers JSA, Toft AD et al (1982) Nocturnal natriuresis in hyperthyroidism. Clin Endocrinol 16:177–182
5. Marvisi M, Zambrelli P, Brianti M et al (2006) Pulmonary hypertension is frequent in hyperthyroidism and normalizes after therapy. Eur J Intern Med 17:267–271
6. Krahn AD, Klein GJ, Kerr CR et al (1996) How useful is thyroid function testing in patients with recent-onset atrial fibrillation? Arch Intern Med 156:2221–2224
7. Forfar JC, Miller HC, Toft AD (1979) Occult thyrotoxicosis: a reversible cause of "idiopathic" atrial fibrillation. Am J Cardiol 44:9–12
8. Sawin CT, Geller A, Wolf PA et al (1994) Low serum thyrotropin concentrations as a risk factor for atrial fibrillation in older persons. N Engl J Med 331:1249–1252
9. Cappola AR, Fried LP, Arnold AM et al (2006) Thyroid status, cardiovascular risk, and mortality in older adults. JAMA 295:1033–1041
10. Auer J, Scheibner P, Mische T et al (2001) Subclinical hyperthyroidism as a risk factor for atrial fibrillation. Am Heart J 142:838–842
11. Beckett GJ, Toft AD (2008) Thyroid dysfunction. In: Marshall WJ, Bangert SK (eds) Clinical biochemistry. Metabolic and clinical aspects. Churchill Livingstone Elsevier, Edinburgh, pp 394–421
12. Spencer C, Eigen A, Shen D et al (1987) Specificity of sensitive assays for thyrotropin (TSH) used to screen for thyroid disease in hospitalized patients. Clin Chem 33:1391–1396
13. Kim D, Smith TW (1984) Effects of thyroid hormone on sodium pump sites, sodium content, and contractility responses to cardiac glycosides in cultured chick ventricular cells. J Clin Invest 74:1481–1488
14. Ngo AS, Lung Tan DC (2006) Thyrotoxic heart disease. Resuscitation 70:287–290
15. Dalan R, Leow MK (2007) Cardiovascular collapse associated with beta blockade in thyroid storm. Exp Clin Endocrinol Diabetes 115:392–396
16. Toft AD, Irvine WJ, Campbell RWF (1976) Assessment by continuous cardiac monitoring of minimum duration of pre-operative propranolol treatment in thyrotoxic patients. Clin Endocrinol 5:195–198
17. Shulkin BL, Peek ME, Utiger RD (1984) Beta-adrenergic antagonist inhibition of hepatic 3, 5, 3?-triiodothyronine production. Endocrinology 115:858–861
18. Page SR, Sheard CE, Herbert M et al (1996) A comparison of 20 and 40 mg per day of carbimazole in the initial treatment of hyperthyroidism. Clin Endocrinol 45:511–515
19. Toft AD, Irvine WJ, Hunter WM et al (1974) Anomalous plasma TSH levels in patients developing hypothyroidism in the early months after 131-I therapy for thyrotoxicosis. J Clin Endocrinol Metab 39:607–608
20. Azizi F, Ataie L, Hedayati M et al (2005) Effect of long-term continuous methimazole treatment of hyperthyroidism: comparison with radioiodine. Eur J Endocrinol 152:695–701
21. Shafer RB, Nuttall FQ (1975) Acute changes in thyroid function in patients treated with radioactive iodine. Lancet ii:635–637
22. Burch HB, Solomon BL, Cooper DS et al (2001) The effect of antithyroid drug pre-treatment on acute changes in thyroid hormone levels after 131I ablation for Graves' disease. J Clin Endocrinol Metab 86:3016–3021
23. Larsen PR (1975) Thyroidal triiodothyronine and thyroxine in Graves' disease: correlation with presurgical treatment, thyroid status and iodine content. J Clin Endocrinol Metab 41:1098–1104
24. Solomon B, Glinoer D, Lagasse R et al (1990) Current trends in the management of Graves' disease. J Clin Endocrinol Metab 70:1518–1524
25. Sabri O, Zimny M, Schulz G et al (1999) Success rate of radioiodine therapy in Graves' disease. J Clin Endocrinol Metab 84:1229–1233
26. Bonnema SJ, Bennedbaek FN, Veje A et al (2006) Continuous methimazole therapy and its effect on the cure rate of

hyperthyroidism using radioactive iodine: an evaluation by a randomized trial. J Clin Endocrinol Metab 91:2946–2951

27. Andrade VA, Gross JL, Maia AL (2001) The effect of methimazole pretreatment on the efficacy of radioiodine therapy in Graves' hyperthyroidism: one-year follow-up of a prospective, randomized study. J Clin Endocrinol Metab 86:3488–3493

28. Imseis RE, Vanmiddlesworth L, Massie JD et al (1998) Pretreatment with propylthiouracil but not methimazole reduces the therapeutic efficacy of iodine-131 in hyperthyroidism. J Clin Endocrinol Metab 83:685–687

29. Bonnema SJ, Bartalena L, Toft AD et al (2002) Controversies in radioiodine therapy: relation to ophthalmopathy, the possible radioprotective effect of antithyroid drugs, and use in large goitres. Eur J Endocrinol 147:1–11

30. Yuen RW, Gutteridge DH, Thompson PL et al (1979) Embolism in thyrotoxic atrial fibrillation. Med J Aust 1:630–631

31. Yipintsoi T, Jirathimopas W, Suntiparpluacha C et al (1992) Embolism and atrial fibrillation. J Med Assoc Thai 75:73–78

32. Kellett HA, Sawers JSA, Boulton FE et al (1986) Problems of anticoagulation with warfarin in hyperthyroidism. Q J Med 58:43–51

33. Nakazawa H, Lythall DA, Noh J et al (2000) Is there a place for the late cardioversion of atrial fibrillation? A long-term follow-up study of patients with post-thyrotoxic atrial fibrillation. Eur Heart J 21:327–333

34. O'Sullivan AJ, Lewis M, Diamond T (2006) Amiodarone-induced thyrotoxicosis: left ventricular dysfunction is associated with increased mortality. Eur J Endocrinol 154:533–536

35. Tanda ML, Piantanida E, Lai A et al (2008) Diagnosis and management of amiodarone-induced thyrotoxicosis: similarities and differences between North American and European thyroidologists. Clin Endocrinol 69:812–818

36. Osman F, Franklyn JA, Sheppard MC, et al (2002) Successful treatment of amiodarone-induced thyrotoxicosis. Circulation 105:1275–1277

37. Keating FR, Parkin TW, Selby JB et al (1961) Treatment of heart disease associated with myxedema. Progr Cardiovasc Dis 3:364–381

38. Toft A (2005) Which thyroxine? Thyroid 15:124–126

39. Hak AE, Pols HA, Visser TJ et al (2000) Subclinical hypothyroidism is an independent risk factor for atherosclerosis and myocardial infarction in elderly women: the Rotterdam Study. Ann Intern Med 132:270–278

40. Parle JV, Maisonneuve P, Sheppard MC et al (2001) Prediction of all-cause and cardiovascular mortality in elderly people from one low serum thyrotropin result: 1 10-year cohort study. Lancet 358:861–865

41. Danese MD, Ladenson PW, Meinert CL et al (2000) Effect of thyroxine therapy on serum lipoproteins in patients with mild thyroid failure: a quantitative review of the literature. J Clin Endocrinol Metab 85:2993–3001

42. Kong WM, Sheikh MH, Lumb PJ et al (2002) A 6-month randomized trial of thyroxine treatment in women with mild subclinical hypothyroidism. Am J Med 112:358–354

43. Biondi B, Fazio S, Palmieri EA et al (2002) Effects of subclinical hypothyroidism on the heart. Ann Intern Med 137:904–914

44. Surks MI, Chopra IJ, Mariash CN et al (1990) American Thyroid Association guidelines for use of laboratory tests in thyroid disorders. JAMA 263:1529–1532

45. Vaidya B, Pearce SHS (2008) Management of hypothyroidism in adults. Br Med J 337:284–289

46. Uzzan B, Campos J, Cucherat M et al (1996) Effects on bone mass of long-term treatment with thyroid hormone: a meta-analysis. J Clin Endocrinol Metab 81:5278–4289

Alessandro Pingitore, Vincenzo Lionetti and Francesca Forini

Abstract Heart failure (HF) should be seen in a unique scenario of altered systemic homeostasis, in which heart dysfunction, peripheral organ dysfunction, and derangement of the neuroendocrine and immune systems represent chronic cross-talking between stress stimuli, with continuous activation of the stress response. The thyroid hormone (TH) system is profoundly involved in cardiovascular and systemic homeostasis. In HF, the most frequent alteration of TH metabolism is a low-triiodothyronine state, which may participate directly in progression of HF. Initial results have shown that TH replacement therapy in patients with HF improves cardiac performance, hemodynamic and exercise performance. It also induces deactivation of the neuroendocrine profile, as a result of the significant reductions in vasoconstrictor/sodium-retaining norepinephrine and aldosterone. It in the plasma levels of their counterpart, N-terminal pro B-type natriuretic peptide (NT-proBNP). Depending on the pathophysiology of the HF, two strategies of TH replacement therapy have been suggested: (1) the cardiosystemic strategy, which involves administration of synthetic T_4 or T_3, and (2) the cardioselective one, using TH analogues, in particular 3,5-diiodothyropropionic acid (DITPA). The rationale of these two approaches is based on the pathophysiology of HF progression, which is linked to progressive impairment of systolic–diastolic cardiac function, but also to systemic disturbance, which frequently progresses independently of deteriorating cardiac function.

Keywords Heart failure • Thyroid hormone • Homeostasis • Triiodothyronine • Thyroxine • Thyroid analogues

20.1 Heart Failure and Systemic Dyshomeostasis: The Role of the Thyroid Hormone System

Cardiac insufficiency is the prime mover of heart failure (HF) syndrome. The left ventricle moves less and too weakly to pump a sufficient amount of blood throughout the body. An increase in atrial pressure and capillary wedge pressure is the local consequence of left ventricular dysfunction; an inadequate circulating blood supply is the systemic one. Neuroendocrine activation is the direct and immediate response to reduced cardiac output and provides a suitable explanation of the systemic involvement in HF. This response is characterized by the activation of different systems that can be divided into two main, counterbalancing arms: the vasoconstrictive sodium water-retaining systems and the vasodilative natriuretic systems. Atrial natriuretic peptide (ANP) is primarily synthesized by the atria in response to atrial distention, whereas brain

A. Pingitore (✉)
C.N.R. Clinical Physiology Institute, S. Cataldo Research Campus, Pisa, Italy

G. Iervasi, A. Pingitore (eds.), *Thyroid and Heart Failure.*
© Springer-Verlag Italia 2009

natriuretic peptide (BNP) is synthesized by the ventricles in response to increased filling pressure and ventricular dilation. Both have vasodilator and natriuretic effects in response to fluid overload induced by cardiac insufficiency, thus antagonizing the vasoconstriction and fluid retention mechanisms of the sympathetic and the renin–angiotensin–aldosterone systems.

More recently, besides those of the neurohormone family, other biologically active molecules have been implicated in the pathophysiology and evolution of HF. In addition to neuroendocrine activation, the so-called cytokine hypothesis implies that overexpression of these molecules – in particular, tumor necrosis factor α (TNF-α) and interleukin-6 (IL-6) – is a maladaptive response favoring progressive cardiac decompensation in HF [1–3]. In experimental studies, cytokines inhibit contractility directly [4], increase apoptosis, and alter interstitial matrix [5]. Clinical studies showed that TNF-α and IL-6 increase in patients as their functional HF classification deteriorates [6] and the levels these factors were independent predictors of mortality [7, 8].

Neuroendocrine activation and increased plasma levels of cytokines represent only a part of the large spectrum of systemic derangement in HF. Kidney involvement was the basis of the hemodynamic model proposed in the past in an attempt to describe the pathophysiology of HF. More recently, the so-called cardiorenal syndrome underscored the high incidence (almost 25% of patients with HF) of renal insufficiency and its negative prognostic impact in patients with HF [9]. In particular, moderate renal insufficiency (glomerular filtration rate $\cong$ 60 ml/min) was shown to increase overall and cardiac death, with every 1 ml/min decrease in estimated glomerular filtration rate, corresponding to a 1% increase in mortality in patients with HF [10, 11]. In addition, anemia is associated with cardiorenal insufficiency in the so-called cardiorenal–anemia syndrome [12]. Renal insufficiency contributes to anemia by reduced production of erythropoietin, in association with diabetes, elevated plasma cytokine levels, malabsorption, and the use of angiotensin-converting enzyme (ACE) inhibitors and angiotensin receptor antagonists [12]. The prevalence of anemia among patients with HF is almost 20% [13], and when it is persistent, it provides independent prognostic information, with higher overall mortality and re-hospitalization rates in patients with HF [14,15].

Depressive disorders are the other relevant clinical aspect of the systemic disturbance in HF. The incidence of depression in chronic HF varies between 11 and 58%; the prognostic relevance of this disorder is still debated [16]. Recently, depression was shown to be independently associated with poor clinical outcomes including all-cause mortality and vascular events (stroke, transitory ischemic attacks, and acute myocardial infarction) in elderly patients with HF [17].

For these reasons, in the pathophysiology of chronic stress stimuli [18], HF should be seen in a unique scenario of altered systemic homeostasis (Fig. 20.1), in which heart dysfunction, peripheral organ dysfunction, and derangement of the neuroendocrine and immune systems represent chronic stress stimuli, with continuous activation of the stress response. This, in turn, predisposes to allostatic load, defined by McEwan as "the cumulative strain on the body produced by repeated ups and downs of physiologic response, as well as by the elevated activity of physiologic systems under challenge and the changes in metabolism and the impact of wear and tear on a number of organs and tissue," which "can predispose the organism to disease" [18]. In other words, "allostatic load" is the price the body pays for being continuously forced to adapt to adverse physical and pathophysiological situations [19]. In the case of HF, this refers to the continuous up-regulation that occurs when neuroendocrine and immunoreactive systems shift their effects from compensatory to unfavorable and, finally, to toxic, as documented by the induction of calcium overload and apoptosis and stimulation of myocardial fibrosis – all promoting left ventricular remodeling [20] and systemic impairment.

In this scenario, left ventricular dysfunction is the most important clinical and prognostic variable in the early phases of HF, when this is still an organ disease, and that in the continuing evolution of HF can progress in two very different arms, cardiac and systemic, in which clinical status and patient outcome are mainly dominated by the progressive left ventricular dysfunction and the systemic derangement, respectively.

The thyroid hormone (TH) system is profoundly involved in cardiovascular and systemic homeostasis. The effects of TH on the heart are mediated either through extranuclear nongenomic or genomic actions [21, 22]. Genomic TH actions regulate the transcription of genes encoding different enzymes

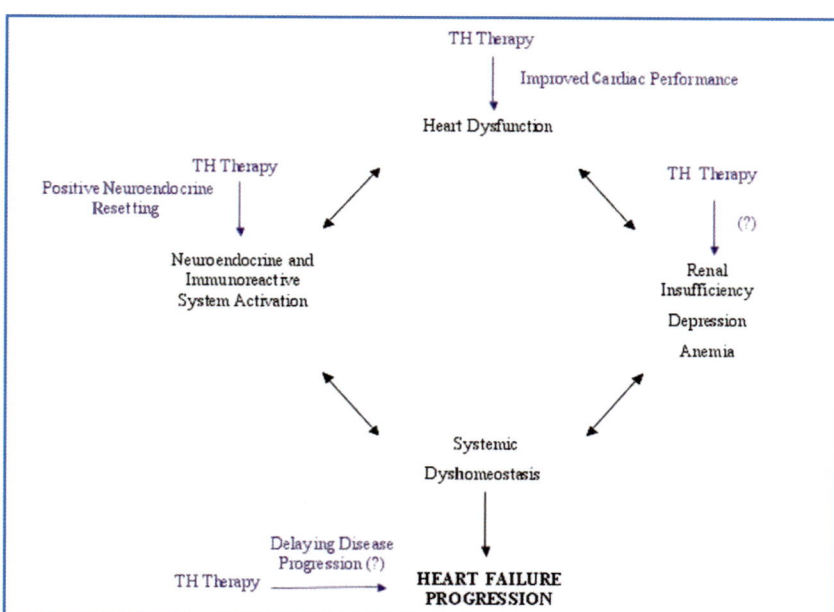

Fig. 20.1 Hypothesized pathophysiological scenario of heart failure (HF) in which heart dysfunction, peripheral organ dysfunction, and neuroendocrine and immune systems act synergetically to impair systemic homeostasis and promote HF progression. This may be delayed by TH therapy, which has positive effects on heart function, neuroendocrine activation, and probably also on peripheral organ function

and functional and structural proteins, such as Na^+-K^+ ATPase, sarcoplasmic reticulum Ca^{++} adenosine triphosphatase (SERCA II), phospholamban, voltage-gated K channels, Na^+/Ca^{++} exchanger, and myosin heavy chains (MHC) [21, 22]. Nongenomic actions include the cellular transport of amino acids and sugars and ion fluxes at the level of the plasma membrane [23]. At the vascular level, TH promotes arterial vasodilation through nongenomic and endothelium-independent mechanisms, but also through a direct and acute endothelial-mediated vasodilating effect on resistance vessels, as shown experimentally and in thyroidectomized patients [24, 25]. The role of the TH system in maintaining systemic homeostasis is determined by its effects on the functions of different organs and systems, that is, the same organs and systems found to be altered in HF, and its interactions with several hormonal pathways. Altered thyroid metabolism leads to renal insufficiency and mood alterations, with symptoms of depression and anxiety. In hypothyroid patients, serum creatinine is higher than in controls, and the severity of thyroid dysfunction correlates with renal function [26]. More interestingly, as discussed in Chapter 17 of this volume, low-T_3 syndrome frequently characterizes end-stage renal failure; in these patients it correlates with the severity of left ventricular dysfunction and is an independent predictor of death [27, 28].

The main psychological symptoms in hypothyroidism are working memory decrement, somatic complaints, anxiety, and depressive features [29, 30]. Moreover, patients with coronary artery disease and depressive symptoms have a higher incidence of HF and lower T_3 circulating levels, suggesting an association between altered thyroid profile, depression, and cardiac dysfunction [31]. The relationship between thyroid system and other hormone pathways is particularly crucial in the HF context, in which neuroendocrine activation plays a pivotal pathophysiological role. Cellular, subcellular, and biohumoral findings reinforce this hypothesis. Thyroid–adrenergic synergy is bidirectional [32], with TH potentiating β_1-adrenergic receptor signals, increasing both the number of receptors and cAMP production through the stimulation of adenylyl cyclase activity [32, 33], whereas the adrenergic system promotes peripheral conversion of T_4 to T_3 by increasing type II iodothyronine 5β-deiodinating activity [34]. The expression of genes encoding angiotensin type I and II receptors, which mediate TH-induced myocardial hypertrophy through transforming growth factor β_1 [35], significantly increased in rats with thyroidectomy-induced hypothyroidism [36]. This result may be interpreted as being part of the fetal gene program induced by low T_3 circulating levels, characterized by changes in MHC proteins, with decreased expression of α-MHC and increased β-MHC expression, and a reduced SERCAII/phospholamban ratio [37, 38].

Cytokines, in particular TNF and ILs 1 and 6, have been implicated in the pathogenesis of low-T_3 syndrome in several groups of patients, especially those with HF [39, 40]. Cytokine induction in low-T_3 syndrome is similar to that documented in HF, i.e., the reduction in peripheral T_4 to T_3 conversion by the inhibition of deiodination activity [41].

TH increases serum levels of BNP, probably through a direct stimulatory effect on its secretion at the level of both atrial and ventricular myocytes [42]. BNP secretion, BNP mRNA levels, and BNP promoter activity increased three- to sixfold following T_3 treatment [43]. In patients with subclinical or overt hyperthyroidism, BNP levels were significantly higher than those of controls [44].

In addition to these close links between TH and other endocrine patterns, which justify the supposition of a central role of TH in preserving systemic homeostasis, other aspect strengthening the role of TH is the finding showing subclinical and reversible alterations of cardiovascular and other organ system functions in mild TH dysfunction, i.e., subclinical hypothyroidism and subclinical hyperthyroidism [26, 45, 46]. A negative prognostic impact of any form of mild TH dysfunction has been observed in cardiac patients [47]. Thus, it is plausible that a normal thyroid status is essential for maintaining systemic and cardiovascular homeostasis; when it is persistently lost, increased whole-body and cardiovascular vulnerability is observed.

20.2 The Low-T3 Syndrome in Heart Failure: The Two Sides of a Coin

The most frequent alteration of TH metabolism in HF is the low-T_3 syndrome, previously interpreted as a merely adaptive mechanism that resulted in the reduction of catabolic processes of illness, thus having beneficial effects through the reduction in metabolic demand [48, 49]. However, as previously described by Danzi and Klein (see Chap. 10), low-T_3 syndrome mimics hypothyroid syndrome, sharing similar cardiovascular and systemic alterations. Accordingly, the new hypothesis is that low-T_3 syndrome participates directly in HF progression. This hypothesis is supported by the observed direct detrimental effect induced by hypothyroidism on cardiac morphology and on the structure, histology, and systolic and diastolic function of the left ventricle, as shown in the experimental setting, and the

reversibility of these alterations after normalization of the TH profile [50]. Further clinical findings showed the negative prognostic impact of low-T_3 syndrome in patients with HF, who had a significantly higher incidence of cardiac and cumulative death than did patient without low-T_3 syndrome [50–54]. Thus, restoration of normal TH metabolism appears to interrupt the vicious cycle of HF, which involves heart dysfunction, systemic impairment, and activation of the neuroendocrine and immune–inflammatory systems, together resulting in impairment of systemic and cardiovascular homeostasis.

In this context, TH replacement therapy may be considered a new therapeutic frontier in patients with HF, in addition to the current neuroendocrine treatment portfolio. The potential therapeutic strategies that can be employed to optimize TH signaling in the presence of HF and nonthyroidal illness syndrome can be summarized by the following points:

- Administration of synthetic L-T_4. By this approach, the main physiological pathway of secretion and peripheral metabolism of TH system is guaranteed.
- Administration of L-T_3, that is, the biologically active form of TH.
- Administration of a TH analogue having a predominantly cardiotropic action, with positive properties similar to those of natural TH, but with lower adverse effects.
- Genetic manipulation of the expression of cardiovascular deiodinases; in this case, the goal is to increase the local production and bioavailability of T_3.
- Genetic manipulation of the cardiovascular TH receptor pattern. Here, the goal is to increase hormonal signaling in the presence of normal or even low levels of bioavailable T_3.

The last two points are discussed in Chapter 22 of this volume. In the present chapter, TH treatment with synthetic L-T_4 and with L-T_3 and TH analogues is discussed.

20.3 Thyroid Hormone Administration in Experimental Settings

During HF progression, a vicious cycle is activated, consisting of cell loss, altered glycemic and lipid metabolism, and abnormal coronary microcirculation [55–59], which reciprocally interact to further left ventricular dilation and dysfunction. Abnormality of TH metabolism – specifically, reduced availability of biologically active T₃ – favors this vicious cycle through a direct detrimental effect on genomic complement, histology, and cardiac morphology and structure [60], and thus on the systolic and diastolic function of the left ventricle. Normalization of the TH profile through the administration of TH may reverse the negative effects of altered thyroid metabolism, potentially interrupting the vicious cycle of HF progression [61]. In experimental settings, the beneficial effects of TH administration have been observed at different levels of the heart system: cellular, metabolic, and vascular [62, 63] (Fig. 20.2).

20.3.1 Myocytes

Alteration of the cardiomyocyte cytoskeleton, a reduced number of myocytes, and increased myocardial fibronecrosis have been documented under various experimental conditions of hypothyroidism (Bio T0-2 hamster model of primitive dilated cardiomyopathy in which subclinical hypothyroidism develops spontaneously and in the rat

model of hypothyroidism induced by 6 weeks of treatment with propylthiouracil [64], and also in a human model of prolonged (10 days) T₃-deprived atrial myocardial cultured tissue [60]). In this latter study, cellular remodeling, consisting of enlargement of myocyte surface area and transverse diameter, led to the disorganization of cultured myocardium and phenotypical remodeling of myocardium [60], which resembled the gross and cellular structural impairment observed during HF progression [50, 65, 66]. These morphological and structural alterations were associated with a significantly reduced expression of α-sarcomeric actin, an essential protein for preserving the cytoskeleton, which has been related to left ventricular remodeling in human HF [67]. Experimental studies showed that T₃ administration reverses cellular degenerative processes, very likely through activation and regulation of the different intracellular signaling pathways involved in cell protection, growth, and proliferation. Among these, P13K-Akt signaling, which exerts a potent antiapoptotic action [68], was shown to be rapidly activated in isolated rat myocytes treated with continuous T₃ administration for 24 h [69, 70]. The evidence that the T₃-induced Akt signaling pathway is mediated through α₁ thyroid

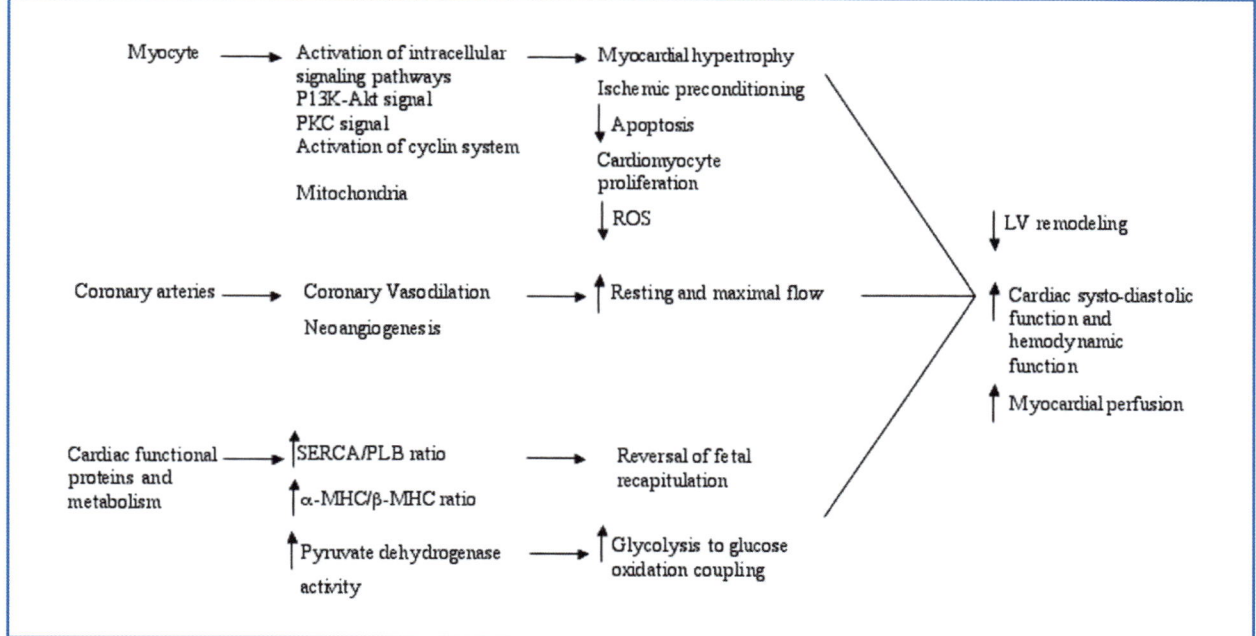

Fig. 20.2 Cardiac effects of synthetic TH administration in the experimental setting of dilated cardiomyopathy and/or hypothyroidism. *SERCA* sarcoplasmic reticulum Ca adenosine triphosphatase, *PLB* phospholamban, *MHC* myosin heavy chains, *ROS* reactive oxygen species, *PKC* protein kinase C, *LV* left ventricle

receptors located in the cytosol [69] supports the hypothesis of cytosolic nongenomic actions of TH that are rapid in onset and able to maintain the hormone's long-term effects.

Protein kinase C (PKC), one of a family of serine–threonine kinases, is involved in several cardiac processes, including left ventricular hypertrophy, regulation of cardiac gene expression, and the modulation of different steps in excitation–contraction coupling [71, 72]. PKC isozymes are differentially expressed in neonatal and adult cardiac rats, with the α, δ, and ϵ forms equally expressed in neonatal heart and ϵ isozymes predominant in the adult heart. TH specifically down-regulates PKC-α and PKC-ϵ in the neonatal heart and PKC-ϵ in the adult heart [73]. TH regulatory activation of PKC signaling may have relevant clinical and therapeutic implications in light of evidence that stable activation of PKC can promote disturbances in the growth and hormone responsiveness of noncardiac cells, and, in particular, that sustained treatment with the selective PKC-ϵ inhibitor attenuates cardiac fibrosis and dysfunction in hypertension-induced HF [74]. Moreover, T_3 administration promotes myocyte proliferation, mediated by the activation of cyclins and cyclin-dependent kinases. Cyclin D1 mRNA cytosolic levels were enhanced in the heart of T_3-treated rats, and, most importantly, also in the nuclear fraction, indicating that T_3 has the ability to induce translocation of the cyclin from the cytoplasm to the nucleus. Moreover, the nuclear translocation of cyclin D1 was associated with increased synthesis of cardiomyocyte DNA, as demonstrated by increased levels of cyclin A, a specific marker of the S phase of the cell cycle [75].

The importance of oxidative stress is increasingly emerging with respect to a pathophysiological mechanism of left ventricular remodeling responsible for progression of HF. Mitochondria are the predominant source of reactive oxygen species in failing hearts, indicating a pathophysiological link between mitochondrial dysfunction and oxidative stress [76]. Mitochondrial injury is reflected by mtDNA damage as well as by a decline in mtRNA transcripts, protein synthesis, and mitochondrial function [77]. The mitochondrial transcription factor A (TFAM) is a nucleus-encoded protein that binds mtDNA and promotes the transcription of mtDNA. Cardiac-specific disruption of the TFAM gene in mice resulted in dilated cardiomyopathy in association with a reduced amount of mtDNA and

mitochondrial transcripts [78]. In addition, a reduction in TFAM expression has been demonstrated in several forms of cardiac failure [79]. However, the forced overexpression of TFAM was able to produce the opposite effect [80], even ameliorating the decline in mtDNA copy number and mitochondrial electron transport function, which may contribute to a decrease in myocardial oxidative stress [81]. Recent investigations conduced by Iervasi's group confirmed that TFAM expression is significantly reduced in the myocardium of the border zone of infarcted rodent hearts, which is related to a severe regional and global impairment of cardiac function. Long-term administration of T_3, starting at 72 h after coronary ligation, maintained myocardial expression of TFAM at normal levels, which was regionally related to ameliorated mitochondrial activity and improved cardiac function [82].

20.3.2 Coronaries, Microcirculation, and Neoangiogenesis

In an ex vivo animal model of ischemia-reperfusion, a reduction of coronary resistance and an increase in coronary flow was documented after T_3 administration [83]. This finding fits well with evidence of a relaxant effect of TH in different vascular districts, including the coronary arteries, which is independent of cAMP and nitric oxide formation [84]. The T_3 vasodilatory effect has both an endothelium-independent component, which is more evident at physiological concentrations of T_3, and an endothelium-dependent component, more evident at supraphysiological concentrations of T_3 [85]. Also, in the hamster cheek pouch microcirculation, T_3 treatment consistently induced a dose-dependent dilation of arterioles more rapid than that induced by T_4 administration [86]. Further, a neoangiogenic response, consisting of capillary proliferation, has been documented after TH treatment. This response is rapid in onset and occurs after a single injection of synthetic T_4 (L-T_4), primarily in the venous capillaries, and is linked to overexpression of β-FGF as well as to mechanical factors, i.e., wall tension, shear stress, and increased capillary flow [87]. Similarly, long-term administration of a TH analogue, 3,5-diiodothyrotropionic acid (DITPA), stimulates coronary arteriolar growth by up-regulating key angiogenic growth factors in normal rats [88] and in post-infarcted rats, in which DITPA-induced angiogenesis was associated with a less pronounced postinfarction remodeling process, a reduction in infarct expansion, and a high left ventricular ejection fraction [89].

20.3.3 Cardiac Functional Proteins and Metabolism

The effects of TH and of TH abnormalities on cardiac metabolism and proteins are extensively discussed in Chap. 11. This section briefly describes the effects of TH treatment on cardiac metabolism and proteins in experimental settings. The improvement in cardiac efficiency and function after ischemia–reperfusion is partially explained by the T_3-induced modulation of glucose metabolism. T_3 administration during reperfusion improves the coupling of glycolysis to glucose oxidation by increasing the activity of pyruvate dehydrogenase. This metabolic effect is associated with a reduced cellular concentration of protons (H^+) produced from glycolysis, which negatively influences cardiac efficiency. Protons are exchanged with extracellular Na^+ via the Na^+/H^+ exchanger, thus reducing Ca^{2+} efflux and resulting in Ca^{2+} overload and cell death [90].

Modulation of calcium handling through the sarcoplasmic reticulum is strongly influenced by TH, which up-regulates protein levels of sarcoplasmic reticulum calcium-ATPase (SERCA2) and down-regulates its inhibitor, phospholamban [22]. This effect has been shown in hypothyroid rat hearts treated with T_3 [91] and after acute myocardial infarction in rats treated with thyroid powder, in which the increased SERCA2/phospholamban ratio, associated with a shift in cardiac MHC isoform expression (with increased expression of α-MHC and decreased expression of β-MHC), attenuated cardiac remodeling, and significantly improved myocardial performance [92]. Also, in the unloaded heart, characterized by reduced cardiac performance and impaired left ventricular relaxation, and at the cellular level, by increased phospholamban activity with a reduced SERCA2/phospholamban protein ratio, treatment with physiological doses of T_3 induced normalization of the SERCA2/phospholamban ratio, improving ventricular relaxation and contractility [93]. Interestingly, neither the MHC isoform shift (from the β to the α isoform) nor induction of left ventricular hypertrophy was observed, suggesting that the observed beneficial

effects of T_3 were partly due to the restoration of calcium handling [94]. Another potential T_3-activated pathway is the overexpression of ryanodine receptors, which are an important protein in the junctional sarcoplasmic reticulum, mediating the release of calcium to trigger muscle contraction [95].

20.3.3 Concluding Remarks for Experimental Settings

All the experimental findings described above offer a mechanistic basis for a TH-system-based therapy in patients with left ventricular dysfunction and low or borderline levels of T_3 [61]. Restoration of a normal TH profile might counteract the progression of HF by (1) positive remodeling through the modulation of myocardial gene expression and cell protection and proliferation, (2) improving cardiac systolic and diastolic function and reducing vascular resistance, with a consequent improvement in hemodynamics, and (3) improving myocardial perfusion, which is known to be impaired in the early stage of dilated cardiomyopathy and leads to progression towards HF and death.

20.4 Thyroid Hormone Treatment in Cardiac Patients Without Heart Failure

Several studies have shown potential benefits of TH replacement therapy in patients with acute cardiac diseases frequently characterized by the presence of a low-T_3 syndrome. In patients undergoing cardiac surgery, both adult and pediatric, with or without left ventricular dysfunction [83], T_3 administration reduces the incidence of postoperative atrial fibrillation [96], improves hemodynamic performance, thus reducing the need for inotropic agents, and reduces troponin I release [97, 98]. T_3 treatment also reduces surgical death in patients at high risk of death during open heart surgery [99]. Treatment of children with T_3 before and after cardiopulmonary bypass operations improves myocardial function, especially in patients with low postoperative cardiac output without adverse events, and reduces the need for postoperative intensive care [100, 101]. In the setting of cardiac transplantation, T_3 treatment induces rapid achievement of hemodynamic stability, allowing significant reduction of inotropic support in human brain-dead organ donors, and also provides excellent hemodynamic function of the cardiac allograft in the recipients [102]. In a case of acute myocarditis complicated by hemodynamic instability, acute renal failure, and low-T_3 syndrome, T_3 treatment, given at a rate of 2 μg/h and in addition to dobutamine and intra-aortic balloon pump, was beneficial in stabilizing hemodynamics without the appearance of arrhythmias or other side effects [103].

20.5 Thyroxine Treatment in Patients with Heart Failure

Synthetic T_4 (L-T_4) was given orally at the "physiological" dose of 100 μg/day in the short term (1 week) and as continuous 3-month treatment [104, 105] to patients with nonischemic dilated cardiomyopathy (Table 20.1). In both studies, L-T_4 was well-tolerated and induced a significant improvement in cardiac pump function, consisting of enhanced resting cardiac output and exercise capacity and reduced systemic vascular resistance. Interestingly, low-dose dobutamine (10 μg/kg per min) induced a higher increase in cardiac output and heart rate in L-T_4-treated than in placebo-treated patients, very likely indicating enhanced cardiac adrenergic sensitivity in agreement with experimental data showing a β_1-adrenergic up-regulating effect of TH [106]. The beneficial hemodynamic effects of intravenous T_4 administration (20 μg/h) were documented in 10 patients with cardiogenic shock who were unresponsive to conventional pharmacological inotropic therapy and intra-aortic balloon counterpulsation. In that study, T_3 was sampled at baseline in three patients only and all of them had low-T_3 syndrome, but T_3 or T_4 levels after T_4 infusion were not reported. The cardiovascular effects of continuous infusion of L-T_4 were maintained for a long enough time to complete definitive surgical treatment, consisting of heart transplantation or left ventricular assist device [107].

20.6 Triiodothyronine Treatment in Patients with Heart Failure

A few studies, with a limited number of patients, assessed the effects of synthetic T_3 replacement therapy in patients with HF and low-T_3 syndrome (Table 20.1) [61, 108, 109]. In one study, T_3 was administered intravenously in a bolus dose followed or not by an infusion of L-T_3 for a few hours, whereas in two other studies L-T_3 was administered continuously for 3 days at an initial dose of 20 μg/m^2 body surface per day, diluted in 100 ml saline; the dose was adjusted, when necessary, in order to maintain circ circulatingevels within the physiological range [61, 109]. Irrespective of the L-T_3 regimen adopted, T_3 was well, tolerated and untoward effects (arrhythmias, myocardial ischemia episodes, hemodynamic instability) were not documented. In the study by Hamilton et al., patients with advanced HF (NYHA functional class III–IV) and low T_3 levels and/or elevated plasma rT_3 values, who received the high dose of T_3 (T_3 bolus of 0.7 μg/kg followed by 6–12 h T_3 infusion to a total dose of 1 or 2 μg/kg) had a significant increase in cardiac output and a reduction in systemic vascular resistance [108]. Although circulating T_3 levels obtained after L-T_3 administration varied widely (but always above the upper limit of the normal range), no side effects were documented.

These results were confirmed in an invasive hemodynamic study, and in a noninvasive study that assessed left ventricular performance using cardiac magnetic resonance. These two studies enrolled patients with ischemic and nonischemic dilated cardiomyopathy and low-T_3 syndrome, with optimized conventional HF therapy, and in stable clinical condition. In the invasive study, constant infusion of L-T_3 induced a progressive reduction in systemic vascular resistance and an increase in ejection fraction and cardiac output, the latter invasively monitored by Swan-Ganz catheter. Urinary output also improved, whereas no changes in heart rate and systemic arterial blood pressure were observed [109]. In the noninvasive study, in which the protocol design was randomized allocation to T_3 treatment versus placebo and controlled, a 3-day continuous T_3 infusion (Fig. 20.3) increased stroke volume in association with increased end-diastolic volume, as documented with cardiac magnetic resonance (Fig. 20.4) [61]. The increased end-diastolic volume can be considered to reflect the recruitment of residual ventricular filling reserve, which is a fundamental compensatory mechanism for maintaining cardiac output in patients with HF [110]. It may have been the result of the positive effects of biologically active T_3 on diastolic relaxation secondary to the

Table 20.1 Results of triiodothyronine (T_3) and thyroxine (T_4) treatment in patients with heart failure

Reference/year of study	No. of patients, study type	DCM type	Clinical status	LVEF (%)	TH type	Administration and dose	Main results protocol	Heart rate	Side effects
Hamilton et al. 1998 [108]	23, uncontrolled	Ischemic, nonischemic	Stable	22 ± 1	T_3 cumulative dose 0.15–2.7 µg/kg	Bolus + continuous infusion (6–12 h)	↓SVR ↑CO	Unchanged	No
Moruzzi et al. 1994 [104]	10, randomized placebo-controlled	Nonischemic	Stable 2	7 ± 8	T_4 100 µg/day	1 week p.o.	↓SVR at dobutamine ↑CO at dobutamine ↑Exercise tolerance and oxygen consumption ↑Resting LVEF	Unchanged	No
Moruzzi et al. 1996 [105]	10, randomized placebo-controlled	Nonischemic	Stable	30 ± 4	T_4 100 µg/day	3 months p.o.	↑Cardiac performance at rest, exercise and dobutamine ↓LVEDD ↓SVR	Unchanged	No
Malik et al. 1999 [107]	10, uncontrolled	Systolic HF (cardiogenic shock)	Unstable	Not available	T_4 20 µg/h infusion (36 h)	Bolus+continuous ↓PCWP and MAP	↑CI	Unchanged	No
Iervasi et al. 2001 [109]	6, uncontrolled	Ischemic, nonischemic		24 ± 3	T_3 initial dose 20 µg/m² body surface per day	Continuous infusion (4 days)	↓SVR ↑CO ↑UO	Unchanged	No
Pingitore et al. 2008 [61]	20, randomized placebo-controlled	Ischemic, nonischemic	Stable	25 18–32	T_3 initial dose 20 µg/m² body surface per day	Continuous infusion (3 days)	↑LFSV ↑LVEDV ↓NT-proBNP ↓Norepinephrine ↓Aldosterone	Reduced	No

DCM dilated cardiomyopathy, *LVEF* left ventricular ejection fraction, *TH* thyroid hormone, T_3 triiodothyronine, T_4 thyroxine, *SVR* systemic vascular resistance, *CO* cardiac output, *LVEDD* left ventricular end-diastolic diameter, *PCWP* pulmonary capillary wedge pressure, *MAP* mean arterial pressure, *LVSV* left ventricular stroke volume, *NT-proBNP* N-terminal pro B-type natriuretic peptide

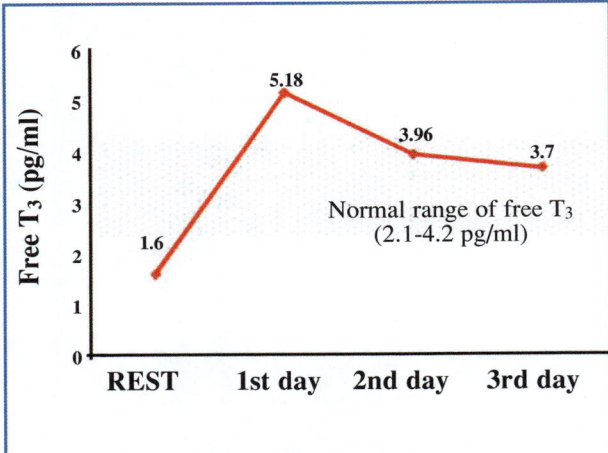

Fig. 20.3 Example of L-T$_3$ circulating levels during 3-day continuous infusion of L-T$_3$. The initial infusion dose of L-T$_3$ was 20 μg/m^2 body surface; during the 3-day infusion, the T$_3$ dose was changed in order to maintain circulating T$_3$ levels within the normal range

increase in calcium ATPase of the SERCA pump [111] and to the inhibition of its counterregulator phospholamban [91, 92]. Our study's results fit well with those observed after normalization of the thyroid state in patients with mild primitive hypothyroidism and normal left ventricular function [112]. In that study, left ventricular stroke volume, ejection fraction, and cardiac index significantly increased after synthetic TH replacement therapy, while blood pressure and heart rate did not change. Importantly, the improvement in cardiac performance induced by T$_3$ did not correspond to increased myocardial oxygen consumption, as indirectly estimated by calculation of the rate pressure product as well as total cardiac work. The ameliorated cardiac metabolism efficiency fits well with the data of Hamilton et al. showing unchanged systemic metabolic demand after T$_3$ infusion, as assessed by indirect calorimetry [108]. Moreover, the benefit of T$_3$ infusion on

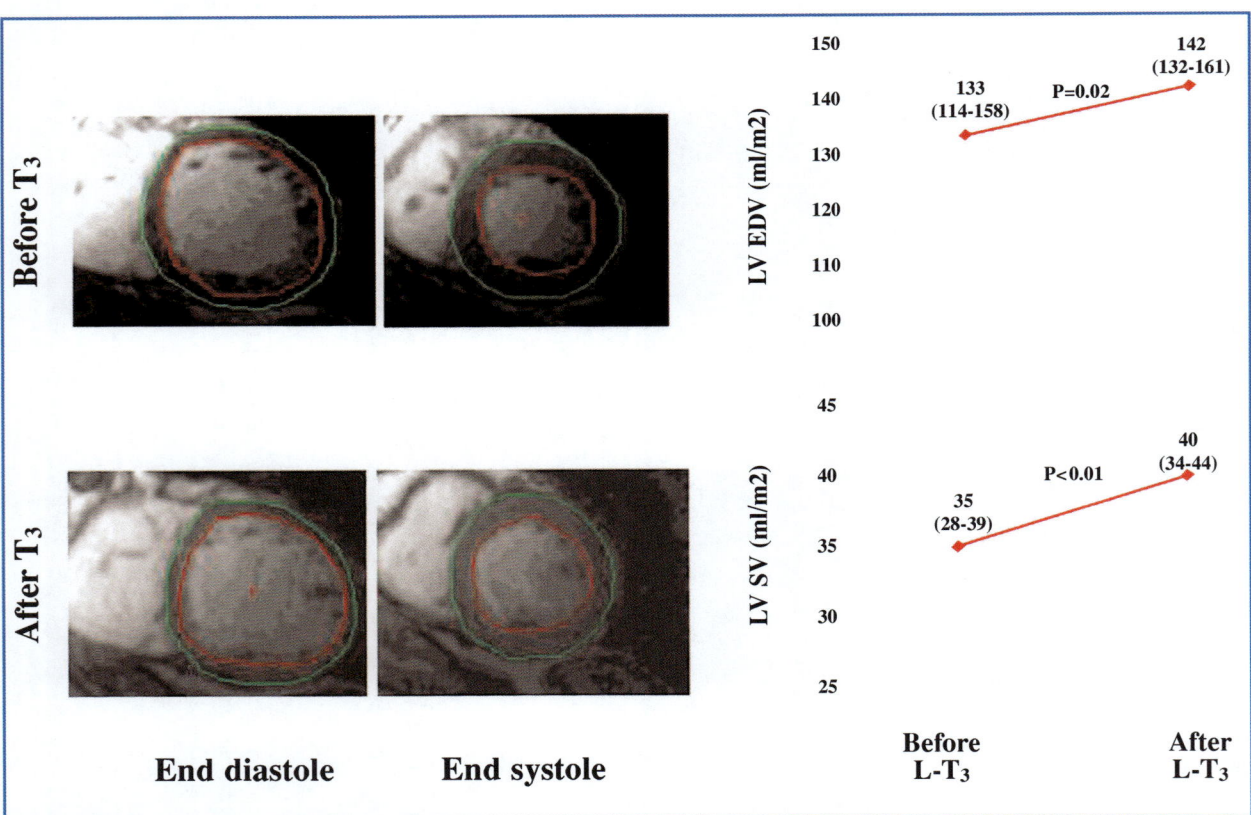

Fig. 20.4 Example of cardiac magnetic resonance performed in a patient with dilated cardiomyopathy and low-T$_3$ syndrome before and after L-T$_3$ treatment. The images show the traced endocardial (*red line*) and epicardial (*green line*) borders of the left ventricle for calculating left ventricular volumes. Histograms show the values of the left ventricular end-diastolic volume (*LVEDV*) and stroke volume (*LVSV*) before and after T$_3$

cardiac function parallels a deactivation of the neuroendocrine profile, as seen from the significant reduction in the vasoconstrictor/sodium-retaining norepinephrine and aldosterone, and in the plasma levels of their counterpart NT-proBNP (Fig. 20.5). It is uncertain whether the neuroendocrine rearrangement is an indirect result of T_3-mediated action, due to improved cardiac performance, rather than a direct result of it. As previously mentioned, THs per se increase rather than decrease catecholamines, BNP, and aldosterone release. However, the potential clinical relevance of T_3-induced neuroendocrine deactivation in patients with left ventricular dysfunction is clearly deducible from an analysis of data reported in the literature that shows highly beneficial effects of aldosterone and β-adrenergic antagonists in terms of survival, rate of hospitalization, symptoms, and cardiac performance [65]. Taken together, the T_3-mediated improvement in cardiac function and positive neuroendocrine reset strongly suggest that normalization of the TH profile inverts the vicious cycle of HF, characterized by progressive cardiac dysfunction, neuroendocrine activation, and systemic disturbance, and thus delays disease progression and restores cardiovascular and systemic homeostasis (Fig. 20.1).

20.7 Which Synthetic Thyroid Hormone and What Dose?

There are no randomized controlled studies documenting which is the better TH treatment – T_3 or T_4 – and the dose for administration in patients with HF. Although T_4 administration may represent the more physiological view of synthetic TH treatment, since the larger part of circulating T_3 derives from the peripheral conversion of T_4 to T_3, several observations suggest that T_3 may in fact be more beneficial than T_4. The physiological pattern of peripheral conversion from T_4 into T_3 is impaired in the presence of a nonthyroidal illness syndrome, and thus the administration of T_3 bypasses this step through direct provision of the biologically active TH. This point becomes all the more critical if we consider that the cardiovascular system predominantly uses circulating T_3. Moreover, experimental findings showed that the restoration of serum-bioactive T_3 by constant infusion of T_4 was unable to normalize tissue levels of T_3, including in the myocardium [112]. This may be even more evident in the presence of impaired peripheral conversion of T_4 into T_3, as in the presence of low-T_3 syndrome.

The dose at which T_3 is given should be adjusted to keep circulating blood levels of T_3 within normal physiological ranges and at a constant blood concentration, avoiding abrupt changes up and down. A constant circulating level of T_3 provides more effective nuclear action and T_3-mediated transcription in the myocardium than do fluctuating T_3 circulating levels [113]. Moreover, the administration of L-T_3 at high doses, mimicking a hyperthy-

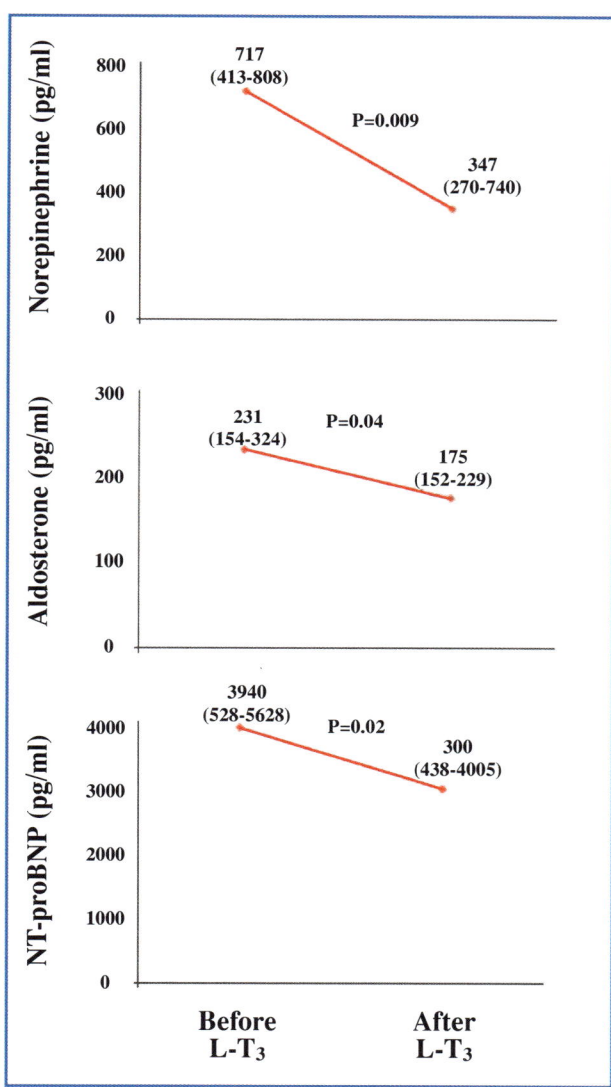

Fig. 20.5 Norepinephrine, aldosterone, and N-terminal pro B-type natriuretic peptide (NT-proBNP) in patients with heart failure before and after L-T_3 treatment

roid status, may be detrimental when the hormone is used long-term. Experimental data have clearly documented that myocardial hypertrophy induced by high doses of T_3 is associated with an improved cardiac performance only initially, followed by a decline after 1 month of treatment [114]. This finding was also associated with the increased expression of uncoupling proteins (UCP2 and 3) that may be responsible for the decrease in mitochondrial efficiency during thyroid hyperfunction [115]. The real question is the mode of administration of T_3 that will maintain constant circulating blood levels of T_3. This is not guaranteed with pills or drops, but probably will require long-acting transdermal patch systems, which are still not commercially available.

20.8 Treatment with TH Analogues in Patients with Heart Failure

The rationale of developing TH analogues is to guarantee organ-selective effects without the potential untoward events of TH. Among the family of TH analogues, diiodothyropropionic acid (DITPA), a thyroxine analogue, has cardiac inotropic and lusitropic selectivity, accompanied by minimal effects on heart rate and oxygen consumption [116]. DITPA binds to T_3 nuclear receptors and induces transcription of genes regulated by T_3 [117]. Although there are numerous experimental studies on the effects of DITPA on systolic and diastolic cardiac function and on coronary arterial growth [118], few studies have assessed the potential beneficial cardiac effects of this compound in patients with HF. In a pilot randomized clinical study of DITPA versus placebo, DITPA was well-tolerated without side effects in patients with NYHA functional class II–III HF. After 4 weeks of treatment, cardiac output significantly increased in association with decreased systemic vascular resistance and improved diastolic function. Interestingly, total serum cholesterol and triglyceride levels also decreased significantly [117]. Because of this limited clinical experience, more data are needed to establish the DITPA dose regimen to be used in patients with HF, and the prognostic and clinical potential benefits of such treatment. However, very recently reported data from a phase 2 randomized controlled trial, presented at the Heart Failure Society of America 2008 scientific meeting, indicated that DITPA is not well-tolerated and fails in the treatment of human HF [119]. Possible explanations are that: (1) a dose-ranging study was not performed prior to the trial, or (2) the use of cardioselective TH analogues may not be the optimal treatment strategy owing to the systemic nature of HF.

20.9 Systemic Effects of Thyroid Hormone Therapy in Patients with Heart Failure

To date, no evidence exists on the systemic effects of TH in patients with HF, with the exception of the positive neuroendocrine resetting mentioned above. However, in patients with hypothyroidism without HF, normalization of the TH profile significantly improves renal function, expressed both as glomerular filtration rate and as serum creatinine concentration [26, 30, 46, 120]. These clinical findings, shown in clinical settings different from HF, are important in view of the systemic dyshomeostasis in HF, which may be further reinforced by low-T_3 syndrome.

20.10 Conclusions

In accordance with the approaches discussed above, two strategies of TH replacement therapy in patients with HF are suggested:
1. Cardiosystemic, administering synthetic T_4 or T_3
2. Cardioselective, using TH analogues, in particular DITPA

The rationale of these two approaches is based on the pathophysiology of HF progression, which is linked to the progressive impairment of systolic–diastolic cardiac function, but also to the systemic disturbance that frequently progresses independently of the worsening of cardiac function. A proof of this is the frequent observation in daily clinical practice of patients with similar cardiac function but differing clinical status and prognosis. These two strategies can be alternated in the context of the patient's clinical status. In the early stages of HF, when it is still an organ disease (specifically cardiac), the cardioselective strategy may be preferable in order to avoid worsening of the cardiac function. When HF becomes a systemic disease, however, in which the cardiac dysfunction parallels the systemic impairment, or when the latter dominates the clinical status, the cardiosystemic strategy of

TH treatment probably is preferable.

Although the systemic effects of TH therapy in HF have not yet been assessed, both the fact that hypothyroidism mimics HF in terms of systemic dyshomeostasis and the positive effects of TH replacement therapy in other clinical settings suggests that hypothyroidism generates a vicious cycle potentially impairing cardiovascular and systemic homeostasis in HF, and also that vicious cycle may be interrupted if the TH profile is normalized.

In conclusion, TH therapy in the setting of HF is still a fully open chapter. Several questions remain unanswered: the mode, dose, and schedule of TH treatment, and the effects of TH therapy on systemic homeostasis. Large, multicenter, prospective, placebo-controlled studies are therefore needed to provide safety and prognostic information about long-term treatment with TH replacement therapy.

Key Points

- Heart failure (HF) should be seen in a unique scenario of altered systemic homeostasis in which heart dysfunction, peripheral organ dysfunction, and derangement of the neuroendocrine and immune systems represent chronic stress stimuli with continuous activation of the stress response.

- The thyroid hormone (TH) system is profoundly involved in cardiovascular and systemic homeostasis. In HF, the most frequent alteration of TH metabolism is a low-triiodothyronine state, which may participate directly in the progression of HF.

- Restoration of normal TH metabolism appears to be useful to interrupt the vicious cycle of HF, which involves heart dysfunction, systemic (multiorgan) impairment, and activation of the neuroendocrine and immune–inflammatory systems.

- Initial results show that TH replacement therapy in patients with HF improves cardiac performance, and hemodynamic and exercise performance, while inducing deactivation of the neuroendocrine profile, as a result of the significant reduction in vasoconstrictor/sodium-retaining norepinephrine and aldosterone, and in the plasma levels of their counterpart NT-proBNP.

- Two strategies of TH replacement therapy in patients with HF are suggested:
  1. Cardiosystemic, administering synthetic T_4 or T_3
  2. Cardioselective, using TH analogues, in particular 3,5-diiodothyropropionic acid (DITPA)

References

1. Seta YJ, Shan K, Bozkurt B et al (1996) Basic mechanisms in heart failure: the cytokine hypothesis. J Card Fail 2:243–249
2. Blum A, Miller H (1998) Role of cytokines in heart failure. Am Heart J 135:181–186
3. Torre-Amione G, Kapadia S, Benedict C et al (1996) Tumor necrosis factor-alpha and tumor necrosis factor receptors in the failing human heart. Circulation 93:704–711
4. Finkel MS, Oddis CV, Jacob TD et al (1992) Negative inotropic effects of cytokines on the heart mediated by nitric oxide. Science 257:387–389
5. Pagani FD, Baker LS, His C et al (1992) Left ventricular systolic and diastolic dysfunction after infusion of tumor necrosis factor-alpha in conscious dogs. J Clin Invest 90:389–398
6. Torre-Amione G, Kapadia S, Lee J et al (1996) Proinflammatory cytokine levels in patients with depressed left ventricular ejection fraction: a report from the Studies of Left Ventricular Dysfunction (SOLVD). J Am Coll Cardiol 27:1201–1206
7. Tsutamoto T, Hisanaga T, Wada A et al (1998) Interleukin-6 spillover in the peripheral circulation increases with the severity of heart failure, and the high plasma level of interleukin-6 is an important prognostic predictor in patients with congestive heart failure. J Am Coll Cardiol 31:391–398
8. Rauchhaus M, Doehner W, Francis DP et al (2000) Plasma cytokine parameters and mortality in patients with chronic heart failure. Circulation 102:3060–3067
9. Damman KJ, Navis G, Smilde TD et al (2007) Worsening renal function and prognosis in heart failure: systematic review and meta-analysis. J Card Fail 13:599–608
10. Dries DL, Exner DV, Domanski MJ, et al (2000) The prognostic implications of renal insufficiency in asymptomatic

and symptomatic patients with left ventricular systolic dysfunction. J Am Coll Cardiol 35:681–689

11. Hillege HL, Nitsch D, Pfeffer MA et al (2006) Renal function as a predictor of outcome in a broad spectrum of patients with heart failure. Circulation 113:671–678

12. Palazzuoli A, Gallotta M, Iovine F et al (2008) Anaemia in heart failure: a common interaction with renal insufficiency called the cardio-renal anaemia syndrome. Int J Clin Pract 62:281–286

13. Tang YD , Stuart DK (2008) The prevalence of anemia in chronic heart failure and its impact on the clinical outcomes. Heart Fail Rev 13:387–392

14. Tang WH, Tong W, Jain A et al (2008) Evaluation and long-term prognosis of new-onset, transient, and persistent anemia in ambulatory patients with chronic heart failure. J Am Coll Cardiol 51:569–576

15. De Silva R, Rigby AS, Witte K et al (2006) Anemia, renal dysfunction, and their interaction in patients with chronic heart failure. Am J Cardiol 98:391–398

16. Pelle AJ, Gidron YY, Szabó BM et al (2008) Psychological predictors of prognosis in chronic heart failure. J Card Fail 14:341–350

17. Macchia A, Monte S, Pellegrini F et al (2008) Depression worsens outcomes in elderly patients with heart failure: an analysis of 48,117 patients in a community setting. Eur J Heart Fail 10:714–721

18. McEwen BS, Stellar E (1993) Stress and the individual. Mechanisms leading to disease. Arch Intern Med 153:2093–20101

19. McEwan BS (2000) The neurobiology of stress: from serendipity to clinical relevance. Brain Res 886:172–189

20. Mann DL, Kent RL, Parsons B et al (1992) Adrenergic effects on the biology of the adult mammalian cardiocyte. Circulation 85:790–804

21. Klein, I, Ojamaa K (2001) Thyroid hormone and the cardiovascular system. N Engl J Med 344:501–509

22. Kahaly, G.J, Dillmann WH (2005) Thyroid hormone action in the heart. Endocrine Rev 26:704–728

23. Davis PJ, Davis FB (2002) Nongenomic actions of thyroid hormone on the heart [review]. Thyroid 12:459–466

24. Napoli R, Guardasole V, Angelini V et al (2007) Acute effects of triiodothyronine on endothelial function in human subjects. J Clin Endocrinol Metab 92:250–254

25. Napoli R, Biondi B, Guardasole V et al (2008) Enhancement of vascular endothelial function by recombinant human thyrotropin. J Clin Endocrinol Metab 93:1959–1963

26. Den Hollander JG, Wulkan RW, Mantel MJ et al (2005) Correlation between severity of thyroid dysfunction and renal function. Clin Endocrinol 62:423–427

27. Zoccali C, Benedetto F, Mallamaci F et al (2006) Low triiodothyronine and cardiomyopathy in patients with end-stage renal disease. J Hypertens 24:2039–2046

28. Zoccali C (2006) Asymmetric dimethylarginine in end-stage renal disease patients: a biomarker modifiable by calcium blockade and angiotensin II antagonism? Kidney Int 70:523–528

29. Samuels MH (2008) Cognitive function in untreated hypothyroidism and hyperthyroidism. Curr Opin Endocrinol Diabetes Obes 15:429–433

30. Gulseren S, Gulseren L, Hekimsoy Z et al (2006) Depression, anxiety, health-related quality of life, and disability in patients with overt and subclinical thyroid dysfunction.

Arch Med Res 37:133–139

31. Bunevicius R, Varoneckas G, Prange AJ Jr et al (2006) Depression and thyroid axis function in coronary artery disease: impact of cardiac impairment and gender. Clin Cardiol 29:170–174

32. Silva JE, Bianco SD (2008) Thyroid-adrenergic interactions: physiological and clinical implications. Thyroid 18:157–165

33. Bumgarner JR, Ramkumar V, Stiles GL (1989) Altered thyroid status regulates the adipocyte A1 adenosine receptor–adenylate cyclase system. Life Sci 44:1705–1712

34. Silva JE, Larsen PR (1983) Adrenergic activation of triiodothyronine production in brown adipose tissue. Nature 305:712–713

35. Diniz GP, Carneiro-Ramos MS, Barreto-Chaves ML.(2007) Angiotensin type 1 (AT1) and type 2 (AT2) receptors mediate the increase in TGF-beta1 in thyroid hormone-induced cardiac hypertrophy. Pflugers Arch 454:75–81

36. Carneiro-Ramos MS, Diniz GP, Almeida J et al (2007) Cardiac angiotensin II type I and type II receptors are increased in rats submitted to experimental hypothyroidism. J Physiol 583:213–223

37. Vergaro G, Emdin M (2008) Cardiac angiotensin receptor expression in hypothyroidism: back to fetal gene programme? J Physiol 1:7–8

38. Kinugawa K, Wayne A, Minobe BS et al (2001) Signaling pathways responsible for fetal gene induction in the failing human heart. Evidence for altered thyroid hormone receptor gene expression. Circulation 103:1089–1094

39. Boelen A, Platvoet-Ter Schiphorst MC, Wiersinga WM (1993) Association between serum interleukin-6 and serum 3,5,3?-triiodothyronine in nonthyroidal illness. J Clin Endocrinol Metab 77:1695–1699

40. Papanas N, Papatheodorou K, Papazoglou D et al (2008) Post-thyroidectomy thyroxine replacement dose in patients with or without compensated heart failure: the role of cytokines. Cytokine 41:121–126

41. Bartalena L, Bogazzi F, Brogioni S et al (1998) Role of cytokines in the pathogenesis of the euthyroid sick syndrome. Eur J Endocrinol 138:603–614

42. Kohno M, Horio T, Yasunari K et al (1993) Stimulation of brain natriuretic peptide release from the heart by thyroid hormone. Metabolism 42:1059–1064

43. Liang F, Webb P, Marimuthu A et al (2003) Triiodothyronine increases brain natriuretic peptide (BNP) gene transcription and amplifies endothelin-dependent BNP gene transcription and hypertrophy in neonatal rat ventricular myocytes. J Biol Chem 278:15073–15083

44. Ertugrul DT, Gursoy A, Sahin M et al (2008) Evaluation of brain natriuretic peptide levels in hyperthyroidism and hypothyroidism. J Natl Med Assoc 100:401–405

45. Ripoli A, Pingitore A, Favilli B et al (2005) Does subclinical hypothyroidism affect cardiac pump performance? Evidence from a magnetic resonance imaging study. J Am Coll Cardiol 45:439–445

46. Caraccio N, Natali A, Sironi A et al (2005) Muscle metabolism and exercise tolerance in subclinical hypothyroidism: a controlled trial of levothyroxine. J Clin Endocrinol Metab 90:4057–4062

47. Iervasi G, Molinaro S, Landi P et al (2007) Association between increased mortality and mild thyroid dysfunction in cardiac patients. Arch Intern Med 167:1526–1532

48. Chopra IJ (1997) Euthyroid sick syndrome: is it a mis-

nomer? J Clin Endocrinol Metab 82:329–334

49. De Groot LJ (1999) Dangerous dogmas in medicine: the nonthyroidal illness syndrome. J Clin Endocrinol Metab 84:151–164

50. Tang YD, Kuzman JA, Said S et al (2005) Low thyroid function leads to cardiac atrophy with chamber dilatation, impaired myocardial blood flow, loss of arterioles, and severe systolic dysfunction. Circulation 112:3122–3130

51. Hamilton MA, Stevenson LW, Luu M et al (1990) Altered thyroid hormone metabolism in advanced heart failure. J Am Coll Cardiol 16:91–95

52. Opasich C, Pacini F, Ambrosino N et al (1996) Sick euthyroid syndrome in patients with moderate-to-severe chronic heart failure. Eur Heart J 17:1860–1866

53. Pingitore A, Landi P, Taddei MC et al (2005) Triiodothyronine levels for risk stratification of patients with chronic heart failure. Am J Med 118:132–136

54. Kozdag G, Ural D, Vural A et al (2005) Relation between free triiodothyronine/free thyroxine ratio, echocardiographic parameters and mortality in dilated cardiomyopathy. Eur J Heart Fail 7:113–118

55. Narula J, Haider N, Arbustini E et al (2006) Mechanisms of disease: apoptosis in heart failure – seeing hope in death. Nat Clin Pract Cardiovasc Med 3:681–688

56. Sharov VG, Kostin S, Todor A et al (2005) Expression of cytoskeletal, linkage and extracellular proteins in failing dog myocardium. Heart Fail Rev 10:297–303

57. Rosca MG, Vazquez EJ, Kerner J, et al (2008) Cardiac mitochondria in heart failure: decrease in respirasomes and oxidative phosphorylation. Cardiovasc Res 80:30–39

58. Stanley WC, Recchia FA, Lopaschuk GD (2005) Myocardial substrate metabolism in the normal and failing heart. Physiol Rev 85:1093–1129

59. Liu PP, Mak S, Stewart DJ (1999) Potential role of the microvasculature in progression of heart failure. Am J Cardiol 84:23L–26L

60. Forini F, Paolicchi A, Pizzorusso T et al (2001) 3,5,3?-Triiodothyronine deprivation affects phenotype and intracellular [Ca2+]i of human cardiomyocytes in culture. Cardiovasc Res 51:322–330

61. Pingitore A, Galli E, Barison A et al (2008) Acute effects of triiodothyronine (T3) replacement therapy in patients with chronic heart failure and low-T3 syndrome: a randomized, placebo-controlled study. J Clin Endocrinol Metab 93:1351–1358

62. Khalife WI, Tang YD, Kuzman JA et al (2005) Treatment of subclinical hypothyroidism reverses ischemia and prevents myocyte loss and progressive LV dysfunction in hamsters with dilated cardiomyopathy. Am J Physiol Heart Circ Physiol 289:H2409–H2415

63. Bauab RC, Perone D, Castro AV et al (2005) Low triiodothyronine (T3) or reverse triiodothyronine (rT3) syndrome modifies gene expression in rats with congestive heart failure. Endocr Res 31:397–405

64. Kopecky J, Houstek J, Szarska E, et al (1986) Thyroxine 5?-deiodinase in brown adipose tissue of myopathic hamsters. Am J Physiol 251:E8–E13

65. Mann DL (1999) Mechanism and model in heart failure. Circulation 100:999–1008

66. Glennon PE, Sudgen PH, Pool-Wilson PA (1995) Cellular mechanisms of cardiac hypertrophy. Br Heart J 73:443–447

67. Hein S, Kostin S, Heling A et al (2000) The role of the cytoskeleton in heart failure. Cardiovasc Res 45:273–278

68. Kato T, Muraski J, Chen Y et al (2005) Atrial natriuretic peptide promotes cardiomyocyte survival by cGMP-dependent nuclear accumulation of zyxin and Akt. J Clin Invest 115:2716–2730

69. Kenessey A, Ojamaa K (2006) Thyroid hormone stimulates protein synthesis in the cardiomyocyte by activating the Akt-mTOR and p70S6K pathways. J Biol Chem 281:20666–20672

70. Kuzman JA, Vogelsang KA, Thomas TA et al (2005) L-Thyroxine activates Akt signaling in the heart. J Mol Cell Cardiol 39:251–258

71. Braun MU, LaRosée P, Schön S et al (2002) Differential regulation of cardiac protein kinase C isozyme expression after aortic banding in rat. Cardiovasc Res 56:52–63

72. Steinberg SF, Goldberg M, Rybin VO (1995) Protein kinase C isoform diversity in the heart. J Mol Cell Cardiol 27:141–153

73. Rybin V, Steinberg SF (1996) Thyroid hormone represses protein kinase C isoform expression and activity in rat cardiac myocytes. Circ Res 79:388–398

74. Inagaki K, Koyanagi T, Berry NC et al (2008) Pharmacological inhibition of epsilon-protein kinase C attenuates cardiac fibrosis and dysfunction in hypertension-induced heart failure. Hypertension 51:1565–1569

75. Ledda-Columbano GM, Molotzu F, Pibiri M et al (2006) Thyroid hormone induces cyclin D1 nuclear translocation and DNA synthesis in adult rat cardiomyocytes. FASEB J 20:87–94

76. Sawyer DB, Colucci WS (2000) Mitochondrial oxidative stress in heart failure: "oxygen wastage" revisited. Circ Res 86:119–120

77. Ide T, Tsutsui H, Hayashidani S et al (2001) Mitochondrial DNA damage and dysfunction associated with oxidative stress in failing hearts after myocardial infarction. Circ Res 88:529–535

78. Wang J, Wilhelmsson H, Graff C et al (1999) Dilated cardiomyopathy and atrioventricular conduction blocks induced by heart-specific inactivation of mitochondrial DNA gene expression. Nat Genet 21:133–137

79. Garnier A, Fortin D, Delomenie C et al (2003) Depressed mitochondrial transcription factors and oxidative capacity in rat failing cardiac and skeletal muscles. J Physiol 551:491–501

80. Montoya J, Perez-Martos A, Garstka HL et al (1997) Regulation of mitochondrial trans-cription by mitochondrial transcription factor A. Mol Cell Biochem 174:227–230

81. Ikeuchi M, Matsusaka H, Kang D et al (2005) Overexpression of mitochondrial transcription factor a ameliorates mitochondrial deficiencies and cardiac failure after myocardial infarction. Circulation 112:683–690

82. Forini S, Lionetti V, Sabatino L et al (2008) Long-term L-triiodothyronine treatment drives myocardial adaptive mechanisms dependent on mitochondrial function and enhances cardiac repair in failing rat hearts. Proceedings of 13th International Congress of Endocrinology, Rio De Janeiro, Brazil (OP37)

83. Klemperer JD, Zelano J, Helm RE et al (1995) Triiodothyronine improves left ventricular function without oxygen wasting effects after global hypothermic ischemia. J Thorac Cardiovasc Surg 109:457–465

84. Ojamaa K, Klemperer JD, Klein I (1996) Acute effects of

thyroid hormone on vascular smooth muscle. Thyroid 6:505–512

85. Park KW, Dai HB, Ojamaa K et al (1997) The direct vaso-motor effect of thyroid hormones on rat skeletal muscle re-sistance arteries. Anesth Analg 85:734–738

86. Colantuoni A, Marchiafava PL, Lapi D et al (2005) Effects of tetraiodothyronine and triiodothyronine on hamster cheek pouch microcirculation. Am J Physiol Heart Circ Physiol 288:H1931–1936

87. Tomanek RJ, Doty MK, Sandra A (1998) Early coronary angiogenesis in response to thyroxine: growth characteris-tics and up-regulation of basic fibroblast growth factor. Circ Res 82:587–593

88. Wang X, Zheng W, Christensen LP et al (2003) DITPA stim-ulates bFGF, VEGF, angiopoietin, and Tie-2 and facili-tates coronary arteriolar growth. Am J Physiol Heart Circ Physiol 284:H613–H618

89. Zheng W, Weiss RM, Wang X et al (2004) DITPA stimu-lates arteriolar growth and modifies myocardial postin-farction remodeling. Am J Physiol Heart Circ Physiol 286:H1994-H2000

90. Liu Q, Clanachan AS, Lopaschuk GD (1998) Acute effects of triiodothyronine on glucose and fatty acid metabolism during reperfusion of ischemic rat hearts. Am J Physiol 275:E392–E399

91. Kiss E, Jakab G, Kranias EG et al (1994) Thyroid hormone-induced alterations in phospholamban protein expression. Regulatory effects on sarcoplasmic reticulum Ca2+ trans-port and myocardial relaxation. Circ Res 75:245–251

92. Pantos C, Mourouzis I, Markakis K et al (2007) Thyroid hormone attenuates cardiac remodeling and improves he-modynamics early after acute myocardial infarction in rats. Eur J Cardiothorac Surg 32:333–339

93. Ito K, Nakayama M, Hasan F et al (2003) Contractile re-serve and calcium regulation are depressed in myocytes from chronically unloaded hearts. Circulation 107:1176–1182

94. Minatoya Y, Ito K, Kagaya Y et al (2007) Depressed con-tractile reserve and impaired calcium handling of cardiac myocytes from chronically unloaded hearts are ameliorat-ed with the administration of physiological treatment dose of T3 in rats. Acta Physiol 189:221–231

95. Jiang M, Xu A, Tokmakejian S et al (2000) Thyroid hor-mone-induced overexpression of functional ryanodine re-ceptors in the rabbit heart. Am J Physiol Heart Circ Phys-iol 278:H1429–H1438

96. Klemperer JD, Klein IL, Ojamaa K et al (1996) Triiodothy-ronine therapy lowers the incidence of atrial fibrillation af-ter cardiac operations. Ann Thorac Surg 61:1323–1327

97. Klemperer JD, Klein I, Gomez M et al (1995) Thyroid hor-mone treatment after coronary-artery bypass surgery. N Engl J Med 333:1522–1527

98. Ranasinghe AM, Quinn DW, Pagano D et al (2006) Glu-cose-insulin-potassium and tri-iodothyronine individually improve hemodynamic performance and are associated with reduced troponin I release after on-pump coronary ar-tery bypass grafting. Circulation 114:I245–I250

99. Novitzky D, Fontanet H, Snyder M et al (1996) Impact of triiodothyronine on the survival of high-risk patients under-going open heart surgery. Cardiology 87:509–555

100. Portman MA, Fearneyhough C, Ning XH et al (2000) Tri-iodothyronine repletion in infants during cardiopulmonary

bypass for congenital heart disease. J Thorac Cardiovasc Surg 120:604–608

101. Bettendorf M, Schmidt KG, Grulich-Henn J et al (2000) Tri-iodothyronine treatment in children after cardiac surgery: a double-blind, randomised, placebo-controlled study. Lancet 356:529–534

102. Novitzky D (1996) Novel actions of thyroid hormone: the role of triiodothyronine in cardiac transplantation. Thy-roid 6:531–536

103. Brokhin M, Klein I (2005) Low T3 syndrome in a patient with acute myocarditis. Clin Cornerstone 7:S28–S29

104. Moruzzi P, Doria E, Agostoni PG et al (1994) Usefulness of L-thyroxine to improve cardiac and exercise performance in idiopathic dilated cardiomyopathy. Am J Cardiol 73:374–378

105. Moruzzi P, Doria E, Agostoni PG et al (1996) Medium-term effectiveness of L-thyroxine treatment in idiopathic dilat-ed cardiomyopathy. Am J Med 101:461–467

106. Hammond HK, White FC, Buxton IL et al (1987) Increased myocardial beta-receptors and adrenergic responses in hy-perthyroid pigs. Am J Physiol 252:H283–H290

107. Malik FS, Mehra MR, Uber PA et al (1999) Intravenous thy-roid hormone supplementation in heart failure with cardio-genic shock. J Card Fail 5:31–37

108. Hamilton MA, Stevenson LW, Fonarow GC et al (1998) Safety and hemodynamic effects of intravenous triiodothy-ronine in advanced congestive heart failure. Am J Cardiol 81:443–447

109. Iervasi G, Emdin M, Colzani RMP et al (2001) Beneficial effects of long-term triiodothyronine (T3) infusion in pa-tients with advanced heart failure and low T3 syndrome. In: Kimchi A (ed) Heart disease: new trends in research, diag-nosis and treatment. Medimond, Bologna, pp 549–553

110. Mano T, Sakamoto H, Fujita K et al (1998) Effects of thy-roid hormone on catecholamine and its metabolite concen-trations in rat cardiac muscle and cerebral cortex. Thyroid 8:353–335

111. Park CW, Shin YS, Ahn SJ et al (2001) Thyroxine treatment induces up-regulation of renin-angiotensin-aldosterone sys-tem due to decreasing effective plasma volume in patients with primary myxoedema. Nephrol Dial Transplant 16:1799–1806

112. Escobar-Morreale HF, Del Rey FE, Obregon MJ et al (1996) Only the combined treatment with thyroxine and tri-iodothyronine ensures euthyroidism in all tissues of the thy-roidectomized rat. Endocrinology 137:2490–2502

113. Danzi S, Dubon P, Klein I (2005) Effect of serum tri-iodothyronine on regulation of cardiac gene expression: role of histone acetylation. Am J Physiol Heart Circ Physiol 289:H1506–H1511

114. Degens H, Gilde AJ, Lindhout M et al (2003) Functional and metabolic adaptation of the heart to prolonged thyroid hormone treatment. Am J Physiol Heart Circ Physiol 284:H108–H115

115. Boehm EA, Jones BE, Radda GK et al (2001) Increased un-coupling proteins and decreased efficiency in palmitate-per-fused hyperthyroid rat heart. Am J Physiol Heart Circ Phys-iol 280:H977–H983

116. Pennock GD, Raya TE, Bahl JJ et al (1992) Cardiac effects of 3,5-diiodothyropropionic acid, a thyroid hormone ana-log with inotropic selectivity. J Pharmacol Exp Ther 263:163–169

117. Morkin E, Pennock G, Spooner PH et al (2002) Pilot studies on the use of 3,5-diiodothyropropionic acid, a thyroid hormone analog, in the treatment of congestive heart failure. Cardiology 97:218–225

118. Morkin E, Ladenson P, Goldman S et al (2004) Thyroid hormone analogs for treatment of hypercholesterolemia and heart failure: past, present and future prospects. J Mol Cell Cardiol 37:1137–1146

119. Goldman S, McCarren M , Morkin E et al (2008) DITPA, a thyroid hormone analog to treat heart failure: phase II Trial VA Cooperative Study. J Card Fail 2008; 14:796

120. Villabona C, Sahun M, Roca M et al (1999) Blood volumes and renal function in overt and subclinical primary hypothyroidism. Am J Med Sci 318:277–280

Thyroid Hormone Supplementation for Infants and Children Undergoing Cardiopulmonary Bypass for Cardiac Surgery

21

Aaron K. Olson and Michael A. Portman

Abstract In infants and children undergoing cardiopulmonary bypass for congenital heart disease surgery, thyroid hormone (TH) levels drop immediately after bypass and reach a nadir 24–48 h postoperatively. A small number of studies have been published evaluating triiodothyronine (T₃) supplementation in this population. T₃ supplementation appears to be safe and to improve some measures of recovery; however, no published studies have clearly shown a clinical benefit for this treatment as these investigations have been significantly limited by low patient numbers. The Triiodothyronine for Infants and Children Undergoing Cardiopulmonary Bypass (TRICC) study, the largest pediatric study on T₃ supplementation, recently completed enrollment but a full evaluation of the results has yet to be published. The TRICC study should provide additional, important safety and efficacy data.

Keywords Cardiopulmonary bypass • Heart surgery • Pediatric • Thyroid hormone supplementation

21.1 Introduction

Thyroid hormones (THs) have important cardiovascular effects [1] including increasing cardiac contractility [2] and lowering systemic vascular resistance [3]. However, cardiac surgery involving cardiopulmonary bypass (CPB) induces a significant and persistent reduction in circulating TH levels in the critical postoperative recovery period in all age groups [4–7]. Depressed TH levels increase post cardiac-surgery morbidity in adults [5]. Controlled, randomized studies have demonstrated that parenteral triiodothyronine (T₃) repletion after adult coronary artery bypass surgery improves postoperative ventricular function, reduces the need for inotropic support and mechanical devices, and reduces myocardial ischemia [5, 8, 9].

Postoperative cardiac dysfunction also contributes to morbidity, mortality, and a requirement for mechanical circulatory support after surgery to treat congenital heart defects in infants and children. Postoperative TH depression may contribute to hemodynamic alterations in this immature patient population [10, 11]. Studies of T₃ repletion in infants and children undergoing cardiac surgery and CPB are hindered by low patient numbers, heterogeneity of disease severity and operative repair, and large variances in the physiological maturation of the study subjects (neonates to postpubertal) [7, 12–15]. Nevertheless, the data indicate that TH replenishment is beneficial if administered to selected high-risk pediatric subjects.

M.A. Portman (✉)
University of Washington, and Children's Hospital and Regional Medical Center, Seattle, WA, United States

G. Iervasi, A. Pingitore (eds.), *Thyroid and Heart Failure*.

21.2 Thyroid Hormone Levels After CPB for Cardiac Surgery in Pediatric Patients

Studies in pediatric patients undergoing CPB for cardiac surgery have consistently demonstrated a severe and prolonged suppression of TH postoperatively [10, 16, 17]. TH levels drop immediately with the initiation of CPB, compatible with a dilution effect from the CPB priming solution. While adults typically show a decline in only T_3, infants and neonates display suppression of T_3, thyroxine (T_4), and thyroid-stimulating hormone (TSH). Based upon multiple studies, total and free T_3 levels reach a nadir between 12 and 48 h after bypass and remain depressed for 5–7 days postoperatively [6, 7, 12–14, 16, 18]. Levels of TSH, free T_4, and total T_4 show a similar pattern of reduction. However, free T_4 levels transiently rise above baseline after the institution of bypass [16]. This phenomenon has been attributed to the effect of heparin on TH-binding proteins, resulting in increased non-protein-bound T_4 [16]. Figure 21.1 shows the TH levels for 72 h postoperatively, measured during Portman et al.'s randomized trial (discussed later) of T_3 supplementation in infants undergoing cardiac surgery [7]. The duration of TH suppression indicates a high likelihood of additional causes beyond hemodilu-

tion from CPB. In neonates with hypoplastic left heart syndrome, the Norwood surgical procedure results in a decline of free T_3 levels to around 40% of baseline [19]. The reduction of T_3 in infants and neonates appears to be greater than that reported in adults [16, 20].

Multiple mechanisms for TH suppression have been proposed. While the initial fall is likely due to dilution, the continued decline appears to be multi-factorial. Commonly used peri- and postoperative medications, such as steroids [21], dopamine [22], and the iodine surgical wash [17], may depress TH levels. CPB imposes a large physiological stress that may disrupt the pituitary–thyroid axis postoperatively. These stressors include circulatory arrest (required for some specific operations), hypothermia, and nonpulsatile blood flow [10]. Postoperative TH levels may also be suppressed by the endogenous release of cellular mediators, such as glucocorticoids [23], tumor necrosis factor [24], and interleukin-6 (IL-6) [25]. Finally, surgery in general creates several insults, including a prolonged fasting state and surgical stress [23]. The precise importance of these various mechanisms has yet to be elucidated and likely varies between patients and over time. Regardless of the mechanism, TH levels drop significantly in infants and children after CBP for cardiac surgery. Whether this

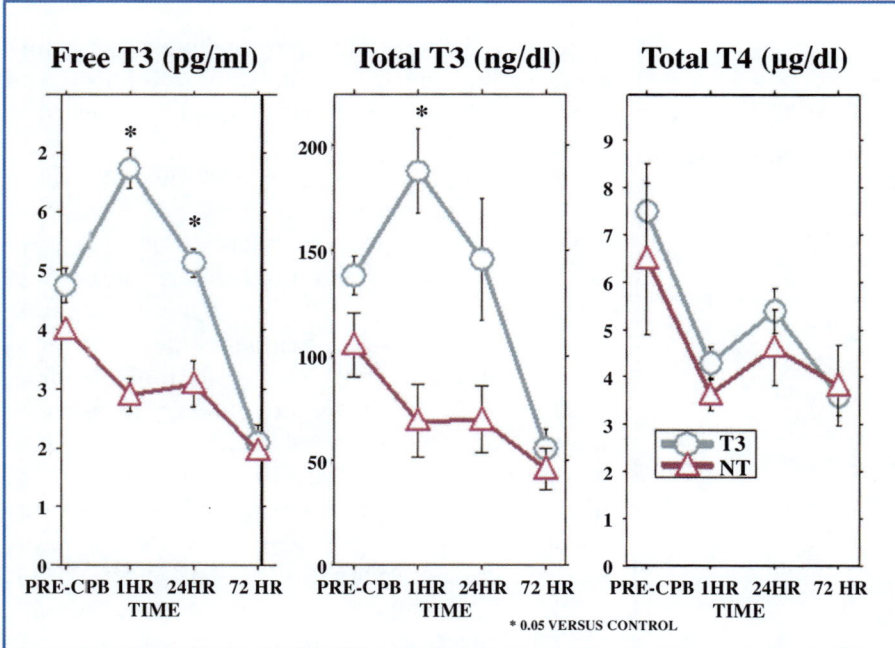

Fig. 21.1 Levels of free T_3, total T_3, and total T_4 prior to cardiopulmonary bypass (CPB) and up until 72 h postoperative. NT patients did not receive thyroid hormone supplementation. T_3 patients received T_3 treatment as discussed in Section 21.3. (Reproduced from [7] with permission)

fall is a clinically important treatment target has yet to be determined.

Postoperative TH levels in children appear to correlate with illness severity. Bettendorf and colleagues compared TH levels with the postoperative course of a heterogeneous group of 132 children (ages 10 days to 16.2 years) undergoing cardiac surgery [10]. Patients were retrospectively divided into two groups based upon lowest plasma T_3 levels, with a cutoff value of 0.6 nmol/l. The lowest T_3 group had a greater postoperative need for cardiac medications, longer period of mechanical ventilation and oxygen supplementation, and a longer hospitalization. However, interpretation of these results is hindered by a lack of analysis for demographic, diagnostic, and surgical data between the two groups. Important differences in the severity of the cardiac lesions, operative difficulty, and duration of CPB may have existed between these groups that would affect the reported outcomes. Dagan and colleagues determined postoperative T_4 and TSH levels in neonates undergoing open-heart surgery requiring CPB [11]. Levels of T_3, the active form of the hormone, were not determined. The patients were divided into two groups based upon the level of postoperative inotropic support (high versus mild). Both groups had a significant reduction in T_4 and TSH in the early postoperative period. However, the high-inotropic-support group had a longer suppression of T_4 that lasted at least 7 days. The high-support group also had a longer duration of mechanical ventilation and higher severity of illness postoperatively. These studies provide additional evidence that T_3 may be beneficial in the postoperative recovery of pediatric patients undergoing cardiac surgery. However, only clinical trials can definitively answer this question.

21.3 Clinical Studies

Several studies have been published that examined T_3 supplementation in the pediatric population during and/or after CPB. Initially, Mainwaring et al. evaluated T_3 supplementation in patients who had undergone a modified Fontan operation [15]. The Fontan operation is usually the final surgery for patients with single-ventricle anatomy and consists of connection of the inferior vena cava or right atrial blood flow directly into the pulmonary artery. These patients usually undergo an earlier procedure

in which the superior vena cava is connected to the pulmonary arteries. Therefore, the Fontan results in all systemic venous blood flowing directly to the pulmonary arteries. In these study patients, with ages between 16 and 78 months, T_3 supplementation reduced the length of hospitalization compared to historical controls. However, flaws in the study design limit the value of these results. The study was nonrandomized and compared a small group of patients ($n = 10$) who had received T_3 supplementation (0.4 μg/kg) following surgery with historical controls ($n = 8$). Substantial modifications in the care of Fontan patients occurred both nationally and at the study institution during the intervening time period, which may have affected outcome parameters. Nevertheless, this nonrandomized study provided justification for future studies.

Bettendorf and colleagues performed a randomized placebo-controlled study that examined T_3 supplementation in 40 pediatric patients after cardiac surgery [6]. Treatment consisted of T_3 2 μg/kg body weight on the day of surgery and then 1 μg/kg daily until discontinuation of dopamine or postoperative day 12. The study population had large variations in age (2 days to 10.4 years) and diagnosis. In treated patients, T_3 levels rose well above accepted normal ranges. Nevertheless, no differences in adverse events, including arrhythmias, were reported. Patients receiving T_3 exhibited greater increases in cardiac index during the early postoperative period and received fewer cumulative doses of the inotropic medications epinephrine and dobutamine. The subject numbers were inadequate to allow assessment of clinically important end points, including length of stay in the intensive care unit and the duration of mechanical ventilation.

Chowdhury et al. evaluated postoperative total T_3 levels in 75 consecutive pediatric patients undergoing cardiac surgery [12]. Patients with serum T_3 levels < 40 ng/dl (or < 60 ng/dl in infants) on postoperative days 0, 1, or 2 were randomized to receive either continuous T_3 infusion at 0.05–0.15 μg/kg body weight per hour to maintain serum levels within normal levels (80–100 ng/dl) or placebo. Of the 75 patients evaluated, 28 met the criteria for randomization. No differences were found between groups for the degree of postoperative care, use of inotropic medications, length of hospital stay, and duration of mechanical ventilation. This study population also had large variations in patient age and, presumably, diagnoses. Chowdhury et al. further analyzed patients less than 1 month old. Nine patients fell within this group, with five receiving treatment and four receiving placebo. T_3-treated neonates displayed significantly lower postoperative management requirements and lower inotropic support scores. Although the difference in length of hospital stay and days of mechanical ventilation did not reach statistical significance, the mean values displayed a trend towards shorter stays in the T_3-treated group. The authors concluded that T_3 treatment in newborn patients undergoing cardiac surgery may be beneficial.

Mackie and colleagues undertook a focused evaluation of the effect of T_3 supplementation on the early postoperative course of neonates undergoing aortic arch reconstruction during either the Norwood procedure (for single-ventricle anatomy) or a two-ventricle repair of interrupted aortic arch/ventricular septal defect [13]. CPB is required for both of these procedures. The study enrolled 42 patients in a randomized, double-blind, placebo-controlled protocol, with patients receiving a continuous infusion of T_3 (0.05 µg/kg per hour) or placebo. Primary end points were a composite clinical outcome score and cardiac index at 48 h. Even though the median clinical outcome scores were the same between groups, the T_3-treated group had a statistically significantly better outcome score due to differences in the distribution of values. All the patients with the worse scores came from the placebo groups. Cardiac index was not altered by T_3 supplementation. The T_3 group had a slightly earlier time to negative fluid balance (2.0 days in the T_3 group vs. 2.5 days in the placebo group). The authors concluded that T_3 treatment in neonatal heart surgery is safe and resultes in an improvement of clinical outcome scores. However, a larger multicenter study would be necessary before the routine use of T_3 supplementation for neonates after cardiac surgery and CPB could be recommended.

Portman et al. also undertook a randomized placebo-controlled trial in children less 1-year-old undergoing surgery for repair of ventricular septal defect or tetralogy of Fallot [7]. Fourteen patients (7 per group) were randomized to receive either a bolus of T_3 (0.4 µg/kg) prior to CPB and after release of aortic cross-clamp or placebo. Heart rate and peak systolic pressure rate (systolic blood pressure × heart rate) were increased in T_3-treated patients at 6 h after termination of CPB. Elevation of the peak systolic pressure rate implies that T_3

repletion improves myocardial oxygen consumption. Length of stay in the intensive care unit and hospitalization were not determined during this investigation. This study was the initial phase of a much larger clinical trial discussed below.

The Triiodothyronine for Infants and Children Undergoing Cardiopulmonary Bypass (TRICC) study was designed to overcome many of the shortcomings noted in the previous studies, including low patient numbers and large variations in age and diagnosis [26]. The study is a multicenter randomized clinical trial designed to determine the safety and efficacy of T_3 supplementation in children below 2 years of age undergoing surgical procedures for congenital heart disease. The six-center study has enrolled 195 patients with 99 randomized to multiple T_3 boluses given over 12 h during and after surgery and 96 to placebo. Randomization was stratified by nine diagnostic and surgical procedures to achieve balance by treatment arm and to alleviate confounding by condition complexity. The primary end point was time to extubation. Enrollment for the TRICC study was recently completed but a full evaluation of the results has yet to be published. Preliminary analyses show that T_3 treatment improved cardiac function, as assessed by ejection fraction, cardiac index, and/or myocardial performance index at 24 h in the low- and high-risk patients. The primary end point, time to extubation, was not changed by T_3 treatment. However, absolute T_3 levels were associated with changes in the chance of extubation in placebo and experimental groups.

21.4 Mechanisms

As noted earlier, THs have important effects on the cardiovascular system, including increasing cardiac contractility and decreasing systemic vascular resistance. Yet, the molecular mechanisms accounting for the improved cardiovascular performance are mostly unknown, especially in infants and children. Danzi and colleagues studied the effect of T_3 on gene transcription in infants undergoing cardiac surgery and CPB [27]. Left ventricular biopsy samples were collected by those investigators before and after CPB during Portman et al.'s study on T_3 supplementation [7]. Adequate tissue was obtained to evaluate one to three genes. Based upon the results of prior studies, this work focused on genes for adenine nucleotide translocator isoform-1 (ANT-1), α-myosin heavy chain (α-MHC), and sodium calcium exchanger-1 (NCX-1). NCX-1 and α-MHC transcription rates were unaffected. However, ANT-1 transcription rate was increased by T_3. ANT-1 is the nuclear gene coding for the mitochondrial protein controlling adenosine diphosphanate/adenosine triphosphate exchange.

ty evaluation of TH supplementation in pediatrics. The specific safety outcome, clinically important tachyarrhythmias, was not different between groups and occurred in 9.4% of placebo-treated and 11.1% of T_3-treated patients ($p = 0.69$). The study did not identify an increase in adverse events between TH-treated and placebo-treated patients for other safety measures.

21.5 Complications

An important consideration for the use of TH supplementation in infants and children undergoing CPB is the number and severity of adverse events. Supplementation has a theoretical side-effect profile similar to that of hyperthyroidism, which would include tachycardia, arrhythmias, and hyperthermia. Tachycardia and arrhythmias are commonly encountered after cardiac surgery in children and can cause clinically detrimental outcomes such as low cardiac output. Prior to the TRICC study, rare episodes of dysrhythmias in patients who had received TH supplementation were reported. The number of adverse events did not appear significantly increased; however, those earlier studies were underpowered.

The large number of patients enrolled in the TRICC study has provided the most thorough safe-

21.6 Conclusions

T_3 supplementation after CPB for cardiac surgery is an effective measure to return levels of the hormone to the normal range. Based upon multiple studies, the treatment appears to be safe for infants and children. The efficacy in improving postoperative recovery is less clear. TRICC, the largest study to date, evaluating this treatment in 195 randomized pediatric patients, has recently been completed. A thorough evaluation of the TRICC results has not yet been published but should be available soon. Preliminary data and previous studies indicate that T_3 supplementation improves postoperative cardiac function in this vulnerable population. However, these improvements may lead to clinically important benefits only in the highest-risk patients, such as neonates and those undergoing complex surgical procedures.

Key Points

- Thyroid hormones have important cardiovascular effects.

- In infants and children undergoing cardiopulmonary bypass for cardiac surgery:

  - Thyroid hormone levels drop immediately with bypass and reach a nadir between 24 and 48 h postoperatively.

  - Few studies have been published on triiodothyronine (T_3) supplementation in infants and children and all have been limited by low patient numbers.

  - T_3 supplementation appears to be safe and improves some measures of postoperative recovery.

  - However, no published studies have clearly shown an improvement in clinical outcomes for this treatment.

  - The Triiodothyronine for Infants and Children Undergoing Cardiopulmonary Bypass (TRICC) study, the largest pediatric study on T_3 supplementation, recently completed enrollment but a full evaluation of the results has yet to be published

References

1. Klein I, Ojamaa K (2001) Thyroid hormone and the cardiovascular system. N Engl J Med 344: 501–509
2. Novitzky D, Human PA, Cooper DK (1988) Inotropic effect of triiodothyronine following myocardial ischemia and cardiopulmonary bypass: an experimental study in pigs. Ann Thorac Surg 45:50–55
3. Park KW, Dai HB, Ojamaa K et al (1997) The direct vasomotor effect of thyroid hormones on rat skeletal muscle resistance arteries. Anesth Analg 85:734–738
4. Bennett-Guerrero E, Jimenez JL, White WD et al (1996) Cardiovascular effects of intravenous triiodothyronine in patients undergoing coronary artery bypass graft surgery. A randomized double-blind placebo- controlled trial. Duke T3 study group. JAMA 275:687–692
5. Klemperer JD, Klein I, Gomez M et al (1995) Thyroid hormone treatment after coronary-artery bypass surgery. N Engl J Med 333:1522–1527
6. Bettendorf M, Schmidt KG, Grulich-Henn J et al (2000) Triiodothyronine treatment in children after cardiac surgery: a double-blind randomised placebo-controlled study. Lancet 356:529–534
7. Portman MA, Fearneyhough C, Ning XH et al (2000) Triiodothyronine repletion in infants during cardiopulmonary bypass for congenital heart disease. J Thorac Cardiovasc Surg 120:604–608
8. Dyke CM, Ding M, Abd-Elfattah AS et al (1993) Effects of triiodothyronine supplementation after myocardial ischemia. Ann Thorac Surg 56:215–222
9. Mullis-Jansson SL, Argenziano M, Corwin S et al (1999) A randomized double-blind study of the effect of triiodothyronine on cardiac function and morbidity after coronary bypass surgery. J Thorac Cardiovasc Surg 117:1128–1134
10. Bettendorf M, Schmidt KG, Tiefenbacher U et al (1997) Transient secondary hypothyroidism in children after cardiac surgery. Pediatr Res 41:375–379
21. Dagan O, Vidne B, Josefsberg Z et al (2006) Relationship between changes in thyroid hormone level and severity of the postoperative course in neonates undergoing open-heart surgery. Paediatr Anaesth 16:538–542
12. Chowdhury D, Ojamaa K, Parnell VA et al (2001) A prospective, randomized clinical study of thyroid hormone treatment after operations for complex congenital heart disease. J Thorac Cardiovasc Surg 122:1023–1025
13. Mackie AS, Booth KL, Newburger JW et al (2005) A randomized double-blind placebo-controlled pilot trial of triiodothyronine in neonatal heart surgery. J Thorac Cardiovasc Surg 130:810–816
14. Mainwaring RD, Nelson JC (2002) Supplementation of thyroid hormone in children undergoing cardiac surgery. Cardiol Young 12:211–217
15. Mainwaring RD, Lamberti JJ, Nelson JC et al (1997) Effects of triiodothyronine supplementation following modified Fontan procedure. Cardiol Young 7:194–200
16. Mainwaring RD, Lamberti JJ, Carter TL Jr et al (1994) Reduction in triiodothyronine levels following modified Fontan procedure. J Card Surg 9:322–331
17. Brogan TV, Bratton SL, Lynn AM (1997) Thyroid function in infants following cardiac surgery: comparative effects of iodinated and noniodinated topical antiseptics. Crit Care Med 25:1583–1587
18. Mainwaring RD, Capparelli E, Schell K et al (2000) Pharmacokinetic evaluation of triiodothyronine supplementation in children after modified Fontan procedure. Circulation 101:1423–1429
19. Mainwaring RD, Healy RM, Meier FA et al (2001) Reduction in levels of triiodothyronine following the first stage of the Norwood reconstruction for hypoplastic left heart syndrome. Cardiol Young 11:295–300
20. Mitchell IM, Pollock JC, Jamieson MP et al (1992) The effects of cardiopulmonary bypass on thyroid function in infants weighing less than five kilograms. J Thorac Cardiovasc Surg 103:800–805
21. Brabant G, Brabant A, Ranft U et al (1987) Circadian and pulsatile thyrotropin secretion in euthyroid man under the influence of thyroid hormone and glucocorticoid administration. J Clin Endocrinol Metab 65:83–88
22. Van den Berghe G, de Zegher F, Lauwers P (1994) Dopamine suppresses pituitary function in infants and children. Crit Care Med 22:1747–1753
23. Dimmick S, Badawi N, Randell T (2004) Thyroid hormone supplementation for the prevention of morbidity and mortality in infants undergoing cardiac surgery. Cochrane Database Syst Rev: CD004220
24. van der Poll T, Romijn JA, Wiersinga WM et al (1990) Tumor necrosis factor: a putative mediator of the sick euthyroid syndrome in man. J Clin Endocrinol Metab 71:1567–1572
25. Butler J, Chong GL, Baigrie RJ et al (1992) Cytokine responses to cardiopulmonary bypass with membrane and bubble oxygenation. Ann Thorac Surg 53:833–838
26. Portman MA, Fearneyhough C, Karl TR et al (2004) The Triiodothyronine for Infants and Children Undergoing Cardiopulmonary Bypass (TRICC) study: design and rationale. Am Heart J 148:393–398
27. Danzi S, Klein I, Portman MA (2005) Effect of triiodothyronine on gene transcription during cardiopulmonary bypass in infants with ventricular septal defect. Am J Cardiol 95:787–789

New Approaches for Treating Heart Disease by Modulating Thyroid Hormone Signaling Using Gene Therapy Approaches

Mark Davis, Maria Giovanna Trivieri and Peter H. Backx

Abstract Heart failure is characterized by changes in gene and protein expression as well as function that mimic the changes observed with hypothyroidism. The changes include impaired contractility, bradycardia, arrhythmias, impaired contractile relaxation, slowed Ca^{2+} transient relaxation, increased lipid metabolism, and hypertension. Acute thyroid hormone (TH) treatment leads to increased contractility, calcium cycling, and heart rates due to changes in TH gene expression targets. Thus, it is not surprising that heart disease can be viewed as a condition of hypothyroidism amenable to treatment with TH. Unfortunately, treatment of heart disease patients with TH and hyperthyroidism, more generally, can have many negative effects on the cardiovascular system such as inducing arrhythmias and increased workloads, leading to increased mortality. These effects are believed to arise, at least in part, from extracardiac actions of thyroid hormone. In this chapter, we discuss new genetic approaches that can modulate the local cardiac hypothyroidism that develops in heart disease. These approaches directly target the myocardium, thereby avoiding the effects of thyroid hormone on extracardiac tissues.

Keywords Thyroid hormone • Gene therapy • Deiodinases • Thyroid hormone receptors • Heart disease • Heart failure • Hypothyroidism • Lentiviruses • Adenoviruses • Adeno-associated viruses • Transgenics • Therapeutics

22.1 Introduction

This chapter discusses new strategies for the cardiac-specific modulation of thyroid hormone signaling in the treatment of heart disease using gene therapy. The following four areas are considered:

- Molecular links between thyroid hormone and heart disease
- Pitfalls of systemic thyroid hormone therapy for treating heart disease
- Potential mechanisms underlying changes in thyroid signaling in heart disease
- Strategies for heart failure treatment by using gene therapy, thereby avoiding the systemic actions of thyroid hormone

22.2 Thyroid Hormone Signaling in the Heart

Thyroid hormone (TH) and thyroid hormone receptors (TRs) are critical for the development and maintenance of normal energy metabolism in several thyroid-dependent tissues including the heart [1–3]. Consequently, hypo- and hyperthyroidism

P.H. Backx (✉)
Departments of Physiology and Medicine,
University of Toronto, Toronto, Canada

G. Iervasi, A. Pingitore (eds.), *Thyroid and Heart Failure*.
© Springer-Verlag Italia 2009

may cause disturbances in cardiac function, thermoregulation, metabolism, hearing, and mental capacity [2–5]. Under normal conditions, TH is tightly regulated by feedback mechanisms involving the thyroid, pituitary, and hypothalamic glands. Although thyroxine (T_4) is the principal circulating TH produced primarily by the thyroid gland, its ability to activate TRs is weak. Nevertheless, T_4 is a prohormone precursor for other THs, and the synthesis of the relatively inactive T_4 occurs almost exclusively within the thyroid gland [6, 7]. By contrast, the production of 85% of the biologically active TH, 3,5,3'-triiodothyronine (T_3), occurs locally within target tissues [8–10]. Thus, TR activation in tissues requires T_4 entry into cells, possibly via a specific T_4 membrane transporter, followed by local metabolism of inactive T_4 into active T_3 by three monodeiodinase isoenzymes (type 1 or D1, type 2 or D2, type 3 or D3) [11–13], each containing the uncommon amino acid selenocysteine at the active site [10, 14]. Regulation of the "local" conversion of T_4 to T_3 relies heavily in most tissues on D2 [2, 9, 15–17]. Although the type 1 deiodinase (D1) can also convert T_4 to T_3, its primary action appears to be the conversion of T_3 to an inactive TH metabolite called reverse T_3 or rT_3 [9, 10]. By contrast, D3 exclusively converts T_4 to rT_3 as well as T_3 to biologically inactive products (Fig. 22.1) [8, 18]. While the degradation of T_3 and T_4 by deiodinases can obviously influence TH signaling by altering active hormone levels, inactive metabolites like rT_3 may also have genomic and nongenomic actions that modulate TH signaling [19–24]. Importantly, the levels of the deiodinases vary between tissues and are regulated during development and in disease, by pre- and post-translational mechanisms [8, 9, 19–22]. For example, D3 is relatively abundant in the developing heart and in the placenta, presumably to protect the fetus against excessive simulation by cardiac TRs [16, 25]. In heart disease, D3 levels rise [8, 16, 26] (Fig. 22.1) and this may be responsible for the reduced cardiac T_3 levels in diseased hearts [8], even when serum T_4 levels are within the normal range (euthyroid). Consistent with a possible role of D3 in heart disease, rT_3 levels are elevated [8, 26–28]. Deiodinases levels can also vary in conditions such as hypothermia, hypothyroidism, and hyperthyroidism as well with elevated intracellular Ca^{2+} [8, 9, 19–22].

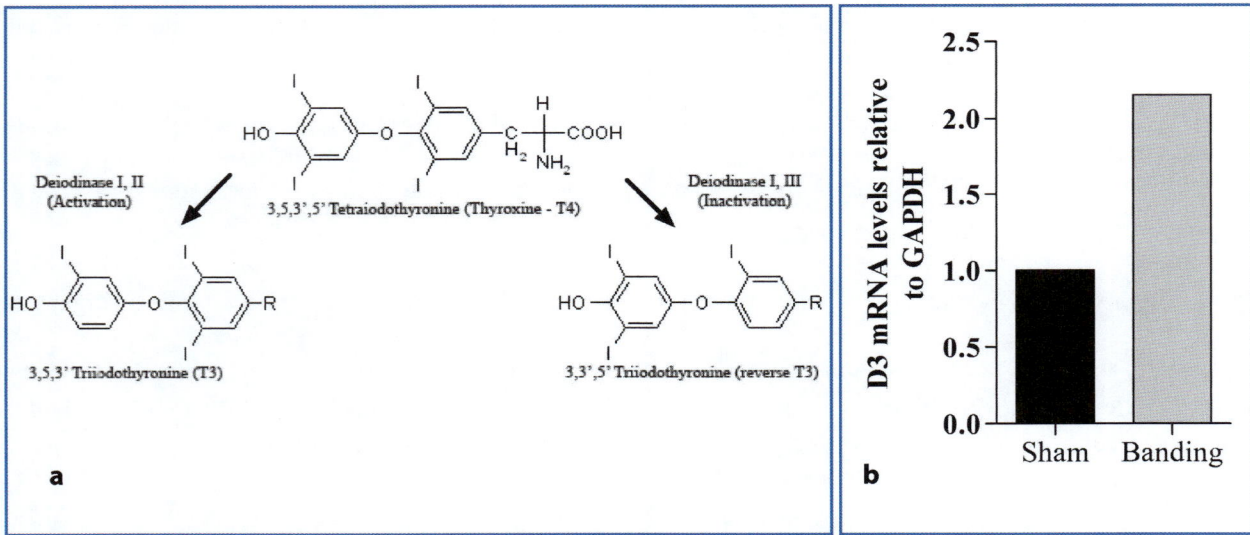

Fig. 22.1 a Deiodinases types 1 and 2 remove the 5' iodine residue on the outer ring of thyroxine, resulting in the activation to triiodothyronine within the cell. The action of deiodinases types 1 and 3 results in the inactivation of thyroxine by removing the 5 iodine residue on its inner ring, forming reverse triiodothyronine. Deiodinase type 3 is highly expressed in the placenta, deactivating thyroxine before it enters the fetus, so as to prevent thyroxine-mediated alterations in gene expression. **b** Deiodinase type 3 expression in the heart in sham and banded mice. Following aortic banding, D3 mRNA levels increase in the ventricle, resulting in the inactivation of thyroid hormone within cardiomyocytes (unpublished data, Backx Lab). This presents a potential area of intervention. By blocking the upregulation of deiodinase type 3 in the heart following banding, the amount of active thyroid hormone within the heart can be increased

Interest in TH signaling in the heart has been fueled by the observation that many important functional genes are regulated by TR [11]. For instance, TR activation transcriptionally up-regulates the expression levels of SERCA, α-MHC, β1-adrenergic receptors/G-proteins, Na/K-ATPase, and L-type calcium channels, hyperpolarization-activated cyclic nucleotide-gated channels (i.e., HCN2 and HCN4), and several potassium channels, including the inward rectifying K^+ channels, Kv1.5, Kv4.2, and Kv4.3 [11, 16, 17, 29], while suppressing expression of β-MHC, phospholamban, the Na^+/Ca^{2+} exchanger, transient outward Kv1.4 channels, and cardiac KATP channels [16, 30–34]. Consequently, acute TH treatment leads to increased heart rates and cardiac contractility, which is associated with enhanced Ca^{2+} cycling, accelerated contraction kinetics, and altered electrical properties of the working myocardium. Increased TH signaling also enhances energy metabolism in cardiomyocytes by altering the expression of cellular and mitochondrial enzymes involved in glucose and fatty acid utilization as well as in oxidative metabolism such as malate dehydrogenase [35, 36].

Consistent with the regulation of many functional genes by TH, hypothyroidism causes impaired cardiac contractility, reduced cardiac output, low heart rates (i.e., bradycardia), diastolic dysfunction, action potential (AP) prolongation, and increased susceptibility to arrhythmias [37]. These functional changes of hypothyroidism are associated with increased β-MHC/α-MHC ratios and Na^+/Ca^{++} exchanger levels, and decreased SERCA2a expression. Hypothyroid hearts also show poor substrate utilization (glucose, lactate, and, especially, free fatty acids) by the mitochondria, as a consequence of decreased enzymes in the citric acid cycle and increased pyruvate dehydrogenase kinase-2 activity, leading to inhibition of the pyruvate dehydrogenase complex [38]. Collectively, these changes lead to a shift away from fatty acid utilization, which might explain the free fatty acid accumulation in the myocardium, particularly in diabetic patients. Altered fat metabolism might also underlie the hyperlipidemia seen in hypothyroid patients which is believed to be responsible for their increased atherosclerosis, coronary artery disease, and myocardial infarction rates [5, 39–41]. Since hypothyroidism is characterized by low levels of circulating T_3 and T_4, restoring the euthyroid state will likely reduce the cardiovascular changes seen in these patients [29, 42, 43].

22.3 Links Between TH and Heart Disease

Remarkably, although most heart failure patients often have normal serum levels of TH, the functional and genetic expression changes seen in heart disease patients closely mimic those of hypothyroidism [2, 11, 41, 43]. In fact, the genetic changes seen in heart disease generally recapitulate those associated with the fetal phenotype, consistent with the known requirement of a TH surge, along with possible changes in cardiac deiodinase expression [16, 31, 44–46]. Collectively these observations suggest that altered TH signaling occurs in disease [33, 47, 48], which is not unexpected since many (if not all) of the cardiac genes involved in heart disease and fetal development have thyroid hormone response elements (TREs) in their promoters [49]. Moreover, an excellent predictor of poor outcomes in heart disease patients is the ratio of levels of T_3 to levels of rT_3 (T_3/rT_3 ratio) [7, 50–52], a reduction of which may result from increased D3 expression (Fig. 22.1), possibly combined with reduced D2 expression in some tissues. Interestingly, abnormal TH signaling and impaired heart function are also often observed following surgery (a condition referred to as "euthyroid sick syndrome") [53, 54].

Based on connections between TH and heart disease, TH treatment has been advocated for cardiovascular patients. Clinical studies have been conducted to test whether patients with heart failure benefit from TH supplementation [42, 55]. Not surprisingly, studies in human patients [35, 42, 43, 55] as well as in animal models [56–58] showed that TH can improve heart function and shift cardiac gene expression towards that seen in normal euthyroid hearts. For example, TH treatment can reverse cardiomyocyte remodeling associated with the onset of heart failure [55] and restore α-MHC to β-MHC ratios as well as the levels of SERCA metabolic enzymes [35]. Some of the beneficial effects of TH might, however, not involve changes in gene expression and genomic effects, since acute intravenous T_3 treatment enhances the cardiac performance and cardiac output of heart failure patients [7, 59, 60].

Although there is a strong rationale for treating heart disease patients with TH, proven benefit of TH administration in patients with heart disease has been difficult to establish. Indeed, while short-term thyroxine and T_3 treatment appears helpful for these patients prolonged (chronic) treatment with TH causes cardiac hypertrophy, elevated heart rates, increased cardiac protein synthesis, atrial arrhythmias, reduced left ventricular ejection fractions (LVEFs), and cardiomyopathy [61]. These detrimental effects of long-term treatment with TH could result from inappropriate dosing levels, since similar changes are seen in hyperthyroidism, although these changes can be partially prevented with propranolol [62, 63]. Alternatively, TH-induced cardiomyopathy observed with prolonged TH treatment of patients with heart disease could result from reduced peripheral resistance [40, 64–66] and the associated increased cardiac workload [67, 68] of the already compromised heart. Indeed, hyperthyroidism does not induce cardiac hypertrophy in unloaded heterotopically transplanted hearts [48, 69, 70].

Thus, treating patients with TH for heart disease can be either beneficial or have harmful consequences, possibly depending on drug dosing [2, 11, 71]. In essence the problem is that, although the heart shows clear signs of impaired TH signaling, patients with heart disease are generally euthyroid (i.e., have normal circulating TH levels), suggesting that the altered thyroid signaling originates from local changes within the myocardium itself. The situation in patients with heart disease is in some ways like the persistent clinical symptoms of the hypothyroidism seen in some patients receiving thyroxine therapy, despite "normal" serum levels of T_3 and T_4 [72]. On the other hand, while treatment of heart disease patients with TH administration may overcome the local impairment of thyroid signaling in the myocardium, the resulting elevations in circulating TH can induce either subclinical hyperthyroidism (low TSH levels for the corresponding TH levels) or overt hyperthyroidism, either of which could have negative effects on the cardiovascular system and other tissues. These problems are exacerbated by the common problems of patients with heart disease such as improper adherence to drug schedules [72].

22.4 Potential New TH-Dependent Approaches for Treating Heart Disease

Successful treatment with TH might best be directed at the underlying "hypothyroidism" within the myocardium itself, which could arise from five different mechanisms: (1) reductions in T_4 uptake into the heart, (2) shifts in TH metabolism leading to reduced active TH (T_3), (3) altered expression profiles of TRs, (4) impaired TR signaling, or (5) altered actions of other hormones that may interfere with or counteract normal hormone signaling. Because several mechanisms may contribute to the cardiac hypothyroidism seen in heart disease, a number of novel strategies may prove effective in correcting TH signaling in a heart-specific manner. In the remainder of this chapter, several interrelated mechanisms for "cardiac hypothyroidism" in heart disease are discussed along with possible strategies for exploiting these mechanisms in treating heart disease.

22.4.1 Alterations in T_4 Uptake by the Heart

A critical step in the cellular actions of TH involves its transport into cells. Consequently, reduced local TH signaling may occur in heart disease as a result of decreased T_3 uptake or decreased T_3 production following reduced T_4 uptake into the myocardium. Although earlier work suggested that T_4 readily crosses lipid bilayers, recent studies have established that T_4 and its metabolites including T_3 enter cells through various organic anion transporters such as Na^+-dependent taurocholate transporters, fatty acid translocases, multidrug-resistance-related proteins, L-type amino acid transporters, organic-anion-transporting polypeptides (OATP), and monocarboxylate transporters (MCT) [11–13, 73]. However, only the OATPs (i.e., OATP1C1) and MCTs (i.e., MCT8 and MCT10) have been shown to selectively transport T_4, T_3, and other TH derivatives with high affinity [12]. OATP1C1 preferentially transports T_4 and MCT8 primarily T_3 [12]. Although the role for selective transport of TH, by transporters like OATP1C1 and MCT8, in the tissue regulation of THs has been primarily described in the vessels and neurons of the brain [9, 13], MCT8 is the only transporter known to be expressed in rat and human hearts. The importance of MCT8 in TH transport into the myocardium is, however, unclear since patients with X-linked MTC8 mutations show severe neurological disorders without obvious cardiovascular symptoms

[12, 13]. Moreover, mice lacking MCT8 were not reported to have either obvious neurological signs or cardiac impairment. Despite the paucity of information on TH transport in the heart, it is conceivable that the local "hypothyroidism" observed in heart disease could originate from impaired T_3 and T_4 entry into the myocardium. If impaired TH transporter activity does occur in heart disease, then a potential strategy for correcting the local hypothyroidism would be to increase TH transport into the myocardium.

22.4.2 Shifts in TH Metabolism Leading to Reduced Active T_3

Levels of active TH are determined locally in many tissues such as the heart by a balance between production and destruction of T_3 [8, 9, 25]. The human heart expresses the D2 and D3 monodeiodinase enzymes [8, 26, 74]. Recent studies have shown that in heart disease the level of D3 rises (Fig. 22.1) in conjunction with elevated cardiac rT_3 levels [8] and reduced T_3 levels [8]. These changes are predicted to alter the expression levels of thyroid-dependent genes. Moreover, the levels of D3 enzyme expression correlate with disease progression [75], while the levels of rT_3 and T_3 and their ratio are powerful predictors of morbidity and mortality in patients with congestive heart failure. Furthermore, overexpression of D2 in the myocardium was able to prevent changes in the expression of SERCA2a, sarcolipin, and selected

markers of pathological hypertrophy, while correcting the impaired Ca^{2+} cycling and contractility induced in hearts subjected to pressure overload hypertrophy (Fig. 22.2) [74]. Based on these observations, strategies for reducing D3 activity with or without increasing D2 actions would be desirable in treating heart disease patients.

Consistent with changes in TH metabolism in the heart, it has recently been shown that other components of TH production, including TSH receptors, are also present within the myocardium [76]. Indeed, the H9c2 "cardiac" cell-line contains all the necessary proteins – thyroglobulin, sodium iodide symporter, pendrin, thyroid peroxidase, and TSH receptor – to produce TH [77]. Although the physiological significance of these observations is unclear, cardiomyoblasts and rat cardiomyocytes increase their T_4 and T_3 production in response to ischemia while thyroglobulin levels increase in the failing myocardium [77]. Moreover, TRH is induced in the left ventricles of rats with heart failure [78]. These findings suggest that, in diseased hearts, cardiomyocytes either induce or locally increase TH production, possibly to compensate for local hypothyroidism or impaired TH-TR-TRE signaling in heart disease.

22.4.3 Disruption in the Thyroid Receptor Profile

As already discussed, TH primarily signals in the nucleus by binding to four major TRs originating

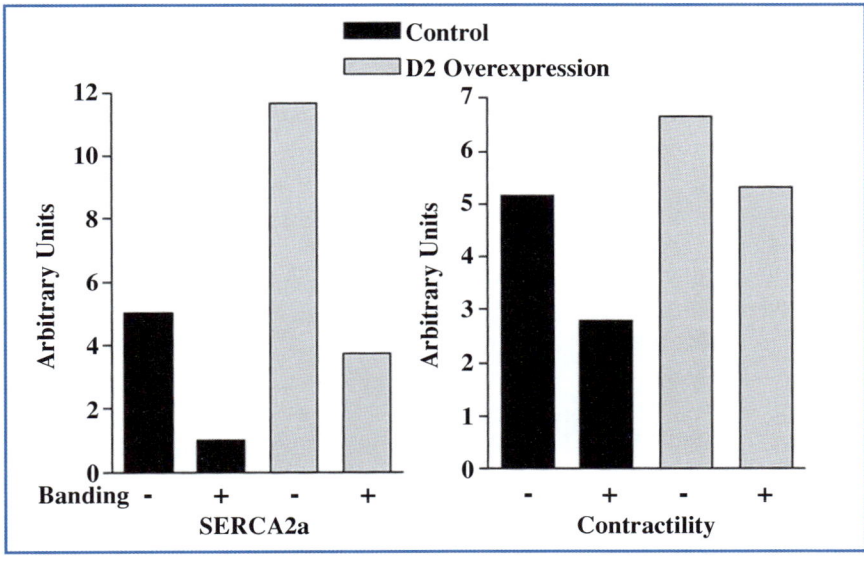

Fig. 22.2 Comparison of SERCA2a and contractile ability of control and D2-overexpressing mice with and without aortic banding. The changes in SERCA2a expression are paralleled by similar changes in contractility. In both cases, D2 overexpression prevents the decrease in SERCA2a levels and decrease in contractility associated with the onset of pressure overload heart failure. (Adapted from [74])

from alternative splicing of two genes (TRα and TRβ). Recently, it has been shown that T_3 treatment induces translocation of TRβ1 from the cytoplasm into the nucleus as well as preferential retention of TRα1 within the nucleus [79]. Shuttling between the cytoplasm and the nucleus supports possible nongenomic actions of TR [17, 23, 79–81]. Of the four main TRs produced by the body, TRα1, TRα2, and TRβ1 are expressed in the myocardium, while TRβ2 is only found largely in the brain and the pituitary [11, 82, 83]. TRs bind to canonical TREs within gene promoters to regulate gene transcription. In general, ligand binding transforms TRs from suppressors to activators of gene transcription, although the expression of many genes is reduced following TH binding to TRs. In addition, occupancy of TREs by unliganded TRs can suppress baseline expression of many thyroid-dependent genes [2, 5, 38]. In this respect, TRα2 uniquely blocks transcriptional activation because of its inability to bind T_3 [11, 16]. In addition, several other alternative splice variants of TRα and TRβ have been identified, some lacking DNA binding domains, but their role in thyroid signaling is poorly defined [84], although some may act as dominant-negative TRs [85]. The concept of gene suppression by unliganded TRs is particularly well-illustrated by the observations that TRα1 deletion is able to largely rescue the postnatal development in mice unable to produce TH (i.e., Pax8-/- mice) [86], and that knockin TRα1 mutations which eliminate ligand binding show a more profound hypothyroidism than mice lacking TRα1 [87, 88]. By contrast, overexpression of dominant-negative TRβ1 leads to changes in gene expression mimicking those of hypothyroidism which cannot be reversed by thyroxine treatment [11]. The majority of T_3 binding (i.e., approx. 70%) in the heart appears to bind to TRα1 with the remainder predominantly binding to TRβ1, consistent with conclusions from mouse studies that T_3 signaling via TRα1 dominates in the heart [89]. This seems particularly relevant in regard to thyroid signaling in heart disease and cardiac hypertrophy, since collectively several studies have shown that TRα1 levels are reduced along with increased TRα2 and TRβ1 [29, 44, 81, 83, 90], leading to decreases in T_3 binding sites [44, 82, 91]. These alterations in TR levels could lead to changes in nuclear as well as cytoplasmic signaling, suggesting that corrections in TR expression will lead to normalization of function in diseased myocardium.

22.4.4 Interference with Thyroid Receptor Signaling

TRs function primarily as homodimers with other TRs or by forming heterodimer partners with retinoid X receptors (RXRs) [11, 16, 17], which in turn dimerize with other receptors such as peroxisome-proliferator-activated receptors (PPARs), retinoic acid receptors (RARs), and others [11, 16, 92]. Thus, changes in thyroid signaling could originate from changes in the expression of RXR or its other binding partners. Moreover, binding of TRs to canonical TREs of thyroid-responsive genes involves their association with numerous co-activators and/or co-repressors in transcriptional complexes [16], that regulate gene transcription in the presence and absence of ligand. Typically, unliganded TRs co-assemble with co-repressors such as nuclear receptor co-repressor (NCoR), silencing mediator for retinoic acid and TR receptor (SMRT), Sin-3, and histone deacetylases to inhibit transcription of thyroid-regulated gene expression [93]. By contrast, transcriptional activation involves co-assembly of TRs with steroid receptor co-activators (SRC) and the vitamin D receptor interacting protein/TR-associated protein (DRIP/TRAP) complexes [94], which can bind with many transcriptional activators including histone acetyltransferases. Involvement of SRC in thyroid signaling was established in SRC-1 knock-out mice, which show altered thyroid-dependent gene expression as well as heart rate [95, 96]. Thus, it is conceivable that changes in interactions between TRs and other transcriptional co-repressors and co-activators lead to altered thyroid signaling in heart disease. This possibility is particularly intriguing since co-activators of TR signaling such as SRC also interact with transcriptional factors such as AP-1 and NF-κB, which are involved in the signaling changes observed in cardiac hypertrophy and heart disease [94, 97]. Clearly the activation of many pathways involved in cardiac hypertrophy and heart disease can lead to altered thyroid signaling as a consequence of direct or indirect modulation of factors that participate in forming the transcriptional complexes containing TRs. In this respect it is interesting to note that changes in thyroid state directly modulate both adrenergic receptor and renin-angiotensin signaling. Moreover, the nongenomic actions of TRα1 and TRβ1 lead to the activation of p38 MAPK, PI3 kinases, PKB, and ERK1/2, all of which play critical roles in alterations in gene transcription in cardiac hypertrophy and heart disease [79, 82].

22.5 Gene Delivery of Thyroid Genes for Treating Heart Disease

Since many observations suggest that the diseased myocardium has reduced or impaired TH signaling, there seems to be a strong rationale for treating heart disease patients with TH [11, 17, 98]. However, as discussed above, one limitation of treating heart disease with exogenous TH is the danger of creating a hyperthyroid state for extracardiac tissues. Clearly, strategies for specifically altering thyroid signaling in the heart are desirable, and possibly necessary. With recent advancements in gene therapy, it seems likely that cardiac-specific alterations in selective targets involved in thyroid signaling are viable approaches for future therapies [29, 99]. Increased TH signaling could be accomplished in multiple ways, and two strategies have already been examined. First, increasing the conversion of T_4 to T_3 by increasing D2 expression within the heart has already been shown to prevent the expression of markers of pathological hypertrophy as well as the reductions in Ca^{2+} transients and associated impaired contractility (Fig. 22.2) induced by mechanical stress, although this approach did not prevent cardiac hypertrophy [74]. Second, TH signaling could conceivably be augmented by normalizing the expression of TRs within the myocardium [29], which appear to be decreased in heart disease. Indeed, overexpression of TRα1 or TRβ1 using adeno-associated viruses (AAVs) improved developed pressure and increased SERCA expression compared to LacZ-treated mice following mechanical stress [29]. As in the D2 overexpression mice, TRα1 or TRβ1 overexpression did not prevent hypertrophy.

A number of other strategies for altering TH signaling might also be effective in treating heart disease, such as increasing the number of TH sarcolemmal transporters or co-activators of TH transcription in the myocardium. Alternatively, reductions in the co-repressors or D3 deiodinases using gene silencing could also be viable approaches. As more molecular information becomes available, additional targets will no doubt emerge. For example, it is conceivable that the heart can be reprogrammed to respond differently to TH stimulation or precursors. One such strategy might originate from the recent recognition that microRNAs, which act as negative regulators of gene expression by inhibiting the translation or promoting the degradation of target mRNAs, transduce the regulation of myosin heavy chain by TH. Moreover, cardiac microRNAs can be genetically silenced via the systemic delivery of anti-microRNAs [100, 101]. These genetic manipulations are most logically delivered using AAV vectors, lentivirus vectors, or adenoviruses.

Adenoviruses remain the most commonly used gene delivery system for experimental animal models, delivering gene products of up to 30 kb [102]. These viruses are trophic for cardiomyocytes, as well as many other cell types [102, 103], and adenoviruses typically initiate strong immunological reactions. Thus, either direct myocardial injection or intracoronary delivery leads to intense inflammatory reactions resulting in damage to endothelial cells and vascular smooth muscle cells combined with a relatively short half-life for delivered genes in the body [102]. At least one death has been directly attributed to the use of adenoviral vectors in clinical trials [102]. Because adenoviruses can infect many types of cells in the body, in addition to cardiomyocytes, these gene delivery vectors are not expected to be tissue- specific, unless the genes being delivered are driven by cardiac-specific promoters such as α-myosin heavy chain or ventricular myosin light chain [102, 103].

Many of the complications observed with adenoviral use for gene delivery are overcome with the use of AAV vectors. Specifically, AAVs evoke a minimal immune response [102, 103], generate minimal cellular damage, and produce stable long-term expression [104, 105]. To date, no reports have linked AAVs to disease or death in humans. The use of these viruses has been limited in humans and animal models due to difficulties in generating high viral titers as well as limitations in the size of the genes that can be delivered using this system (i.e., < 4.8 kb) [102]. Furthermore, since AAV vectors use single-stranded DNA, gene expression is slower than with other vector systems, although methods have been developed to accelerate expression rates [103, 106]. In addition, the ability to target cardiomyocytes has been improved by the identification of cardiac-specific serotypes (i.e., AAV8 and AAV9) [107, 108]. AAVs have been used to deliver TRα and TRβ in a rodent model, while two clinical trials are investigating the ability of increased SERCA2a expression to benefit heart failure patients (run from Imperial College London, ClinicalTrials.gov identifier: NCT00534703, and the Celladon Corporation, ClinicalTrials.gov identifier: NCT00454818). The results of these trials are much anticipated, as proof of safety and therapeutic efficacy will allow further AAV-mediated cardiac gene therapy for heart failure.

Retroviral vectors were used in clinical trials as early as 20 years ago. A major shortcoming of the earlier retroviruses was their preference/requirement for mitotically active cells, which effectively excluded adult cardiomyocytes [102, 103]. More recently, retroviruses derived from type 1 human immunodeficiency virus (HIV-1), called lentiviruses, have become popular [102, 103], although their use has been largely confined to animal models. Lentiviral vectors can efficiently transfect postmitotic cells like cardiomyocytes and can readily deliver inserts close to 10 kb in size [102]. Although many HIV-1 accessory proteins have been removed to prevent replication of these viruses, issues with biological safety have and undoubtedly will continue to limit their use in humans.

22.6 Conclusions

TH has a plethora of actions on the cardiovascular system, and recent results show that changes in TH signaling are important components in the pathophysiology of heart disease. Indeed, the changes in gene expression that occur in heart disease (i.e., the "fetal switch") mimic those in hypothyroidism. Moreover, primary diseases involving thyroid metabolism are associated with cardiovascular disease. Accordingly, TH and its analogs are already being tested and used in the treatment of heart disease. However, treatment with exogenous thyroid drugs increases the risk of inducing hyperthyroidism in other tissues of the body as well as the heart. Recent advances in our understanding of the molecular mechanisms of TH metabolism and signaling combined with new approaches for tissue-specific gene delivery provide unprecedented opportunities for correcting the alterations in TH signaling in heart disease.

Key Points

- Impaired TH signaling is a key feature of heart disease.

- Impaired TH signaling in heart disease may be due to altered T_3 and T_4 metabolism in the myocardium, possibly as a result of elevated levels of D3 and reductions of D2.

- The beneficial effects of TH in heart disease are complicated by differential organ responses to systemic TH treatment.

- Targeted treatments to combat impaired TH signaling in heart disease include: (1) enhancing TH uptake into the heart, (2) altering local TH metabolism to increase the levels of active T_3, (3) differential activation of TR subtypes, and (4) correcting TR profiles and downstream transcriptional signaling.

- Adeno-associated virus vectors 8 and 9 are promising vectors for cardiac-specific gene delivery.

References

1. Zhang J, Lazar MA (2000) The mechanism of action of thyroid hormones. Annu Rev Physiol 62:439–466
2. Klein I, Danzi S (2007) Thyroid disease and the heart. Circulation 116:1725–1735
3. Cutler MJ, Rosenbaum DS, Dunlap ME (2007) Structural and electrical remodeling as therapeutic targets in heart failure. J Electrocardiol 40:S1–S7
4. Johansson C, Gothe S, Forrest D et al (1999) Cardiovascular phenotype and temperature control in mice lacking thyroid hormone receptor-beta or both alpha1 and beta. Am J Physiol 276:H2006–2012
5. Biondi B, Palmieri EA, Lombardi G, Fazio S (2002) Effects of subclinical thyroid dysfunction on the heart. Ann Intern Med 137:904–914
6. Levey GS, Klein I (1994) Disorders of the thyroid. In: Stein J (ed) Stein's textbook of medicine. Little Brown, Boston, pp 1383–1397

7. Gomberg-Maitland M, Frishman WH (1998) Thyroid hormone and cardiovascular disease. Am Heart J 135:187–196

8. Olivares EL, Marassi MP, Fortunato RS et al (2007) Thyroid function disturbance and type 3 iodothyronine deiodinase induction after myocardial infarction in rats: a time course study. Endocrinology 148:4786–4792

9. Bianco AC, Kim BW (2006) Deiodinases: implications of the local control of thyroid hormone action. J Clin Invest 116:2571–2579

10. St Germain DL, Galton VA (1997) The deiodinase family of selenoproteins. Thyroid 7:655–668

11. Kahaly GJ, Dillmann WH (2005) Thyroid hormone action in the heart. Endocr Rev 26:704–728

12. Visser WE, Friesema ECH, Jansen J, Visser TJ (2008) Thyroid hormone transport in and out of cells. Trends Endocrinol Metab 19:50–56

13. Jansen J, Friesema ECH, Milici C, Visser TJ (2005) Thyroid hormone transporters in health and disease. Thyroid 15:757–768

14. Larsen PR (1997) Update on the human iodothyronine selenodeiodinases, the enzymes regulating the activation and inactivation of thyroid hormone. Biochem Soc Trans 25:588–592

15. Burmeister L.A, Pachucki J, St. Germain DL (1997) Thyroid hormones inhibit type 2 iodothyronine deiodinase in the rat cerebral cortex by both pre- and posttranslational mechanisms. Endocrinology 138:5231–5237

16. Pantos C, Mourouzis I, Xinaris C et al (2008) Thyroid hormone and "cardiac metamorphosis": potential therapeutic implications. Pharmacol Ther 118:277–294

17. Dillmann WH (2002) Cellular action of thyroid hormone on the heart. Thyroid 12:447–452

18. Sato M, Fuller SJ, Hajjar RJ, Harding SE (2005) Targeting genes and cells in the progression to heart failure. Heart Fail Clin 1:287–301

19. Wagner MS, Morimoto R, Dora JM et al (2003) Hypothyroidism induces type 2 iodothyronine deiodinase expression in mouse heart and testis. J Mol Endocrinol 31:541–550

20. Chan S, Kachilele S, McCabe CJ et al (2002) Early expression of thyroid hormone deiodinases and receptors in human fetal cerebral cortex. Brain Res Dev Brain Res 138:109–116.

21. Yonemoto T, Nishikawa M, Matsubara H et al (1999) Type 1 iodothyronine deiodinase in heart – effects of triiodothyronine and angiotensin II on its activity and mRNA in cultured rat myocytes. Endocr J 46:621–628

22. Hosoi Y, Murakami M, Mizuma H et al (1999) Expression and regulation of type II iodothyronine deiodinase in cultured human skeletal muscle cells. J Clin Endocrinol Metab 84:3293–3300

23. Leonard JL (2008) Non-genomic actions of thyroid hormone in brain development. Steroids 73:1008–1012

24. Dubuis JM, Sanchez-Menegay C, Burger AG (1992) Effects of thyroxine triiodothyronine and reverse triiodothyronine on the neonatal hypothyroid rat cerebellum. Acta Med Austriaca 19 Suppl 1:106–109

25. Dumitrescu AM, Refetoff S (2007) Novel biological and clinical aspects of thyroid hormone metabolism. Endocr Dev 10:127–139

26. Wassen FW, Schiel AE, Kuiper GG et al (2002) Induction of thyroid hormone-degrading deiodinase in cardiac hypertrophy and failure. Endocrinology 143:2812–2815

27. Wu S-Y, Green WL, Huang W-S et al (2005) Alternate pathways of thyroid hormone metabolism. Thyroid 15:943–958

28. Friberg L, Werner S, Eggertsen G, Ahnve S (2002) Rapid down-regulation of thyroid hormones in acute myocardial infarction: is it cardioprotective in patients with angina? Arch Intern Med 162:1388–1394

29. Belke DD, Gloss B, Swanson EA, Dillmann WH (2007) Adeno-associated virus-mediated expression of thyroid hormone receptor isoforms-{alpha}1 and -{beta}1 improves contractile function in pressure overload-induced cardiac hypertrophy. Endocrinology 148:2870–2877

30. Cernohorsky J, Kolar F, Pelouch V et al (1998) Thyroid control of sarcolemmal Na+/Ca2+ exchanger and SR Ca2+-ATPase in developing rat heart. Am J Physiol 275:H264–273

31. Reed TD, Babu GJ, Ji Y, Zilberman A et al (2000) The expression of SR calcium transport ATPase and the Na+/Ca2+ exchanger are antithetically regulated during mouse cardiac development and in hypo/hyperthyroidism. J Mol Cell Cardiol 32:453–464

32. Light P, Shimoni Y, Harbison S et al (1998) Hypothyroidism decreases the ATP sensitivity of KATP channels from rat heart. J Membr Biol 162:217–223

33. Wickenden AD, Kaprielian R, You XM, Backx PH (2000) The thyroid hormone analog DITPA restores I(to) in rats after myocardial infarction. Am J Physiol Heart Circ Physiol 278:H1105–1116

34. Wickenden AD, Kaprielian R, Parker TG et al (1997) Effects of development and thyroid hormone on K+ currents and K+ channel gene expression in rat ventricle. J Physiol 504:271–286

35. Maitra N, Adamson C, Greer K et al (2007) Regulation of gene expression in rats with heart failure treated with the thyroid hormone analog 3,5-diiodothyropropionic acid (DITPA) and the combination of DITPA and captopril. J Cardiovasc Pharmacol 50:526–534

36. Athéa Y, Garnier A, Fortin D et al (2007) Mitochondrial and energetic cardiac phenotype in hypothyroid rat. Relevance to heart failure. Pflugers Arch 455:431–442

37. Ojamaa K, Balkman C. Klein IL (1993) Acute effects of triiodothyronine on arterial smooth muscle cells. Ann Thorac Surg 56:S61–66; discussion S66–67

38. Portman MA (2008) Thyroid hormone regulation of heart metabolism. Thyroid 18:217–225

39. Biondi B, Palmieri EA, Lombardi G, Fazio S (2002) Effects of subclinical thyroid dysfunction on the heart. Ann Intern Med 137:904–914

40. Fazio S, Palmieri EA, Lombardi G, Biondi B (2004) Effects of thyroid hormone on the cardiovascular system. Recent Prog Horm Res 59:31–50

41. Grover GJ, Egan DM, Sleph PG et al (2004) Effects of the thyroid hormone receptor agonist GC-1 on metabolic rate and cholesterol in rats and primates: selective actions relative to 3,5,3'-triiodo-L-thyronine. Endocrinology 145:1656–1661

42. Pingitore A, Galli E, Barison A et al (2008) Acute effects of triiodothyronine (T3) replacement therapy in patients with chronic heart failure and low-T3 syndrome: a randomized placebo-controlled study. J Clin Endocrinol Metab 93:1351–1358

43. Thomas TA, Kuzman JA, Anderson BE et al (2005) Thyroid hormones induce unique and potentially beneficial changes

in cardiac myocyte shape in hypertensive rats near heart failure. Am J Physiol Heart Circ Physiol 288:H2118–2122

44. Kinugawa K, Minobe WA, Wood WM et al (2001) Signaling pathways responsible for fetal gene induction in the failing human heart: evidence for altered thyroid hormone receptor gene expression. Circulation 103:1089–1094

45. Mai W, Janier MF, Allioli N et al (2004) Thyroid hormone receptor {alpha} is a molecular switch of cardiac function between fetal and postnatal life. Proc Natl Acad Sci 101:10332–10337

46. Rajabi M, Kassiotis C, Razeghi P, Taegtmeyer H (2007) Return to the fetal gene program protects the stressed heart: a strong hypothesis. Heart Fail Rev 12:331–343

47. Ladenson PW, Sherman SI, Baughman KL et al (1992) Reversible alterations in myocardial gene expression in a young man with dilated cardiomyopathy and hypothyroidism [published erratum appears in Proc Natl Acad Sci U S A (1992) 89:8856]. Proc Natl Acad Sci U S A 89:5251–5255

48. Ojamaa K, Samarel AM, Kupfer JM et al (1992) Thyroid hormone effects on cardiac gene expression independent of cardiac growth and protein synthesis. Am J Physiol 263:E534–540

49. Litwin SE, Zhang D, Roberge P, Pennock GD (2000) DITPA prevents the blunted contraction-frequency relationship in myocytes from infarcted hearts. Am J Physiol Heart Circ Physiol 278:H862–870

50. Iervasi G, Pingitore A, Landi P et al (2003) Low-T3 syndrome: a strong prognostic predictor of death in patients with heart disease. Circulation 107:708–713

51. Hamilton MA, Stevenson LW, Luu M, Walden JA (1990) Altered thyroid hormone metabolism in advanced heart failure. J Am Coll Cardiol 16:91–95

52. Hamilton MA, Stevenson LW (1996) Thyroid hormone abnormalities in heart failure: possibilities for therapy. Thyroid 6:527–529

53. Wartofsky L, Burman KD (1982) Alterations in thyroid function in patients with systemic illness: the "euthyroid sick syndrome". Endocr Rev 3:164–217

54. Utiger RD (1995) Altered thyroid function in nonthyroidal illness and surgery. To treat or not to treat? [editorial; comment]. N Engl J Med 333:1562–1563

55. Pantos C, Mourouzis I, Markakis K et al (2008) Long-term thyroid hormone administration reshapes left ventricular chamber and improves cardiac function after myocardial infarction in rats. Basic Res Cardiol 103:308–318

56. Pennock GD, Raya TE, Bahl JJ et al (1992) Cardiac effects of 3,5-diiodothyropropionic acid, a thyroid hormone analog with inotropic selectivity. J Pharmacol Exp Ther 263:163–169

57. Pennock GD, Raya TE, Bahl JJ et al (1993) Combination treatment with captopril and the thyroid hormone analogue 3,5-diiodothyropropionic acid. A new approach to improving left ventricular performance in heart failure. Circulation 88:1289–1298

58. Morkin E, Pennock GD, Raya TE et al (1996) Development of a thyroid hormone analogue for the treatment of congestive heart failure. Thyroid 6:521–526

59. Katz AM (2008) The "modern" view of heart failure: how did we get here? Circ Heart Fail 1:63–71

60. Katz D, Reginato MJ, Lazar MA (1995) Functional regulation of thyroid hormone receptor variant TR alpha 2 by phosphorylation. Mol Cell Biol 15:2341–2348

61. Forfar JC, Muir AL, Sawers SA, Toft AD (1982) Abnormal left ventricular function in hyperthyroidism: evidence for a possible reversible cardiomyopathy. N Engl J Med 307:1165–1170

62. Hu LW, Benvenuti LA, Liberti EA et al (2003) Thyroxine-induced cardiac hypertrophy: influence of adrenergic nervous system versus renin-angiotensin system on myocyte remodeling. Am J Physiol Regul Integr Comp Physiol 285:R1473–1480

63. Klein I (1988) Thyroxine-induced cardiac hypertrophy: time course of development and inhibition by propranolol. Endocrinology 123:203–210

64. Dernellis J, Panaretou M (2002) Effects of thyroid replacement therapy on arterial blood pressure in patients with hypertension and hypothyroidism. Am Heart J 143:718–724

65. Dagre AG, Lekakis JP, Papaioannou TG et al (2005) Arterial stiffness is increased in subjects with hypothyroidism. Int J Cardiol 103:1–6

66. Toruner F, Altinova AE, Karakoc A et al (2008) Risk factors for cardiovascular disease in patients with subclinical hypothyroidism. Adv Ther 25:430–437

67. Zhu WX, Johnson SB, Brandt R et al (1997) Impact of volume loading and load reduction on ventricular refractoriness and conduction properties in canine congestive heart failure. J Am Coll Cardiol 30:825–833

68. Sun H, Gaspo R, Leblanc N, Nattel S (1998) Cellular mechanisms of atrial contractile dysfunction caused by sustained atrial tachycardia. Circulation 98:719–727

69. Klein I, Hong C (1986) Effects of thyroid hormone on cardiac size and myosin content of the heterotopically transplanted rat heart. J Clin Invest 77:1694–1698

70. Ojamaa K, Petrie JF, Balkman C et al (1994) Posttranscriptional modification of myosin heavy-chain gene expression in the hypertrophied rat myocardium. Proc Natl Acad Sci U S A 91:3468–3472

71. Klein I, Ojamaa K (2001) Thyroid hormone and the cardiovascular system. N Engl J Med 344:501–509

72. Walsh JP (2002) Dissatisfaction with thyroxine therapy – could the patients be right? Curr Opin Pharmacol 2:717–722

73. Friesema ECH, Jansen J, Visser TJ (2005) Thyroid hormone transporters. Biochem Soc Trans 33:228–232

74. Trivieri MG, Oudit GY, Sah R et al (2006) Cardiac-specific elevations in thyroid hormone enhance contractility and prevent pressure overload-induced cardiac dysfunction. Proc Natl Acad S 103:6043–6048

75. Wassen FWJS, Schiel AE, Kuiper GG et al (2002) Induction of thyroid hormone-degrading deiodinase in cardiac hypertrophy and failure. Endocrinology 143:2812–2815

76. Drvota V, Janson A, Norman C et al (1995) Evidence for the presence of functional thyrotropin receptor in cardiac muscle. Biochem Biophys Res Commun 211:426–431

77. Meischl C, Buermans HP, Hazes T et al (2008) H9c2 cardiomyoblasts produce thyroid hormone. Am J Physiol Cell Physiol 294:C1227–1233

78. Jin H, Fedorowicz G, Yang R et al (2004) Thyrotropin-releasing hormone is induced in the left ventricle of rats with heart failure and can provide inotropic support to the failing heart. Circulation 109:2240–2245

79. Davis PJ, Davis FB, Lin H-Y (2008) Promotion by thyroid hormone of cytoplasm-to-nucleus shuttling of thyroid hormone receptors. Steroids 73:1013–1017

80. Kuzman JA, Vogelsang KA, Thomas TA, Gerdes AM (2005) L-Thyroxine activates Akt signaling in the heart. J Mol Cell Cardiol 39:251–258

81. Pantos C, Xinaris C, Mourouzis I et al (2007) Thyroid hormone changes cardiomyocyte shape and geometry via ERK signaling pathway: potential therapeutic implications in reversing cardiac remodeling? Mol Cell Biochem 297:65–72

82. Kinugawa K, Jeong MY, Bristow MR, Long CS (2005) Thyroid hormone induces cardiac myocyte hypertrophy in a thyroid hormone receptor {alpha}1-specific manner that requires TAK1 and p38 mitogen-activated protein kinase. Mol Endocrinol 19:1618–1628

83. Pantos C, Mourouzis I, Saranteas T et al (2005) Thyroid hormone receptors a1 and b1 are downregulated in the post-infarcted rat heart: consequences on the response to ischaemia-reperfusion. Basic Res Cardiol 100:422–432

84. Williams GR (2000) Cloning and characterization of two novel thyroid hormone receptor beta isoforms. Mol Cell Biol 20:8329–8342

85. Plateroti M, Gauthier K, Domon-Dell C et al (2001) Functional interference between thyroid hormone receptor alpha (TRalpha) and natural truncated TRDeltaalpha isoforms in the control of intestine development. Mol Cell Biol 21:4761–4772

86. Wikström L, Johansson C, Saltó C et al (1998) Abnormal heart rate and body temperature in mice lacking thyroid hormone receptor alpha1. EMBO J 17:455–461

87. Tinnikov A, Nordström K, Thorén P et al (2002) Retardation of post-natal development caused by a negatively acting thyroid hormone receptor alpha1. EMBO J 21:5079–5087

88. Kaneshige M, Suzuki H, Kaneshige K et al (2001) A targeted dominant negative mutation of the thyroid hormone alpha 1 receptor causes increased mortality infertility and dwarfism in mice. Proc Natl Acad Sci U S A 98:15095–15100

89. Gloss B, Trost S, Bluhm W et al (2001) Cardiac ion channel expression and contractile function in mice with deletion of thyroid hormone receptor alpha or beta. Endocrinology 142:544–550

90. d'Amati G, di Gioia CR, Mentuccia D et al (2001) Increased expression of thyroid hormone receptor isoforms in end-stage human congestive heart failure. J Clin Endocrinol Metab 86:2080–2084

91. Modesti PA, Marchetta M, Gamberi T et al (2008) Reduced expression of thyroid hormone receptors and beta-adrenergic receptors in human failing cardiomyocytes. Biochem Pharmacol 75:900–906

92. Li D, Yamada T, Wang F, Vulin AI, Samuels HH (2004) Novel roles of retinoid X receptor (RXR) and RXR ligand in dynamically modulating the activity of the thyroid hormone receptor/RXR heterodimer. J Biol Chem 279:7427–7437

93. Harvey CB. Williams GR (2002) Mechanism of thyroid hormone action. Thyroid 12:441–446

94. McKenna NJ O'Malley BW (2002) Minireview: nuclear receptor coactivators – an update. Endocrinology 143:2461–2465

95. Takeuchi Y, Murata Y, Sadow P et al (2002) Steroid receptor coactivator-1 deficiency causes variable alterations in the modulation of T3-regulated transcription of genes in vivo. Endocrinology 143:1346–1352

96. Sadow PM, Chassande O, Gauthier K et al (2003) Specificity of thyroid hormone receptor subtype and steroid receptor coactivator-1 on thyroid hormone action. Am J Physiol Endocrinol Metab 284:E36–46

97. Hall G, Hasday JD, Rogers TB (2006) Regulating the regulator: NF-kappaB signaling in heart. J Mol Cell Cardiol 41:580–591

98. Pantos C, Dritsas A, Mourouzis I et al (2007) Thyroid hormone is a critical determinant of myocardial performance in patients with heart failure: potential therapeutic implications. Eur J Endocrinol 157:515–520

99. Dieterle T, Meyer M, Gu Y et al (2005) Gene transfer of a phospholamban-targeted antibody improves calcium handling and cardiac function in heart failure. Cardiovasc Res 67:678–688

100. Krek A, Grün D, Poy MN et al (2005) Combinatorial microRNA target predictions. Nat Genet 37:495–500

101. van Rooij E, Sutherland LB, Qi X et al (2007) Control of stress-dependent cardiac growth and gene expression by a microRNA. Science 316:575–579

102. Ly H, Kawase Y, Yoneyama R, Hajjar RJ (2007) Gene therapy in the treatment of heart failure. Physiology 22:81–96

103. Lyon AR, Sato M, Hajjar RJ, Samulski RJ, Harding SE (2008) Gene therapy: targeting the myocardium. Heart 94:89–99

104. Jiang H, Pierce GF, Ozelo MC et al (2006) Evidence of multiyear factor IX expression by AAV-Mediated gene transfer to skeletal muscle in an individual with severe hemophilia B. Mol Ther 14:452–455

105. Zhu T, Zhou L, Mori S et al (2005) Sustained whole-body functional rescue in congestive heart failure and muscular dystrophy hamsters by systemic gene transfer. Circulation 112:2650–2659

106. Wang Z, Ma HI, Li J et al (2003) Rapid and highly efficient transduction by double-stranded adeno-associated virus vectors in vitro and in vivo. Gene Ther 10:2105–2111

107. Kaspar BK, Roth DM, Lai NC et al (2005) Myocardial gene transfer and long-term expression following intracoronary delivery of adeno-associated virus. J Gene Med 7:316–324

108. Vandendriessche T, Thorrez L, Acosta-Sanchez A et al (2007) Efficacy and safety of adeno-associated viral vectors based on serotype 8 and 9 vs. lentiviral vectors for hemophilia B gene therapy. J Thromb Haemost 5:16–24

Subject Index

Printed in April 2009